CUSHING'S
DISEASE

———

CUSHING'S DISEASE

AN OFTEN MISDIAGNOSED AND NOT SO RARE DISORDER

Edited by

EDWARD R. LAWS, JR., M.D., F.A.C.S.
Professor of Neurosurgery, Harvard Medical School
Director, Neuro-Endocrine/Pituitary Program
Department of Neurosurgery
Brigham and Women's Hospital
Boston, Massachusetts, United States

With an Introduction by Louise Pace,
Founder and President of the Cushing's Support
and Research Foundation

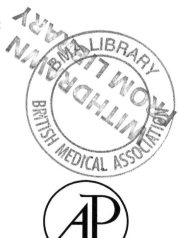

ELSEVIER

AMSTERDAM • BOSTON • HEIDELBERG • LONDON
NEW YORK • OXFORD • PARIS • SAN DIEGO
SAN FRANCISCO • SINGAPORE • SYDNEY • TOKYO
Academic Press is an imprint of Elsevier

Academic Press is an imprint of Elsevier
125 London Wall, London EC2Y 5AS, United Kingdom
525 B Street, Suite 1800, San Diego, CA 92101-4495, United States
50 Hampshire Street, 5th Floor, Cambridge, MA 02139, United States
The Boulevard, Langford Lane, Kidlington, Oxford OX5 1GB, United Kingdom

Notices
Knowledge and best practice in this field are constantly changing. As new research and experience broaden our understanding, changes in research methods, professional practices, or medical treatment may become necessary.

Practitioners and researchers must always rely on their own experience and knowledge in evaluating and using any information, methods, compounds, or experiments described herein. In using such information or methods they should be mindful of their own safety and the safety of others, including parties for whom they have a professional responsibility.

To the fullest extent of the law, neither the Publisher nor the authors, contributors, or editors, assume any liability for any injury and/or damage to persons or property as a matter of products liability, negligence or otherwise, or from any use or operation of any methods, products, instructions, or ideas contained in the material herein.

Library of Congress Cataloging-in-Publication Data
A catalog record for this book is available from the Library of Congress

British Library Cataloguing-in-Publication Data
A catalogue record for this book is available from the British Library

ISBN: 978-0-12-804340-0

For information on all Academic Press publications
visit our website at https://www.elsevier.com/

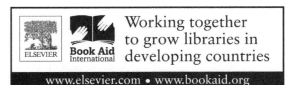

Working together
to grow libraries in
developing countries

www.elsevier.com • www.bookaid.org

Publisher: Mica Haley
Acquisition Editor: Tari Broderick
Editorial Project Manager: Lisa Eppich
Production Project Manager: Julia Haynes
Designer: Maria Inês Cruz

Typeset by Thomson Digital

*This book is dedicated, by the physicians, surgeons, and scientists who work
tirelessly on the myriad problems related to Cushing's disease,
to the patients, past, current, and future. They are the heroes
who struggle with the difficulties of diagnosis, testing, treatment,
and recovery from this illness, often following paths littered
with frustrations, delays, difficult decisions, and struggles
to regain their health.*

To my mother who saw me through all of the ups and downs of Cushing's.

*To Jane, my best friend for over 50 years, who diagnosed me just as I was about
to give up and who helped to make this book possible.*

Contents

9. Posttreatment Management of Cushing's Disease

A. PRETE, MD, R. SALVATORI, MD

10. Coping with Cushing's Disease: the Patients' Perspectives

A. SANTOS, MPsy, PhD, S.M. WEBB, MD, PhD

11. Cushing's Disease in Children and Adolescents: Diagnosis and Management

E.J. RICHMOND, MD, MSc, A.D. ROGOL, MD, PhD

List of Contributors

G. Barkhoudarian, MD Pacific Brain Tumor Center and Pituitary Disorders Center, Providence Saint John's Health Center and John Wayne Cancer Institute, Santa Monica, CA, United States

B.M.K. Biller, MD Harvard Medical School; Neuroendocrine Unit, Massachusetts General Hospital, Boston, MA, United States

M. Fleseriu, MD Department of Medicine (Endocrinology), Department of Neurological Surgery, and Northwest Pituitary Center, Oregon Health & Science University, Portland, OR, United States

S. Hopkins, MD Department of Medicine (Endocrinology), Northwest Pituitary Center, Oregon Health & Science University, Portland, OR, United States

J.A. Jane, Jr., MD Department of Neurological Surgery, University of Virginia Health System, Charlottesville, VA, United States

L. Katznelson, MD Pituitary Center, Stanford School of Medicine, Stanford, CA, United States

D.F. Kelly, MD Pacific Brain Tumor Center and Pituitary Disorders Center, Providence Saint John's Health Center and John Wayne Cancer Institute, Santa Monica, CA, United States

E.R. Laws, Jr., MD, FACS Harvard Medical School; Neuro-Endocrine/Pituitary Program, Department of Neurosurgery, Brigham and Women's Hospital, Boston, MA, United States

L. Nieman, MD, FACP Diabetes, Endocrine, and Obesity Branch, The National Institute of Diabetes and Digestive and Kidney Diseases; Endocrinology Consultation Service, National Institutes of Health, Bethesda, MD, United States

A. Prete, MD Unit of Endocrinology, Faculty of Medicine, Catholic University of the Sacred Heart, Rome, Italy

E.J. Richmond, MD, MSc Pediatric Endocrinology, National Children's Hospital, San Jose, Costa Rica

A.D. Rogol, MD, PhD Emeritus, Department of Pediatrics, University of Virginia, Charlottesville, VA, United States

R. Salvatori, MD Pituitary Center, Department of Medicine, Division of Endocrinology, Diabetes, and Metabolism, Johns Hopkins University School of Medicine, Baltimore, MD, United States

A. Santos, MPsy, PhD Endocrinology/Medicine Department, Centro de Investigación Biomédica en Red de Enfermedades Raras (CIBERER, Unidad 747), ISCIII, Research Center for Pituitary Diseases, Hospital Sant Pau, IIB-Sant Pau, and Universitat Autònoma de Barcelona (UAB), Barcelona, Spain

W. Sivakumar, MD Department of Neurosurgery University of Utah, Salt Lake City, UT, United States

N.A. Tritos, MD, DSc Harvard Medical School; Neuroscience Unit, Massachusetts General Hospital, Boston, MA, United States

M.L. Vance, MD Departments of Medicine and Neurological Surgery, Division of Endocrinology and Metabolism, University of Virginia Health System, Charlottesville, VA, United States

S.M. Webb, MD, PhD Endocrinology/Medicine Department, Centro de Investigación Biomédica en Red de Enfermedades Raras (CIBERER, Unidad 747), ISCIII, Research Center for Pituitary Diseases, Hospital Sant Pau, IIB-Sant Pau, and Universitat Autònoma de Barcelona (UAB), Barcelona, Spain

Preface

More than a 100 years ago, Dr. Harvey Cushing treated his famous 23-year-old patient, "Minnie G," who had been suffering from a complex combination of symptoms and signs that Dr. Cushing had not previously recognized. He believed that she suffered from what he called a "polyglandular syndrome," which affected more than one body system. It was not until 1932, however, that a significant number of patients with similar presentations had appeared in the literature. It was then that Dr. Peter Bishop in England reported a series of such patients, many of whom had small benign basophilic tumors in the pituitary gland. It was he who suggested naming this "Cushing's Syndrome." We still marvel at this unique disease and still wonder about its prevalence, etiology, and management.

Those who recognize and treat the many typical manifestations of Cushing's realize that it is more common than the reported cases would imply. It is also clear that patients may have different sets of symptoms and signs and different presentations. They also have different struggles in finding the correct diagnosis and effective treatment, both of the disease and of the additional morbidities that accompany untreated Cushing's Syndrome and Cushing's Disease.

This book is designed to clarify many of the confounding issues regarding Cushing's Disease. It is important to note at the outset that Cushing's Syndrome is a more generic term that describes the results of excess exposure of the body to cortisol, regardless of the source. Cushing's Disease is more narrowly defined as excess cortisol secretion caused by tumors that secrete adrenocorticotropic hormone (ACTH), and secondarily results in excess cortisol secretion from the adrenal glands. This condition is usually the result of a very small, benign tumor in the pituitary gland, involving the cells called corticotrophs that release ACTH and stimulate cortisol secretion.

Our hope is that the readers will gain confidence in understanding this extraordinary illness. Recognizing the symptoms and signs, making the diagnosis, confirming it with laboratory and imaging tests, and evaluating the various therapies are all complex subjects. The experts who have collaborated in producing this volume are examples of the intellect, energy, and expertise that are currently focused on Cushing's Disease. Continuing progress is being made in every aspect of this condition. Surely, it is more common than previously suspected. Even more certainly, with the multidisciplinary collaboration of dedicated physicians, surgeons, and basic science investigators, the mysteries of Cushing's Disease will progressively become unraveled, and more effective diagnostic methods and novel and lasting treatments will ultimately emerge.

Edward R. Laws, Jr.
Boston, MA

List of Abbreviations

A
ACTH   Adrenocorticotropic hormone
ADH   Antidiuretic hormone
AIP   Aryl-hydrocarbon receptor interacting protein
ALT   Alanine transaminase
AST   Aspartate aminotransferase
AVP   Arginine vasopressin

B
BLA   Bilateral adrenalectomy
BMAH   Bilateral macronodular adrenal hyperplasia
BMD   Bone mineral density
BMI   Body mass index

C
cAMP   Cyclic adenosine monophosphate
CBG   Corticosteroid-binding globulin
CI   Confidence interval
COE   Centers of Excellence
CNS   Central nervous system
CREB   Cyclic adenosine monophosphate response element–binding protein
CRH   Corticotropin-releasing hormone
CSF   Cerebrospinal fluid
CSRF   Cushing's Support and Research Foundation
CT   Computed tomography
CVO   Circumventricular organ

D
DDAVP   1-Amino-8-D-arginine vasopressin (or desmopressin)
DEXA   Dual energy X-ray absorptiometry
DHEA   Dehydroepiandrosterone
DHEAS   Dehydroepiandrosterone sulfate
DPP-4   Dipeptidyl-peptidase-4
DST   Dexamethasone suppression test

E
EAS   Ectopic ACTH secretion
ECG   Electrocardiogram
EGFR   Epidermal growth factor receptor
EMA   European Medicines Agency
ERK1/2   Extracellular signal–regulating kinases 1 and 2

F
FDA   Food and Drug Administration
FDG PET ^{18}F-fluorodeoxyglucose positron emission tomography
FIPA   Familial isolated pituitary adenoma
fMRI   Functional magnetic resonance imaging
FSH   Follicle-stimulating hormone

G
GGT   Gamma-glutamyl transferase
GH   Growth hormone
GHRH   Growth hormone–releasing hormone
GLP-1   Glucagon-like peptide-1
GnRH   Gonadotropin-releasing hormone
GSPN   Greater superficial petrosal nerve

H
Hb   Hemoglobin
HbA1c   Hemoglobin A1c
HC   Hydrocortisone acetate
HCG   Human chorionic gonadotropin
H&E   Hematoxylin and eosin stains
11β-HSD   11β-Hydroxysteroid dehydrogenase
HPA   Hypothalamic-pituitary axis
HPAA   Hypothalamic-pituitary-adrenal axis

I
ICU   Intensive care unit
IFG   Impaired fasting glucose
IGF-1   Insulin-like growth factor 1
IM   Intramuscular
IPSS   Inferior petrosal sinus sampling
IV   Intravenous

L
LC   Liquid chromatography
LFT   Liver function test
LH   Luteinizing hormone
LLN   Lower limit of normal
LT$_4$ Levothyroxine

M
MEN 1   Multiple endocrine neoplasia 1
miRNA   microRNA
MSH   Melanocyte-stimulating hormone
MRI   Magnetic resonance imaging

N
NS   Nelson's syndrome

O
OCT   Ocular computed tomography
OMIM   Online Mendelian Inheritance in Man (online database)
OSA   Obstructive sleep apnea

P
PCOS   Polycystic ovary syndrome
PET   Positron emission tomography
PIF   Prolactin inhibitory factor
PKC   Protein kinase C
POMC   Proopiomelanocortin
PPNAD   Primary pigmented nodular adrenocortical disease
PSA   Prostate-specific antigen
PST   Pasireotide suppression test
PTSD   Posttraumatic stress disorder

R
RhGH   Recombinant human growth hormone
RS   Radiosurgery
RT   Radiotherapy

S
SC   Subcutaneous
SEISMIC   Study of the Efficacy and Safety of Mifepristone in the Treatment of Endogenous Cushing's
                  Syndrome
SHBG   Sex hormone–binding globulin
SIADH   Syndrome of inappropriate antidiuretic hormone secretion
SMR   Standardized mortality ratio
SPGR   Spoiled-gradient recalled (acquisition MRI)
SRS   Stereotactic radiosurgery
SRT   Stereotactic radiotherapy
SSTR1–SSTR5   Somatostatin receptor subtypes 1–5

T
T1SE   T1 spin-echo
T$_4$ Thyroxine
TRH   Thyrotropin-releasing hormone
TSH   Thyroid-stimulating hormone

U
UFC   Urinary free cortisol
ULN   Upper limit of normal

V
vmPFC   Ventromedial prefontal cortex

Introduction[a]

The story of Harvey Cushing's (1869–1939) discovery of what came to be known as Cushing's syndrome is, of course, familiar. He, while preparing for a lecture series in 1930, discovered a photograph of a patient with "basophil adenoma," in a 1924 paper from Czechoslovakia. This patient was "strikingly similar" to several of Cushing's own patients, whom he had previously described (in 1912) as having "polyglandular syndrome." These patients presented with "significant fat deposits, backache, weakness, fatigue, weakening of the bones, skin discoloration and streaking, facial hair, high blood pressure, high blood sugar, and sexual dystrophy." Cushing then "scoured the literature and his own patient records" and published a paper in 1932 describing a syndrome that was "caused by a basophil pituitary adenoma," which, in turn, caused "hypersecretion from the adrenal cortex." Medical journals were quick to label this Cushing's syndrome. Cushing himself stated at the time, "In its milder forms, it is apparently not an uncommon disorder." And yet, almost a century later the diagnosis still remains elusive to many physicians.

As the Founder and President of the Cushing's Support and Research Foundation (CSRF) for the past 22 years and a former Cushing's patient, I have been privy to many, many stories of people with Cushing's whose diagnostic odysseys resemble my own. While some sources claim that time for diagnosis averages only 1–2 years, many patients wait 5–10 years before a diagnosis and go through myriad visits to multiple physicians. That there is *any* delay in diagnosis for individual patients intensifies suffering and worsens physical and cognitive disabilities that may be lifelong and life-altering.

In my own experience as a Cushing's patient, I visited a large number of physicians in many different specialties, looking for an answer to my changing physical and mental status (Figs. 1–3). My symptoms were largely viewed individually within the narrow focus of each specialty with no physician putting together the whole picture. One of the several internists diagnosed a vitamin K deficiency when consulted about skin issues; another internist thought I had a parasitic infection picked up from my travels to Nepal; a gynecologist thought I was going through early menopause when consulted about amenorrhea; an infectious disease specialist decided I had contracted a strange infection, no doubt from worms, from a trip to Africa, when consulted about the striae; a gastroenterologist said I ate too much and had food allergies when consulted about my extraordinary weight gain; a hematologist suggested that the bruising I exhibited was probably leukemia; a dermatologist felt that the rashes and striae were from an abusive husband who I was unwilling to accuse; an orthopedist tested me for lupus because I had difficulty walking; and a psychiatrist felt that I was having a hard time accepting

[a]Quotations taken from: Michael Bliss, Harvey Cushing: a life in surgery. New York: Oxford University Press; 2005, p. 476–478.

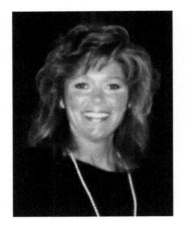 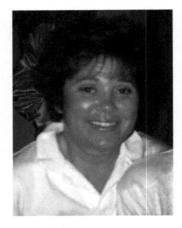 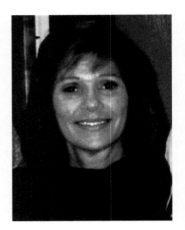

Cushing's disease—"before during after" successful treatment.

the normal aging process when consulted for anxiety, depression, and inability to sleep. This went on for more than 5 years. I ran out of options, and as is obvious now, neither I nor my physicians ever considered an endocrine disorder or an endocrinologist.

In the end, I was not diagnosed by a physician but rather by a medical editor and friend, who Iived 1500 miles away (and thus had not seen me recently). Since I was seriously considering suicide when my symptoms continued to escalate, she asked for a list of my symptoms and told me to "hold on" for 24 h while she researched them. Clued by an offhand comment of mine that a coworker "did not recognize me in the parking lot," she consulted the pituitary chapter of *Harrison's Principles of Internal Medicine*, as she knew that pituitary tumors could "change your looks." There she found a table with 13 symptoms of Cushing's disease; I had 11 of them. She consulted her physician husband before calling me back, and he advised her not to "get me all worked up about Cushing's, the possibility of which was nil." Ignoring his warning, she called back the next day with instructions to "get your cortisol checked now," which led to a definitive diagnosis.

Unfortunately, consulting multiple physicians is not rare, but rather the norm among Cushing's patients. Universally, friends, family, and physicians all think such patients are crazy, lazy, and eating too much. Therefore, the intended audience of this book is all providers, especially physicians, nurse practitioners, physician assistants, nurses, and medical students, whether in primary care or any of the nonendocrinology specialties. Reaching all of these providers to encourage them to think of the Cushing's diagnosis and to let patients teach them about their disease has been a dream of mine for the past 15 years. Edward Laws, MD, the editor of this text, and all of the contributors, many of whom have served on the CSRF medical advisory board, have made this dream come true.

The CSRF has had a booth at many annual medical meetings for numerous specialties across the United States since our inception (1995) to spread the word about Cushing's disease. At these meetings, there is ample opportunity to chat with physicians who visit our booth. Here the conversations are illustrative. One internist, for example, proudly stated that he had "thirty Cushing's patients," while another stated that he had "never seen a Cushing's patient." Was the first physician witness to a strange cohort of Cushing's patients or was the second missing the diagnosis? While this is an interesting question, it has no easy answer. As many patients relate that they are "the first Cushing's patient their physician had ever seen," educating physicians about Cushing's seems especially important.

Almost all internists and primary care providers when confronted by an overweight or obese patient automatically order certain tests, such as a thyroid-stimulating hormone level. Is it too much of a stretch to think that a cortisol level or other Cushing's test could be added to the "must-have tests" for patients with diabetes or obesity or even those who are simply overweight without an obvious cause? With obesity a worldwide epidemic, it is important for physicians to listen carefully to their patients' complaints so as to distinguish between obesity caused by overeating and that caused by some other disorder, especially an endocrine disorder. In particular, physicians should be clued by a round, moon face (steroid face), bruising, characteristic abdominal striae, and reported weakness and personality changes in addition to the weight gain.

Diagnosis is just one of the many problems facing Cushing's patients (Chapter 5). Equally important is proper treatment (Chapters 6 and 7) as is the recognition of the lifelong physical and cognitive deficits experienced by patients, even after being "cured" (Chapters 4 and 10). In 2014, when attending the annual endocrine meeting in San Diego, CA, I had a chance to hear Susan M. Webb, MD, speak about the lifelong cognitive problems experienced by most Cushing's patients. I was very surprised but also thrilled to finally hear a cogent explanation for the memory processing and focusing issues that I had been experiencing for 15 years after successful surgery.

I am hopeful that this text will be read by physicians and other providers who may be consulted for symptoms of Cushing's or encounter these patients in the course of their daily work, but do not know it yet. This text has not been written just for physicians and other providers. It has also been written for patients who suspect that they may have Cushing's or who may want a better understanding of their disease and its treatment. Finally, I hope that professors in medical, nursing, and physician assistant schools will use this text to teach their students how to recognize a symptom complex that may indicate a serious and rare, or maybe not so rare, disorder.

Louise Pace
Founder and President
Cushing Support and Research Foundation
Plymouth, MA, United States

The Pituitary Gland: Anatomy, Physiology, and its Function as the Master Gland

G. Barkhoudarian, MD, D.F. Kelly, MD

Pacific Brain Tumor Center and Pituitary Disorders Center, Providence Saint John's Health Center and John Wayne Cancer Institute, Santa Monica, CA, United States

1 INTRODUCTION

The human body functions best in a state of homeostasis. This balance is necessary for energy management and consumption, temperature control, electrolyte and fluid levels, and blood pressure regulation to name a few. Most of this control is managed by circulating hormones produced by a variety of endocrine organs, such as the adrenal glands and the thyroid gland. Given their importance for survival, there is a need for interaction with the central nervous system (CNS). This interface is mediated by the pituitary gland.

Cushing's Disease. http://dx.doi.org/10.1016/B978-0-12-804340-0.00001-2

No other single organ in the human body is as vital, gram-for-gram, for survival than the pituitary gland. This small structure, situated deep in the skull, protected in its own vault, and surrounded by critical neurovascular structures, lies truly at the nexus of brain, metaphorically acting as the gate-keeper of the blood–brain barrier. Understanding the normal anatomy and function of the pituitary gland is requisite to being able to manage pituitary dysfunction, such as Cushing's disease. This chapter reviews the anatomy and physiology of the pituitary gland, its role in homeostasis, and the discoveries that led to our understanding of this incredible organ.

2 HISTORY

Though the pituitary gland is widely known to be the "master gland," little was known of its true function until the 20th century. This is primarily related to the limited understanding of endocrinology before that time. The word "hormone" was coined by Ernest Starling in 1905 and is derived from the Greek, "to arouse" [1]. For centuries, the pituitary gland was thought to be a conduit for removal of brain mucus. Andreas Vesalius was the first to name *glandula pituitaria*, derived from the Greek *pituita* or "slime" [2]. This "slime or phlegm gland" was also known by the diminutive term, *hypophysis*, coined by Samuel Thomas von Sömmerring [3]. It has even been considered the appendix of the brain, *appendix cerebri* [4].

Martin Rathke was one of the first to describe the development of the pituitary gland, characterizing the evagination of the anterior foregut with the diencephalon during embryogenesis [5]. Hubert von Luschka, in 1860, added to the understanding of the posterior pituitary gland, noting its similarity to the neuronal structures of the spinal cord. He also described the drainage of the cavernous sinuses via the inferior petrosal sinuses and elucidated the portal system and pituitary blood supply [6]. He was the first to identify epithelial cell rests in Rathke's cleft, which led to the understanding of craniopharyngioma pathophysiology [7].

Much of the early discovery of pituitary gland function came from studying disorders that were linked to the pituitary. The first of these were acromegaly (gigantism), attributed to an enlarged pituitary by Oscar Minkowski in 1887 [8]. It was not until 1910, when Harvey Cushing postulated the possibility of a "hormone of growth" [9]. Similarly, adrenocorticotropic hormone (ACTH) induced hypercortisolism, later coined "Cushing's disease," was not postulated to be of pituitary etiology until after Cushing's series was published in 1932 [10]. Diabetes insipidus, though a known and distinct entity, was linked to the posterior pituitary in 1912 [11].

Although purification of hormones (e.g., adrenalin or secretin) had occurred early in the 20th century, the first pituitary hormone to be isolated was prolactin, in 1933 [12]. In 1942, ACTH was isolated, and luteinizing hormone (LH) followed in 1959 [13,14]. These advances helped further the understanding of pituitary disease and provided treatment options for patients with pituitary deficiencies.

Surgery for tumors of the pituitary gland has also developed greatly in the 20th century, with major advances achieved in the first two decades of the 21st century as well. These advances relied on the introduction of new technologies in neurosurgery. The transsphenoidal approach to the pituitary gland, which is the workhorse of pituitary surgery, was first successfully performed in 1907 by Hermann Schloffer [15]. Harvey Cushing embraced and popularized this approach for most of his pituitary tumors. Because of poor visualization, increased complications with reoperations, and improved outcomes with craniotomies, Cushing essentially abandoned the transsphenoidal approach in 1927 at the twilight of his surgical career. In a series of his pituitary tumor operations, he noted using the transsphenoidal approach in 15% of his brain tumor operations and was almost apologetic for its use [16].

By 1965, with the introduction of the operative microscope, bipolar electrocautery, microsurgical instruments, and video fluoroscopy, the transsphenoidal approach was repopularized by Gerard Guiot and his pupil, Jules Hardy [17]. Advances in neuroimaging with computed tomography (CT) and magnetic resonance imaging (MRI) improved the diagnostic capabilities and expanded the ability to perform microadenoma resection safely [18]. As instrumentation improved, larger and more complex tumors could be removed with the extended endonasal approaches [19]. The introduction of neuroendoscopy to these approaches expanded the ability to resect large and invasive tumors safely [20,21]. The implementation of pedicled vascular mucosal flaps, introduced by Haddad and Bassagasteguy, significantly decreased the incidence of postoperative cerebrospinal fluid (CSF) rhinorrhea, improving the safety of these more complex operations [22,23].

3 EMBRYOLOGY

The pituitary gland is essentially two separate structures fused together. The adenohypophysis and neurohypophysis are derived embryologically from different tissues, reflected in the pituitary's mechanisms of function. Ultimately, the pituitary gland originates from the developing ectoderm. An outpouching of the ectoderm that ultimately develops into the nasopharynx, the stomodeum, migrates dorsally and develops into the anterior lobe of the pituitary gland [24]. In concert, the developing diencephalon, originating from the neuroectoderm, generates an outpouching from the floor of the developing third ventricle that ultimately becomes the posterior lobe of the pituitary gland (Fig. 1.1).

During the development of the adenohypophysis, the ectodermal outpouching is known as Rathke's pouch. This ultimately buds off the ectoderm with regression of the primitive craniopharyngeal duct. The junction between Rathke's pouch and the neurohypophysis defines Rathke's cleft. This potential space is well characterized in a cadaveric specimen (Fig. 1.2). This cleft can also be identified and manipulated during surgery, particularly during exploration of the pituitary gland for microadenomas. Certain pathology can arise from aberrant development of this structure, including Rathke cleft cysts and craniopharyngiomas [25,26].

Rathke's pouch forms by 28 days of gestation and maintains an anterior–posterior relation with regard to the developing infundibulum [27]. The anterior pouch develops robustly, becoming the pars distalis and pars tuberalis [28]. The posterior pouch has minimal development and becomes the vestigial pars intermedia. Interestingly, embryonic cells are committed to become adenohypophyseal cells very early in gestation, mediated by homeotic gene expression (e.g., *Otx-2*, *Wnt-2*, and *Pax* in lower mammals) [29,30]. Specific adenohypophyseal

Pituitary development

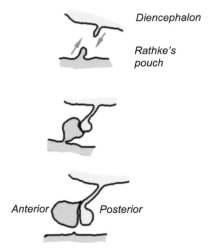

FIGURE 1.1   Schematic of pituitary gland development with ectodermal stomodeum *(pink)* joining neuroecto-derm *(yellow)* with a resultant Rathke's cleft.

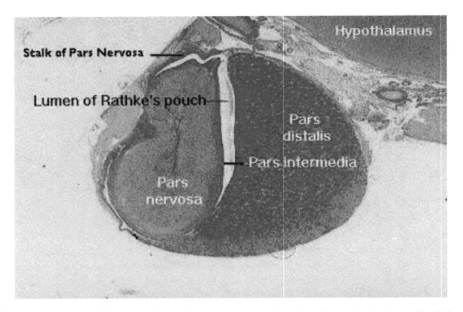

FIGURE 1.2   Histology slide of pituitary gland, demonstrating adenohypophysis (pars distalis), neurohy-pophysis (pars nervosa), infundibulum (stalk), and Rathke's cleft (pouch).

cell types appear together, fitting with the anticipated ontogeny. Somatotrophs, gonado-trophs (alpha-subunit expression) and corticotrophs appear at 8 weeks of gestation [31]. Thy-rotrophs and lactotrophs appear at 13 weeks of gestation [32]. There are numerous regulatory proteins that are thought to help with this differentiation including Pit-1, thyrotroph embry-onic factor, and GHF-1 [33].

4 ANATOMY

The pituitary gland is situated in the center of the skull at the base of the brain. It is housed in the pituitary fossa, a dura-lined space at the top of the sphenoid bone. This region of the sphenoid sinus, the sella turcica—named for its resemblance to an archaic horse saddle—is bound anteriorly by the tuberculum sella, inferiorly by the floor of the sella and posteriorly by the dorsum sella (Fig. 1.3). Lateral bony prominences of these structures include the ante-rior and posterior clinoid processes. The pituitary fossa is bordered laterally by the cavern-ous sinuses, separated by two layers of dura [34,35]. There is a layer of dura overlying the sella—the diaphragma sella—separating the pituitary fossa from the intracranial subdural and subarachnoid spaces [36].

The pituitary fossa is surrounded by critical neurovascular structures (Fig. 1.4). Each of these structures can be affected by pituitary and parasellar pathology, explaining the variety of clinical presentations of pituitary tumors. Laterally, within the cavernous sinuses, course the internal carotid arteries, including the C3, C4, and C5 segments. Just lateral to the ca-rotid artery, is the abducens nerve (cranial nerve VI). Running along the lateral wall of the

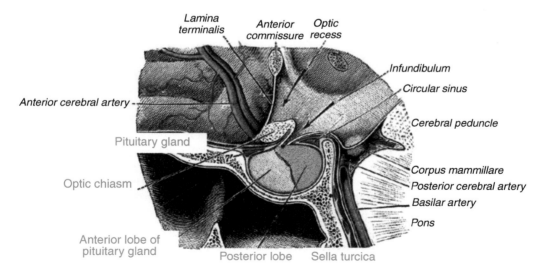

FIGURE 1.3 Sagittal parasellar anatomy demonstrating the pituitary gland sitting within the sella beneath the third ventricle and optic chiasm.

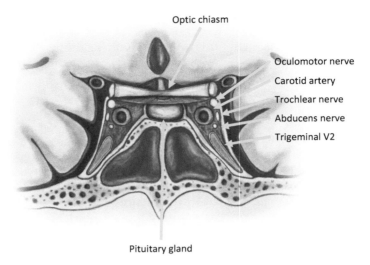

FIGURE 1.4 **Coronal parasellar anatomy demonstrating carotid arteries and cavernous cranial nerves.** *Source: Reprinted with permission from D.F. Kelly, Neurosurgical, Inc.*

cavernous sinus are the oculomotor nerve (CN III), trochlear nerve (CN IV), and the V1 and V2 branches of the trigeminal nerve (CN V) [34]. Superior to the sella is the optic chiasm, with the infundibulum of the pituitary gland traveling adjacent to the posterior midpoint of the chiasm. Superior to the optic chiasm, is the floor of the third ventricle with its lateral walls encompassing the hypothalamus. Prominent structures at the floor of the third ventricle are the mammillary bodies (components of the hypothalamus) [37]. Dorsal to the sella is the brainstem, in particular, the midbrain and upper pons.

The pituitary gland can be divided histologically into the pars distalis, pars tuberalis, pars intermedia, and pars nervosa. Regionally, there is a distinction between the pars distalis and pars tuberalis, but histologically, they are similar and function together as the adenohypophysis (anterior lobe) (Fig. 1.5). The pars nervosa is the neurohypophysis (posterior lobe) and is an extension of the hypothalamus. The pars intermedia is histologically unique but likely a remnant of Rathke's pouch from embryogenesis. Rathke's cleft separates the pars distalis and the pars intermedia. The pars tuberalis is an extension of the adenohypophysis along the infundibulum, wrapping around the pars nervosa. Often, there is an extension of the third ventricle with CSF within the infundibular pars nervosa. This is correlative of the infundibular recess as viewed dorsally (Fig. 1.6) [38].

4.1 Histology

Histologically, the adenohypophysis can be organized based on histochemical staining [39]. These can be divided into acidophils, basophils, and chromophobes. For the common

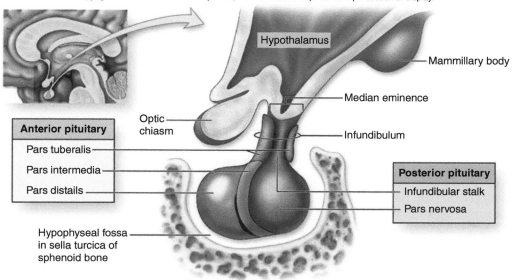

FIGURE 1.5 Diagram of normal pituitary anatomy, including pars distalis and pars tuberalis comprising the adenohypophysis. The infundibular stalk and pars nervosa comprise the neurohypophysis. *Source: Reprinted with permission from Mescher AL. Junqueira's basic histology. text and atlas. 12th ed. New York: McGraw-Hill; 2009, Figure 20.2.*

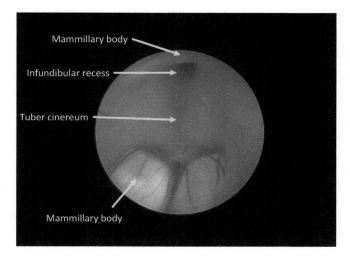

FIGURE 1.6 Endoscopic intraventricular view of the floor of the third ventricle. Note the red blush of the proximal pituitary portal system within the infundibular recess.

hematoxylin and eosin stains (H&E), acidophils take up eosin and basophils take up hematoxylin. Chromophobes have little histological staining uptake with H&E and are thought to be degranulated cells that no longer secrete hormones. Alternatively, they may represent pituitary stem cells that have yet to differentiate. These cells have an acinar arrangement, supported by an extracellular collagen matrix. This is nicely demonstrated with the reticulin (silver) stain.

Immunohistochemical analysis of the adenohypophysis can further characterize the hormone production and secretion within each cell type. The acidophil cells can stain for either growth hormone (GH) or prolactin. Hence, GH-secreting cells are somatotrophs and prolactin-secreting cells are lactotrophs or mammatrophs. A rare cell type in the normal pituitary gland is the mammosomatotroph (0.1–0.2% of cells), which stains for both GH and prolactin [40]. This cell type is thought to be a precursor of mature lactotrophs and somatotrophs. Alternatively, it has been thought to be a transitional cell converting from GH to prolactin secretion or vice versa.

Basophil cells can stain for either ACTH, thyroid-stimulating hormone (TSH), follicle-stimulating hormone (FSH), or LH. As such, ACTH cells are the corticotrophs, TSH cells are the thyrotrophs, and FSH/LH cells are the gonadotrophs.

The pars intermedia can stain for melanocyte-stimulating hormones (MSH) and has a potential interaction with ACTH secretion. Conversely, corticotrophs can potentially secrete MSH in addition to ACTH [41]. Such corticotrophs have been described in animal pituitary glands but much less commonly in humans [42,43].

The pars nervosa has its cell bodies in the hypothalamus—specifically the supraoptic and paraventricular nuclei—and comprises most of the infundibular stalk, terminating in the infundibular process (posterior pituitary lobe) [44]. It is essentially an extension of the brain and, as such, is comprised of neurons, glial cells, and pituicytes. Interestingly, at the capillary junction within the terminal boutons of the nerves, Herring bodies are seen. These structures contain oxytocin and antidiuretic hormone (ADH) and are essentially storage sites for these two hormones [45].

4.2 Hypothalamus

One cannot study the pituitary gland without recognizing its intimate relationship with the hypothalamus. The very name, hypophysis, is from the Greek meaning "outgrowth from below," referring to the hypothalamus just above it. The hypothalamus regulates many homeostatic processes among other functions, such as memory, olfaction, appetite, and emotion. Despite being a relatively small structure, the organization of the hypothalamus is amazingly complex.

The hypothalamus is bordered anteriorly by the lamina terminalis, posteriorly by the mammillary bodies, inferiorly by the median eminence/floor of the third ventricle, and laterally by the internal capsule and basal ganglia. Its superior (dorsal) limit is the hypothalamic sulcus, delineating it from the thalamus. Perhaps the best way to orient one's understanding of hypothalamic anatomy is based on the axial and sagittal plane anatomy of the third ventricle (Figs. 1.7 and 1.8). On either side of the third ventricle are three layers of hypothalamic nuclei: the periventricular nuclei, the medial hypothalamic nuclei, and the lateral hypothalamic nuclei. The medial forebrain bundle courses through the lateral hypothalamic region,

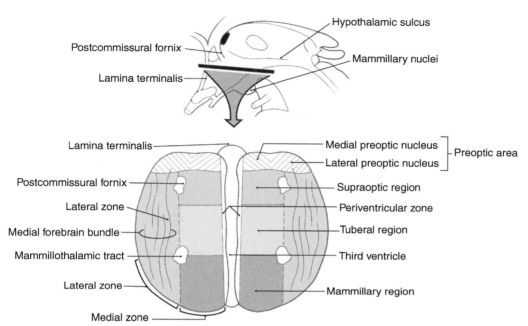

FIGURE 1.7 **Axial cross-section of the hypothalamus, demonstrating periventricular zone, medial hypothalamic nuclear groups and lateral hypothalamic nuclei.** *Source: Reprinted with permission from Haines, D. Fundamental neuroscience for basic and clinical applications. San Diego: Elsevier, Chapter 30, Figure 30.4.*

connecting the basal olfactory regions, the nucleus accumbens, and the ventral tegmental area. The periventricular nuclei, which are distinct from the paraventricular nuclei, are found in a thin subependymal lining of the third ventricle. Although the periventricular and lateral nuclei are broadly situated along the ventrodorsal aspect of the hypothalamus, the medial nuclei can be divided sagittally as well [46].

In the sagittal plane, the hypothalamus can be divided into the preoptic, supraoptic, tuberal, and mammillary regions. The preoptic region, which abuts the lamina terminalis, contains the medial and lateral preoptic nuclei. The supraoptic region has four distinct nuclei, including the supraoptic, paraventricular, suprachiasmatic, and anterior nuclei. The paraventricular and supraoptic nuclei send axons via the tuberohypophyseal tract to the neurohypophysis. The tuberal region has three distinct nuclei, including the dorsomedial, ventromedial, and arcuate nuclei. The mammillary region has two distinct structures, including the posterior nuclei and the mammillary bodies. A discussion of the function of these structures can be found in the physiology section.

4.3 Vascular Anatomy

The gross architecture of pituitary vasculature can be separated into intrinsic and extrinsic vessels [47]. The primary blood supply to the pituitary gland arises from the internal carotid arteries. The superior hypophyseal arteries supply the pituitary infundibulum and, through

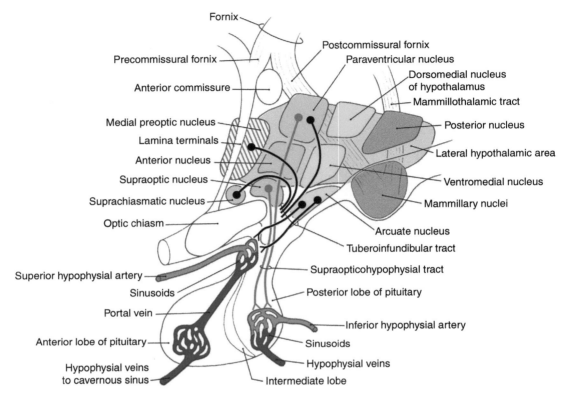

FIGURE 1.8 **Sagittal view of the hypothalamus demonstrating the pre-optic, supraoptic, tuberal, and mammillary groups of medial hypothalamic nuclei.** *Source: Reprinted with permission from Haines, D. Fundamental neuroscience for basic and clinical applications. San Diego: Elsevier, Chapter 30, Figure 30.5.*

the pituitary portal system, supply the anterior pituitary gland. These arteries arise from the supraclinoid carotid and can be duplicated at times. They typically are quite small when compared to the larger posterior communicating and anterior choroidal arteries. These arteries also supply the optic chiasm (Fig. 1.9).

The inferior hypophyseal arteries arise from the meningohypophyseal trunks of the cavernous carotid arteries. They primarily supply the posterior lobe of the pituitary gland. The meningohypophyseal trunk also sends off branches to the tentorial dura (via the arteries of Bernasconi and Casanari) and the clivus. The cavernous internal carotid artery also provides branches to the pituitary pseudocapsule (capsular artery of McConnell) [34].

The portal system is intrinsic to the pituitary gland and courses from the arcuate eminence and infundibulum to the anterior pituitary gland [48]. This vascular system transmits hypothalamic-releasing hormones to the pituitary gland, helping to regulate pituitary hormone secretion. These vessels vary in size and orientation, though larger vessels are found along the infundibulum and in the pars intermedia region. The venous outflow from the pituitary gland drains into the cavernous sinuses bilaterally.

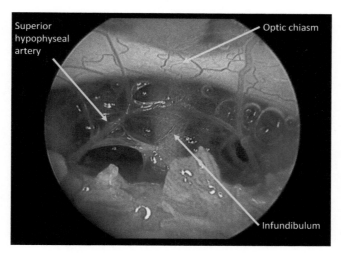

FIGURE 1.9   Endoscopic endonasal intraoperative view of pituitary vasculature, specifically the superior hypophyseal arteries supplying both the infundibulum and the optic nerves.

The pituitary gland releases its hormones into the venous system via draining veins into the cavernous sinuses, located lateral to the pituitary gland [49]. The cavernous sinuses are part of a larger dural–venous complex, draining blood from the brain. The venous sinuses are valveless vessels, the walls of which are comprised of dura mater. Typically, blood drains from the cavernous sinuses via the inferior petrosal sinus to the jugular vein, ultimately returning to the heart via the superior vena cava. There is redundancy built into this system with venous egress from each cavernous sinus via the superior intercavernous sinus (circular sinus), the inferior intercavernous sinus, the clival venous plexus, and the superior petrosal sinus [34].

4.4 Surgical Anatomy

The pituitary gland is most commonly reached surgically via an endonasal transsphenoidal approach. The surrounding anatomy is relevant to the management of pituitary and parasellar tumors and cysts. These tumors can distort the surrounding structures. Hence, a keen understanding of the normal anatomy is critical for safe surgical resection and avoidance of complications. The endonasal approach can be divided into various phases starting with the nasal cavity phase, followed by the sphenoidal and sellar phases, culminating with the tumor or lesional phase (Fig. 1.10).

4.4.1 Nasal Cavity Anatomy

The nasal cavity phase includes the nasal turbinates and nasal septum. The posterior nasal bony septum is commonly resected, carefully sparing the overlying septal mucosa. The bony septum includes the vomer and perpendicular plate of the ethmoid with small components from the palatal bone and sphenoid bone. The vomer and ethmoid contributions articulate with the cartilaginous nasal septum.

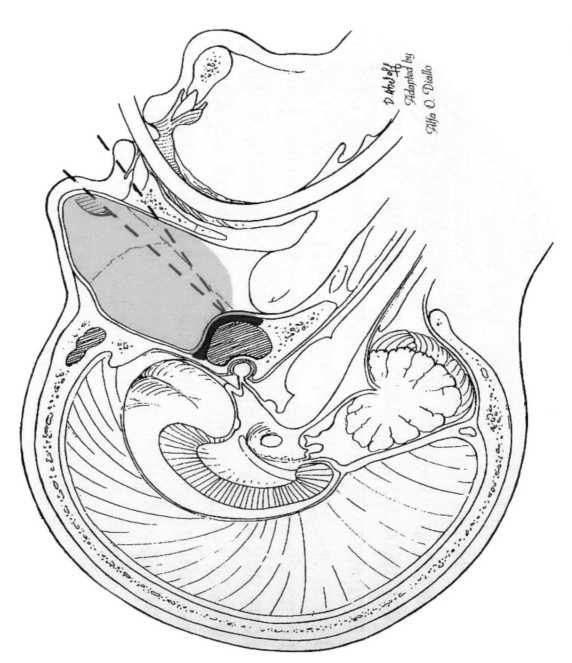

FIGURE 1.10   Schematic of the different phases of pituitary surgery, including sinonasal phase (*green*), sphenoidal (*pink/black*), intrasphenoid (*gray*), and sellar (*white*).

The nasal septum receives blood supply from branches of the sphenopalatine artery (nasal septal branches) and the anterior and posterior ethmoidal arteries. These vessels have anastomoses with each other, allowing for a redundant blood supply. A nasoseptal flap can be elevated and used to augment dural repair, which is pedicled based on the nasal septal branches of the sphenopalatine artery [22,23].

There are commonly three turbinates on either side of the nasal septum. The superior and middle turbinates originate from the ethmoid bone, and the inferior turbinate originates from the medial maxillary sinus. The bone within each turbinate is trebeculated and pneumatized. These structures, thought to help create laminar airflow and warm the inspired air, are typically lateralized and compressed to achieve access to the sphenoid sinus. In unusual cases, one or two of the turbinates can be resected to improve lateral access for larger tumors. The blood supply of these turbinates is also shared between the sphenopalatine artery and ethmoidal arteries. In particular, the blood supply of the middle turbinate originates from the base of the sphenopalatine artery, and care must be taken to preserve the main trunk if resecting this turbinate. The middle turbinate mucosa can be used as a pedicled vascular flap as well to reinforce lateral or anterior skull-base defects.

Olfactory nerve fibers course down from the cribriform plate approximately 1 cm along the nasal septum and the superior and middle turbinates. Hence, a mucosal-sparing technique that prevents the destruction of this mucosa can help preserve olfactory function following surgery (Fig. 1.11) [50]. In some patients, the olfactory fibers can be visualized along the mucosa, allowing the surgeon to preserve this tissue selectively.

4.4.2 Sphenoid Sinus Anatomy

The pituitary fossa resides within the sphenoid sinus, and one must create a sphenoidotomy to access the pituitary gland and surrounding structures. The rostrum of the sphenoid sinus (face of the sinus) is bound superiorly by the planum sphenoidale, inferiorly by the choana, and laterally by the orbital apex. There are two sphenoidal ostia that drain the sinus, located superolaterally, close to the planum sphenoidale. The choana (entrance to the nasopharynx) is a reliable landmark of the floor of the sphenoid sinus, which can be used to guide the surgeon even when the anatomy is distorted. The sphenoid ostia are typically found approximately 1.5 cm directly above the choana (Fig. 1.12). The superior turbinate often obstructs or obscures the sphenoid ostia and must be lateralized for good visualization. Many patients have a small supreme turbinate, which often lies directly over the sphenoid ostium.

The sphenopalatine artery pedicle originates laterally along the rostrum of the sphenoid sinus. This is reliably about 9 mm from the top of the choana [20,51]. The artery exits the sphenopalatine foramen but then courses within the palatovaginal canal before branching into its subsidiaries, including the nasal septal and middle turbinate arteries [52,53]. The sphenoid ostia receive two or three small branches, which must be cauterized during surgical exposure.

The mucosa is typically elevated off the sphenoid rostrum, exposing the sphenoid ostia and the "keel" of the sphenoid. This "keel" is the remnant of the bony nasal septum, typically including part of the vomer and sphenoid bone. This structure is a reliable marker of the midline sagittal plane and very rarely deviates. As the sphenoid rostrum is entered and a wide sphenoidotomy is performed, attention to the sphenopalatine canal is necessary to prevent damage to the vascular pedicle. This can result in either sacrifice of the blood supply of pedicled mucosal flaps or can increase the risk of postoperative arterial epistaxis [50].

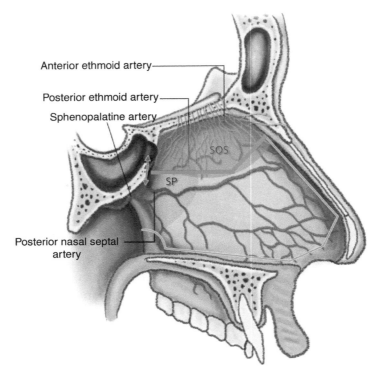

FIGURE 1.11   **Diagram depicting typical incision of "rescue flaps" performed to preserve olfaction and the sphenopalatine pedicle with a horizontal incision** *(red line)*. This is the top incision of the typical nasoseptal flap *(green line)* and can easily be converted intra-operatively or upon repeat surgery. *Source: Reprinted with permission from D.F. Kelly Neurosurgical, Inc.*

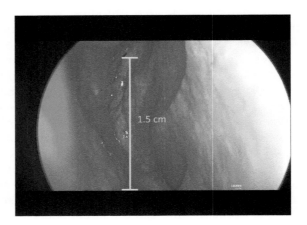

FIGURE 1.12   **Intraoperative endoscopic photograph demonstrating sphenoid ostium and its distance from choana (approximately 1.5 cm).**

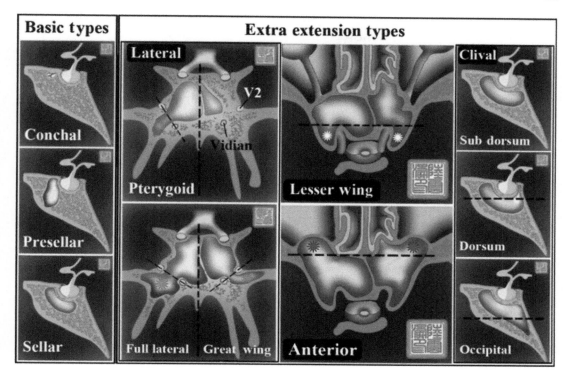

FIGURE 1.13 Diagram demonstrating variable pneumatization of the sphenoid sinus, including conchal (no pneumatization), presellar (partial pneumatization, but no obvious sellar bulge), sellar (full sagittal plane pneumatization). *Source: Reprinted with permission from Yuntao L, Jun P, Songtao Q, et al. Pneumatization of the sphenoid sinus in Chinese: the differences from Caucasian and its application in the extended transsphenoidal approach. J Anat 2011; 219(2):132–142.*

Once the sphenoid sinus is exposed, the sphenoid sinus septations are identified. Typically, two or three septations are seen, although there are numerous anatomical variations, and some patients may have significantly trebeculated sphenoid sinuses. Although one of these septations usually originates from the midline nasal septum, there is a high rate of deviation, often to one or both carotid arteries. A cadaveric study reported 85% of specimens with at least one septation, leading to a carotid artery, and 41% with both carotid arteries involved [54].

The posterior wall of the sphenoid sinus covers the critical structures, including the pituitary gland (sella), the carotid arteries, and the optic nerves. The sella is situated in the midline, extending from the planum sphenoidale to the clivus. The superior junction is the tuberculum sella, and the inferior junction is the clival recess. There is variable pneumatization of the sphenoid sinus, with sellar, presellar, and conchal patterns (Fig. 1.13) [35,55,56].

The carotid artery segments within the sphenoid sinus include the petrous, cavernous, and clinoidal segments. In the lateral walls of the sphenoid sinuses, there is considerable variation of the carotid arteries, including the inter-carotid distance as well as the course and angles of the petrous and cavernous segments. The average inter-carotid distance is 14–17 mm, though distances less than 1 cm are not uncommon [57]. Commonly, the entire sphenoidal courses of the carotid arteries are covered by bone, but bony dehiscence over the vessels has been reported in up to 30% of cadaveric specimens [58].

The inferomedial optic canals are easily seen in most patients. Rarely, a bony dehiscence is identified here. The lateral junction of the optic nerve with the carotid artery is the lateral optico-carotid recess [59]. This correlates to the optic strut seen from the cranial approach. Variations in sphenoid sinus pneumatization can result in pneumatized clinoid processes, Onodi cells, or aberrant posterior ethmoid sinuses, which are important to recognize preoperatively to maximize exposure and minimize complications.

The sphenoid sinus has two pairs of nerves running in the anteroposterior direction along its floor. Medially the Vidian nerve is present (nerve of the pterygopalatine canal). This nerve is the combination of the greater superficial petrosal nerve (GSPN)—a branch of the facial nerve—and the deep petrosal nerve. These nerves form an anastomosis at the foramen lacerum. The GSPN carries parasympathetic preganglionic nerves to the pterygopalatine ganglion. The postganglionic nerves innervate the lacrimal gland as well as mucosal glands within the nasal, palatine, and pharyngeal mucosa. Injury to the GSPN can result in diminished lacrimation and xerophthalmia (dry-eyes) [60]. The sympathetic nerves innervate the nasal cavity, paranasal sinuses, orbit, and face. A specific function is mydriasis of the pupil. Injury to the Vidian nerve can result in a partial or complete Horner's syndrome (i.e., ptosis, meiosis, and anhydrosis of the ipsilateral face) [61]. Surgically, this nerve is a landmark at the inferolateral sphenoid sinus, arising from the junction of the vertical and horizontal petrous carotid artery.

The other set of nerves identified at the lateral floor of the sphenoid sinus (lateral to the Vidian nerve) are the maxillary branches of the trigeminal nerve (V2). This nerve exits Meckel's cave via the foramen rotundum and courses along the floor of the orbit, exiting the infraorbital foramen to provide sensory innervation to the face. The variations of pneumatization respect the location of these two sets of nerves, nearly always contained within their bony canals (Fig. 1.13) [55].

The pituitary fossa is situated between the cavernous sinuses. During surgery, the dura mater (that covers the normal gland and typically contains intrasellar pathology) is incised. This is performed after the carotid arteries are localized with micro-Doppler ultrasound [62]. Tumors of the pituitary gland can alter this normal anatomy, resulting in a significantly expanded sella and, in some cases, invasion into the sphenoid sinus, the cavernous sinuses, the suprasellar/supradiaphragmatic region, and ultimately the third ventricle, frontal lobe, temporal lobe, and brainstem.

To minimize damage to the pituitary gland and resultant hypopituitarism, its location with respect to the tumor or cyst must be assessed before surgery. Often, the pituitary gland is compressed and pushed to one side. In these cases, the interface between the tumor, and normal gland should be identified and used for dissection [63]. For most pituitary adenomas (the most common type of pituitary tumor), the gland has a different color and texture from the tumor. It is usually yellow-pink in color and often thickens and turns purple-red as tumor is resected and blood flow is restored to the gland. The gland has a thicker consistency compared to adenomas, as a result of its retained extracellular collagen reticular structure.

In some cases, the pituitary gland is anterior to the tumor, and commonly an incision is made into the gland to access the tumor or cyst. This incision is performed in a vertical orientation as this is parallel to the pituitary vasculature (particularly the portal venous system). Counterintuitively, this incision does not cause increased pituitary dysfunction and may be protective as this prevents unnecessary laceration of and traction on the normal gland [64].

Other pathologies, such as some craniopharyngiomas, chordomas, and meningiomas, maintain more normal pituitary anatomy, which helps with tumor dissection. In these cases, particularly where the pathology sits on top of the normal gland, careful identification and dissection of the vasculature are necessary to preserve pituitary function and improve visual outcomes. Most important are the superior hypophyseal arteries, which supply both the infundibulum and the optic nerves (Fig. 1.9) [65].

For specific (rare) pathology involving the region anterior to the midbrain, one approach is the transsphenoidal, transsellar avenue. To reach this region involves dissecting the normal pituitary gland off the floor of the sella and from the walls of the cavernous sinus. The gland is then transposed to one side, allowing the dorsum sella to be drilled and the dura incised. The anterior midbrain is just dorsal to this region, including the basilar artery bifurcation and the oculomotor nerves [66]. This approach when carefully used appears to have minimal impact on normal pituitary function [67].

4.5 Radiographic Anatomy

Pituitary gland pathology is often difficult to characterize without advanced neuroimaging. One must fully understand the appearance of a normal pituitary gland and parasellar structures to discern subtle differences. Although no longer common, the first neuroimaging performed of the pituitary was with x-ray roentgenograms. A lateral view x-ray has specific imaging features, including the pneumatized sphenoid sinus, the floor of the anterior skull base and clivus in addition to the anterior sella (Fig. 1.14). Although CT and MRI have greatly improved pituitary imaging, plain x-ray and video fluoroscopy are still used intraoperatively at some institutions for localization when performing speculum-based microscopic transsphenoidal procedures. Historically, roentgenograms have been enhanced with pneumoencephalography to improve contrast of the subarachnoid and ventricular systems [68,69]. This technology has been phased out because of its invasive nature and associated morbidity.

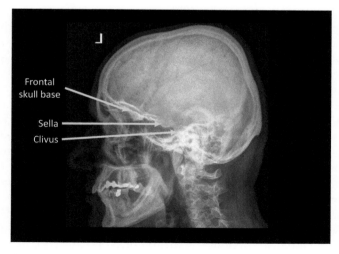

FIGURE 1.14   Lateral skull radiogram demonstrating typical findings helpful for intraoperative fluoroscopic navigation, including the sella, frontal skull-base and clivus.

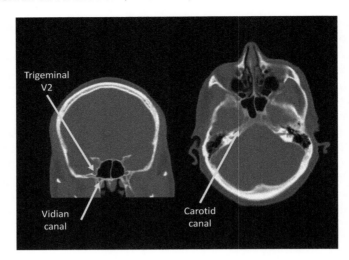

FIGURE 1.15 Coronal and axial computed tomography of the head (bone windows), demonstrating bony canals of the Vidian and trigeminal V2 nerves as well as the petrous horizontal carotid canal.

Cerebral angiography as an isolated imaging modality can also provide some hint of pathology in the suprasellar region with vascular distortion [70]. Though no longer a primary modality for pituitary imaging, digital subtraction angiography still has a role in certain patients with distorted vasculature that needs further characterization, as well as in patients who may benefit from preoperative embolization of large, vascular tumors. It is also necessary if there is any suspicion of an arterial aneurysm in or near the sella.

In the 1970s, CT was introduced and significantly advanced sellar and parasellar imaging. Although MRI is the workhorse of pituitary imaging, CT imaging plays a large role for preoperative planning, postoperative management, and for those patients who cannot have MRIs because of metallic implants. The normal CT scan performed with high-resolution coronal and sagittal reformats delineates numerous bony structures, often better than MRI. The optic canals are reliably identified, along with the Vidian nerve canal and the maxillary nerve canal. The petrosal carotid canals are also well visualized (Fig. 1.15). Sinus anatomy, particularly sphenoid sinus septations are well highlighted. This is most relevant for sphenoid sinus septations, Onodi cells, and aberrant posterior ethmoid and variable sphenoid sinus pneumatization (Fig. 1.16) [71]. These are all structures that are helpful to identify for surgical planning.

The best modality to evaluate pituitary pathology and normal pituitary anatomy is MRI [72]. Each of the main sequences (T1, T2, fat-suppressed, contrast enhanced) adds significantly to the understanding of the gland and adjacent anatomy. "Pituitary protocols" have been established to include these sequences. The field of view is focused on the sella and parasellar structures, and thinner slices are obtained (2–3 mm thick), allowing for improved resolution of the pituitary structures.

The normal gland is best evaluated with T1 noncontrast sequences. The anterior pituitary gland has similar T1 signal intensity as with gray matter. The normal posterior pituitary gland has significant signal shortening (i.e., bright on T1) (Fig. 1.17), resulting in the "bright spot" of the pituitary gland. As the posterior pituitary gland is essentially a storage facility for

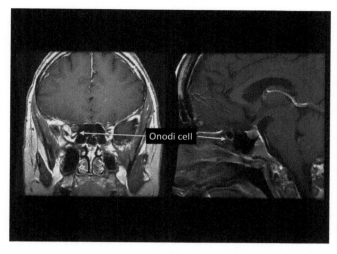

FIGURE 1.16   Coronal and sagittal post-contrast magnetic resonance imaging, demonstrating Onodi cells, typical variant of sinonasal pneumatization.

ADH, the bright spot is thought to be a result of signal shortening by the ADH molecule. This "bright spot" has shown an inverse correlation with diabetes insipidus, whether iatrogenic or caused by other pathology [73,74].

The anterior pituitary gland enhances homogeneously with the administration of gadolinium intravenous contrast. These sequences rarely show a distinction between the anterior and posterior lobes, relying on the precontrast sequences to draw this delineation. Occasionally, Rathke's cleft can be identified, though frequent imaging findings include small Rathke

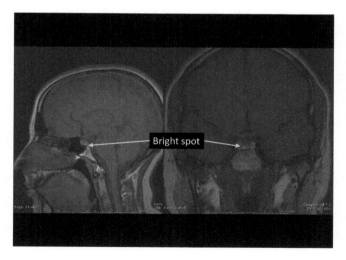

FIGURE 1.17   Sagittal and coronal non-contrast magnetic resonance imaging, demonstrating T1 shortening (bright spot) of the posterior pituitary gland.

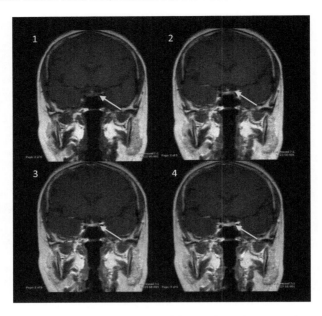

FIGURE 1.18   Dynamic magnetic resonance imaging of the pituitary demonstrating sequential (1–4) filling of contrast in the normal gland (patient's right side) and a delayed filling of the hypoenhancing left sellar microadenoma *(yellow arrow).*

cleft cysts [75]. Fat-saturated T1 post-contrast sequences are helpful to suppress the clival fat signal, which can blur the distinction of the normal gland from the surrounding bone.

The T2 sequence is helpful in identifying surrounding neurovascular structures, most notably the optic chiasm. Even when the chiasm is compressed by a large mass, this sequence shows the location of the chiasm well. Additionally, the T2 signal is helpful when differentiating between small cysts and solid masses. The intensity of the T2 signal can help differentiate between CSF signal and pathological fluid.

Dynamic pituitary series obtain rapid coronal T1 slices timed with the administration of gadolinium contrast [76]. The normal gland should begin to enhance homogeneously. In the setting of a microadenoma or cyst, this enhancement can be delayed and becomes incongruous with the surrounding normal gland (Fig. 1.18). Hence, this is a very helpful sequence for specific pathology, such as Cushing's disease or mild hyperprolactinemia.

5 PHYSIOLOGY

The pituitary gland is known as the "master gland," owing to its governance over a multitude of target organs. This unique gland relies on a set of signal feedback loops to appropriately regulate each of the hormone systems. The function of the pituitary gland can be divided along anatomical differences, primarily between the anterior and posterior pituitary glands (adenohypophysis and neurohypophysis). The main distinction is the pituitary portal venous system involved in the regulation of the adenohypophysis. The neurohypophysis is controlled directly by hypothalamic neurons with axons terminating in this gland.

The anterior pituitary gland is regulated by the hypothalamus, and each hormone system is considered a hypothalamic-pituitary axis (HPA) [77]. These hormone systems include the adrenal axis, governing cortisol production and the stress response; the thyroid axis, regulating metabolism; the gonadotropin axis, regulating reproduction, sexual function, and anabolism; the growth hormone axis, regulating growth and tissue health; and the prolactin axis, regulating lactation. With some exceptions, each of these systems has intermediary target organs that produce a secondary hormone that casts a wider effect on the body and its organ systems. Most of these intermediary hormones regulate the pituitary gland with negative feedback loops. The main exception is prolactin, which does not have an intermediary hormone and is tonically inhibited by dopamine from the hypothalamus.

Three of the pituitary hormones are glycoproteins that exist as heterodimers with alpha and beta subunits. The alpha glycoprotein subunit (α-SU) is a common subunit of TSH, FSH, LH, and human chorionic gonadotropin (HCG), produced by the placenta). Each of these four hormones has a specific beta subunit, conferring receptor specificity (β-TSH, β-FSH, β-LH, and β-HCG) [78]. Both subunits are necessary for proper binding to the respective receptors. Free beta subunits are degraded intracellularly and require the alpha subunit for stability and extracellular secretion [79].

These feedback loops (Fig. 1.19) help establish homeostasis of the hormone system and are influenced by a multitude of factors at each level. A basic understanding of this system

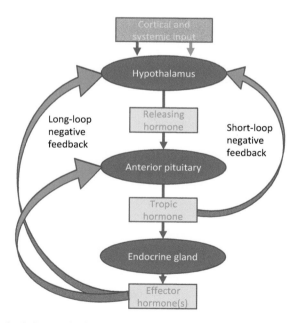

FIGURE 1.19   **Schema depicting typical negative feedback loops.** Not all hypothalamic-pituitary axes follow this exact pattern

TABLE 1.1   Hypothalamic, Pituitary, and End-Organ Hormones and Regulation

	Pituitary axis				
	Corticotrope	Thyrotrope	Gonadotrope	Somatotrope	Lactotrope
Primary hypothalamic regulation	CRH: 41-amino acid peptide, stimulatory	TRH: tripeptide, stimulatory	GnRH: decapeptide, stimulatory	GHRH: 44-amino acid peptide, stimulatory; somatostatin: tetradecapeptide, inhibitory	Dopamine (catecholamine), inhibitory; TRH, stimulatory
Tropic hormone secreted	ACTH: 4.5-kDa protein	TSH: 28-kDa glycoprotein hormone	FSH and LH: 28- and 33-kDa glycoprotein hormones	GH: ≈22-kDa protein	Prolactin: ≈23-kDa protein
Target endocrine gland	Adrenal cortex	Thyroid epithelium	Ovary/testis	Liver	No target gland
Peripheral hormone (negative feedback)	Cortisol	Triiodo-thyronine	Estrogen, progesterone, testosterone, and inhibin	IGF-I	None

ACTH, Adrenocorticotropic hormone; CRH, corticotropin-releasing hormone; FSH, follicle-stimulating hormone; GH, growth hormone; GHRH, growth hormone-releasing hormone; GnRH, gonadotropin-releasing hormone; IGF-1, insulin-like growth factor 1; LH, luteinizing hormone; TRH, thyrotropin-releasing hormone; and TSH, thyroid-stimulating hormone.

is necessary to any clinician aiming to diagnose and treat patients with pituitary disorders and tumors. Each system is discussed in depth, including function and regulation (Table 1.1).

5.1 Hypothalamic Physiology

The physiology of the pituitary gland cannot fully be understood without a discussion of hypothalamic physiology. The hypothalamus has numerous cerebral functions, including its role in the limbic system, memory generation, systemic homeostasis, autonomic function, and endocrine regulation. It is difficult to generalize hypothalamic function, but a good rule-of-thumb is a distinction between the caudolateral and rostromedial hypothalamic nuclei, regulating anxiety/stress versus contentment/relaxation, respectively.

Certain hypothalamic nuclei can be conceptually paired as opposing forces, regulating systemic bodily functions. The anterior nucleus of the supraoptic hypothalamic region governs parasympathetic activation and dissipates heat via thermoregulation. Conversely, the posterior nucleus of the mammillary hypothalamic region governs sympathetic activation and conservation of heat via thermoregulation. Additionally, it is adjacent to the periaqueductal gray zone, which controls pain and anxiety. Similarly, the dorsomedial nuclei of the tuberal hypothalamic region regulates aggressiveness. Stimulation of this nucleus can result in "sham rage" [80–82].

The lateral hypothalamic nuclei are the hunger regions (feeding center) and reward centers of the hypothalamus. These are regulated by paracrine and endocrine hormones, such as leptin [83,84] for hunger and orexin [85] for reward. Lesions of the lateral hypothalamic area can result in anorexia and starvation [86,87]. Conversely, the ventromedial nuclei of the tuberal hypothalamic region regulate satiety. Lesions of these nuclei can result in obesity [88]. Intuitively, this is a potential target for deep brain stimulation to aid in weight loss for obese patients [89–92].

The mammillary nuclei (within the mammillary bodies) are essentially a major ganglion of the limbic system. The cell bodies of the mammillothalamic axons originate in this structure. The postcommissural forniceal axons synapse with these neurons. This is an important relay in the circuit of Papez and the limbic system [93–95]. The mammillothalamic tract connects the mammillary nuclei with the anterior nuclei of the thalami. Lesions to this structure can result in Korsakoff's syndrome with impairment of long-term potentiation and memory generation [96,97]. In addition, the circuit of Papez is involved in emotion and behavior, affecting memory and learning as well [98,99].

The suprachiasmatic nuclei of the supraoptic region regulate circadian rhythm. The anatomical location of this nucleus directly adjacent to the optic chiasm appears to explain this function. This relation has been demonstrated with light stimulation and excitation of the suprachiasmatic nucleus [100]. Efferent output of this nucleus emanates to numerous hypothalamic and extrahypothalamic regions, the most prominent of which include the paraventricular nuclei and the periventricular nuclei [101]. This is the likely pathway for circadian regulation of ACTH, GH, and gonadotropin release. The suprachiasmatic nuclei regulate the pineal gland and melatonin release [102]. Interestingly, the removal of the pineal gland in animals does not significantly affect circadian rhythm. The likely connection between the suprachiasmatic nuclei and the pineal gland is mediated through the sympathetic innervation of the gland via efferent fibers to the posterior hypothalamic nuclei [103,104].

The direct pituitary-endocrine control by the hypothalamus is divided between the anterior pituitary gland, mediated by releasing hormones, and the posterior pituitary gland with efferent axonal fibers from the hypothalamus. The arcuate nuclei, preoptic nuclei, and periventricular nuclei collectively send axons to the median eminence to release their hormones into the pituitary portal system. Additionally, the tuberoinfundibular pathway, one of the four major dopamine systems, originates with the arcuate and periventricular nuclei, regulating prolactin secretion by pituitary lactotrophs [105,106].

The paraventricular and supraoptic nuclei of the supraoptic hypothalamic region both regulate and release ADH (vasopressin or arginine vasopressin [AVP]) as well as oxytocin. These are discussed in further detail in the section on the physiology of the posterior lobe. The regulation of ADH release is affected primarily by osmoreceptors in specific circumventricular organs (CVOs).

The CVOs are unique structures within the CNS, which lack a distinct blood–brain barrier, allowing for neuronal interaction with intravascular contents. The most notable CVO is the chemoreceptor zone in the brainstem, which triggers the nausea centers in the setting of noxious chemical stimuli. The posterior pituitary gland and the arcuate eminence are also considered CVOs. However, the CVOs that regulate the posterior pituitary gland are the subforniceal organ and the organum vasculosum of the lamina terminalis. Together, these structures regulate the paraventricular and supraoptic nuclei [107,108]. Both structures contain osmoreceptors to detect intravascular osmolality.

5.1.1 *Hypothalamus-Pituitary-Adrenal Axis*

Arguably, of all the hormones regulated by the pituitary, cortisol is the most vital for survival. The adrenal glands produce cortisol, so named because of the location of production—the adrenal cortex. Overall, the adrenal glands produce a number of hormones, each regulated by a different system. These include epinephrine and norepinephrine (adrenalin and noradrenalin), directly stimulated by the preganglionic sympathetic nerves from the T5–T11 nerve roots via the sympathetic chain. These hormones are produced in the adrenal medulla.

The adrenal cortex is divided histologically into three layers: zona glomerulosa, zona fasciculata, and zona reticularis. The outermost layer, the zona glomerulosa, produces the corticosteroid, aldosterone. This is a mineralocorticoid, which regulates systemic blood pressure and electrolyte balance via the renin-angiotensin-aldosterone system. There is an indirect involvement of the pituitary gland as angiotensin II, the active metabolite of angiotensinogen/angiotensin I, stimulates the posterior pituitary gland to secrete ADH [109]. This is likely via receptors on the subforniceal organ, a circumventricular structure, and may regulate hypothalamic control of the posterior pituitary gland [110]. Additionally, angiotensin II receptors regulate corticotroph release of ACTH as well as hypothalamic release of corticotropin-releasing hormone (CRH) [111,112].

The innermost layer of the adrenal cortex, the zona reticularis, produces androgens—primarily dehydroepiandrosterone (DHEA), DHEA sulfate, and androstenedione. These have little direct androgenous effect but are regulated by the testes to convert to the more potent testosterone.

The middle cortical layer, the zona fasciculata, is the primary site of glucocorticoid secretion, such as cortisol. Cortisol production is directly controlled by pituitary corticotroph cells secreting ACTH. In turn, ACTH is directly stimulated by CRH, vasopressin, and other peptides. Corticotropin-releasing hormone is produced in the paraventricular nuclei and regulated by neurons from the suprachiasmatic nucleus, solitary tract, and the hippocampi. Cortisol confers negative feedback to both ACTH and CRH production. Vasopressin and angiotensin II positively regulate ACTH. It is negatively regulated by elevations in serum glucose levels. Any systemic stressor also triggers cortisol production, likely through the hypothalamic pathways previously described.

The ACTH protein is derived from the larger precursor protein, proopiomelanocortin (POMC). This protein can also be cleaved into γ-lipotropin, β-endorphin, and MSH— including all three subunits (alpha, beta, and gamma). In settings of ACTH excess (Addison's disease, Nelson's syndrome), there is resultant elevation of α-MSH, effecting increased skin pigmentation (though there is some cross-reactivity of ACTH itself with the MSH receptor).

Cortisol production is directly tied to the individual's circadian rhythm, as regulated by the suprachiasmatic nuclei. Serum cortisol levels peak upon waking and reach a nadir at the onset of sleep [113,114]. Interestingly, the time to peak cortisol becomes earlier as the population ages. However, this does correlate with alterations in bed-times, possibly contributing to this variation [114].

Cortisol and the other glucocorticoids are vital for survival. In the setting of stress, cortisol is essential to increase serum glucose levels by stimulating gluconeogenesis and glycogenolysis in the liver and other tissues, converting circulating molecules, and glycogen into glucose and other sugars [115]. This is primarily regulated via glucagon sensitization [116]. Insulin resistance is also enhanced, mediated primarily through downstream modulation of the insulin receptor [117]. Cortisol is also involved in the catabolism of proteins and lipids as well [118]. Prolonged cortisol release can result in proteolysis [119].

Cortisol helps sensitize cells to catecholamines. It mediates the vasoactive effect of norepinephrine on the vascular system [120]. In addition to the vasopressor effects, cortisol helps activate glycogen phosphorylase, increasing epinephrine's effect on glycogenolysis [121]. This interaction plays an important role in numerous physiologic and pathophysiologic conditions (e.g., posttraumatic stress disorder) [122–124].

Cortisol has a profound role on the immune system, primarily as an immunosuppressant. This effect is mediated on a number of levels, including the lymphocytic, interleukin, and even enzymatic levels. Cortisol decreases certain interleukin levels (i.e., interleukin 12 [IL-12], interferon-γ, and tumor-necrosis factor) while increasing others (i.e., IL-4, IL-10, IL-13) [125]. This allows a shift to the TH2 pathway, possibly limiting overactivity of the immune system [126]. It also can directly activate immune cells, such as the natural killer cells [127]. Cortisol regulates copper-enzyme function, such as superoxide dismutase, which is necessary for bactericidal activity [128].

Cortisol directly affects electrolyte and fluid balance by affecting the glomerular filtration rate (GFR), renal plasma flow, sodium and potassium retention, and intestinal fluid resorption [129]. Cortisol, along with aldosterone, increases the sodium-potassium pump activity in the renal distal tubules, resulting in sodium retention and potassium excretion [130]. Hence, patients with hypocortisolism can have mild hyponatremia. Conversely, patients with hypocortisolism and diabetes insipidus may not have significant diuresis until cortisol is administered, given the interaction between sodium retention and urine concentration [131].

There are numerous pharmacological glucocorticoids that are used to treat a variety of disorders. It is important to note the nuances of these medications, as they can influence the practitioner to prescribe the appropriate agent for the specific patient. This is quite relevant in treating endocrinopathies. The most physiologic glucocorticoid available is hydrocortisone, which is available as enteric, parenteric, and topical formulations. Hydrocortisone has a short biological half-life of about 8–12 h and has mild mineralocorticoid activity (1:150 relative to fludrocortisone and 1:400 relative to aldosterone). Intermediate-acting agents (biological half-life of 12–36 h) include prednisone, prednisolone (i.e., active hepatic metabolite of prednisone, which is ideal for patients with hepatic dysfunction), and methylprednisolone (available intravenously). Long-acting glucocorticoids (biological half-life of 36–54 h) include dexamethasone and betamethasone. These are the least physiologic, but they have the best antiinflammatory activity. Table 1.2 demonstrates equivalent potency and activity [132]. Commonly prescribed glucocorticoid equivalents are:

hydrocortisone 20 mg = prednisone 5 mg = dexamethasone 0.75 mg.

5.1.2 Hypothalamus-Pituitary-Thyroid Axis

The thyroid gland synthesizes thyroid hormone production, which regulates systemic metabolism. Thyroxine is synthesized in the follicular cells, which surround the follicles (a storage site for iodine along with thyroglobulin). The parafollicular cells are interspersed among the follicles and secrete calcitonin to help regulate serum calcium levels. Thyroxine (T_4) is

TABLE 1.2 Comparison Chart of Corticosteroids with Equivalent Glucocorticoid and Mineralocorticoid Dosage

	Potency relative to hydrocortisone half-life			
	Equivalent glucocorticoid dose (mg)	Mineral-corticoid	Plasma (minutes)	Duration of action (hours)
Short-acting				
Hydrocortisone (Cortef, Cortisol)	20	1	90	8–12
Cortisone acetate	25	0.8	30	8–12
Intermediate-acting				
Prednisone	5	0.8	60	12–36
Prednisolone	5	0.8	200	12–36
Triamcinolone	4	0	300	12–36
Methylprednisolone	4	0.5	180	12–36
Long-acting				
Dexamethasone	0.75	0	200	36–54
Betamethasone	0.6	0	300	36–54

formed by the cleavage of tyrosine residues from thyroglobulin, which is linked to iodine at the 3′ and 5′ sites of the benzene ring. Two diiodotyrosine molecules combine to form T_4. This process is stimulated by TSH, secreted by the adenohypophysis. Deiodinase enzymes are responsible for converting T_4 to T_3 (active) and RT_3 (inactive). This occurs primarily in peripheral tissues, though 10–20% is secreted by the thyroid gland. The T_3 crosses the cell membrane (either passively or via transporters, primarily in the CNS) and binds to the nuclear protein, thyroid receptor, which activates numerous genes with the thyroid hormone response element sequence in the promotor region [133–136]. In certain cell types, thyroid hormone function is mediated via the phospholipase C/protein kinase C (PKC) system, activating extracellular signal–regulating kinases 1 and 2 (ERK1/2). This has been seen in the erythrocyte calcium pump as well as cardiac myocardium sarcomere regulation [137].

Thyrotropin, or TSH, is stimulated by thyrotropin-releasing hormone (TRH), secreted by the hypothalamus (paraventricular nucleus). Secretion of TSH is in a pulsatile fashion, with increased production during sleep; then TSH stimulates T_4 production. There is a negative feedback loop by T_4, downregulating TRH secretion and TSH secretion [138]. Somatostatin also inhibits release of TSH, among other hormones [139]. This hormone is secreted by periventricular hypothalamic neurons and transported to the adenohypophysis via the portal system [140].

Cold exposure upregulates TRH [141]. This is mediated by the pontomedullary release of catecholamines (norepinephrine/epinephrine) from the locus ceruleus [142]. Conversely, starvation (or the conversion from the fed state to the starved state) results in down-regulation of TRH and ultimately systemic metabolism to preserve energy stores. This may be regulated by downregulation of TRH related to a fasting-induced increase of glucocorticoids [143]. As expected, leptin upregulates TRH in response to dietary intake [144,145].

Triiodothyronine (T_3), the active metabolite of thyroxine, has numerous systemic effects. Perhaps the most prevalent effect is an increased basal metabolic rate [146,147]. In specific tissue, thyroid hormone can potentiate adrenergic action in white fat as well as adaptive thermogenesis in brown adipose tissue [148,149]. This is mediated through mitochondrial activity and "basal proton leakage" [150]. The effects on the cardiovascular system include increased myocardial contractility, increased heart rate, and systemic vasodilatation [151]. Thyroid hormone has an important effect on neurodevelopment, in part mediated by microtubule regulation of the cytoarchitecture [152,153]. Catabolism, also mediated adrenergically, is regulated by thyroid hormone as well [154].

There are various formulations of thyroid hormone available for patients with thyroid deficiency. The most common medication, levothyroxine, is a synthetic L-enantiomer of T_4. This formulation can be finely titrated to treat the patient's symptoms and laboratory levels. Also, T_3 is available enterally or parenterally as liothyronine. This is useful in patients who have a diminished ability to convert T_4 into T_3. Additionally, given its quick but short half-life, this can be useful in patients with profound hypothyroidism who need a faster-acting agent than T_4, which can take up to a week to reach homeostasis. There are animal thyroid extracts available as well. These agents contain both T_4 and T_3 but do contain other thyroid hormone variants as well.

5.1.3 Hypothalamus-Pituitary-Growth Hormone Axis

The hypothalamic-pituitary-growth hormone axis is unique in that the pituitary hormone has systemic effects. Growth hormone-releasing hormone (GHRH) is secreted by the arcuate nucleus and transported to the adenohypophysis via the portal system. It induces GH synthesis and release by the somatotrophs. The GHRH is secreted in a pulsatile fashion and, along with the inhibitory effect of somatostatin, regulates GH secretion and pulsatility [155,156]. Growth hormone is at highest concentrations in the neonatal and juvenile ages. This does change at puberty, with more prominent GH bursts in men [157]. In adults, there is variation in GH secretion and pulsatility based on gender and age [158,159]. Sleep has a marked effect on GH secretion, with the largest secretory bursts occurring in the first sleep cycle [160].

Growth hormone is an anabolic hormone that affects nearly every organ system. Its target organ is the liver, where it stimulates gluconeogenesis, protein synthesis, and insulin-like growth factor (IGF) secretion. Together, IGF-1 and GH induce skeletal muscle protein synthesis; growth, bone, and cartilage linear growth; and visceral organ growth and health [161,162]. Growth hormone appears to be the predominant factor for adipose lipolysis, though IGF-1 does have some effect on adipogenesis [163,164]. Insulin-like growth factor 1 (and the other IGFs) are transported bound to insulin-like growth factor-binding proteins conjugated with acid labile subunits. Both of these proteins are also synthesized in the liver and induced by GH [165,166].

Both GH and IGF-1 have negative feedback on GH secretion. Growth hormone directly inhibits GHRH secretion and simultaneously stimulates somatostatin release in the hypothalamus [167]. Interestingly, IGF-1 appears to function by stimulating somatostatin release alone at the level of the hypothalamus. Simultaneously, GH and IGF-1 both suppress GH secretion by the somatotrophs [168,169].

Other molecules that regulate GH secretion include ghrelin and dopamine. Ghrelin is an appetite-stimulating neuropeptide secreted by ghrelinergic cells in the gastrointestinal tract and suppressed by stomach stretch [170]. Ghrelin stimulates GH secretion in conjunction with GHRH [171]. Dopamine receptors are also found on somatotrophs. L-Dopa and dopamine agonists have been shown to decrease growth hormone secretion [172,173]. There also appears to be cross-talk between ghrelin and dopamine molecules on GH secretion [174].

For patients with GH deficiency, there are numerous pharmacological agents that are used for replacement. The current formulations are synthesized via recombinant DNA techniques and are injectable agents. Most of these are administered daily, though some formulations are longer lasting, typically requiring monthly injections [175]. Somatostatin analogues are commercially available to modulate GH secretion, particularly in acromegaly [176,177].

5.1.4 Hypothalamus-Pituitary-Gonadal Axis

The regulation of the reproductive system is closely regulated by the hypothalamus and pituitary gland. The release of the gonadotropins, FSH and LH, is regulated by gonadotropin-releasing hormone (GnRH), secreted by the parvocellular region of the arcuate nucleus in the hypothalamus. The gonadotroph cell secretes both FSH and LH, which are stored in separate secretory granules. There is differential control of these vesicles, resulting in nonparallel secretion of these hormones [178]. These hormones regulate the secretion of reproductive hormones (testosterone in men and estrogen/progesterone in women) by the gonads/corpus luteum. They also regulate gametogenesis (spermatogenesis and oogenesis) [179]. Given the notable difference in hormonal regulation between genders, these will be discussed separately. However, a unifying feature is the negative feedback on gonadotropin secretion by prolactin. Although this is physiologically beneficial in women, the effects are identical in men [180].

5.1.4.1 EFFECTS ON MEN

In men, LH regulates testosterone production by the Leydig cells of the testes. Testosterone and other androgens confer systemic effects as well as gender-specific effects. An anabolic steroid, testosterone induces increased muscle mass, bone density, and stimulation of linear bony growth [181]. It also increases erythropoiesis due to bone marrow stimulation [182]. Its androgenic effects include maturation of the primary sex organs during development as well as development of secondary sexual characteristics at puberty (e.g., deepening of voice, growth of facial and axillary hair, and facial bony prominence). It also increases aggressiveness and libido [183].

Testosterone, a lipophilic molecule, has its main mechanism of action by binding to the androgen receptor activating PKC and MAP kinase pathways, initiating transcription of genes regulated by the cyclic adenosine monophosphate (cAMP) response element-binding protein (CREB) [184]. Testosterone also confers negative feedback, decreasing LH and FSH production by the pituitary gland [185].

Follicle-stimulating hormone has its primary effect on the Sertoli cells in men. It stimulates the production of androgen-binding protein, which increases intraluminal testosterone concentration, resulting in spermatogenesis. It also stimulates production of inhibin, which functions as a negative feedback signal to decrease FSH secretion from the pituitary gland [186].

5.1.4.2 EFFECTS ON WOMEN

In women, because of the process of menstruation, the hormonal regulation is more complex (Fig. 1.20). Gonadotropin-releasing hormone pulsatile secretion is essential to induce

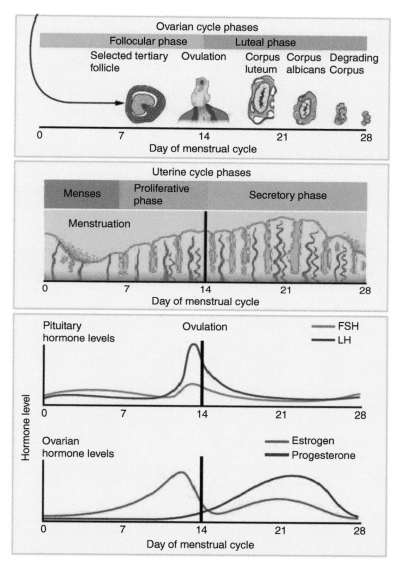

FIGURE 1.20   Diagram of menstrual cycle with respect to gonadotropins, estrogen, and progesterone secretion.

both FSH (slow pulses) and LH (fast pulses) secretion. Kisspeptin (metastin) neurons of the anterior ventral periventricular nuclei stimulate GnRH [187]. At the beginning of the menstrual cycle, FSH concentrations slowly rise, stimulating a growing follicle to develop. This follicle, in turn, secretes estrogens (estradiol), which function as a negative feedback molecule at low concentrations, regulating kisspeptin, GnRH, and FSH secretion. The secretion of estrogen relies on both FSH and LH activity. Luteinizing hormone induces Theca cells (female counterpart to Leydig cells) to convert cholesterol to androgens. These androgens are then converted into estrogens by aromatase (CYP19) or estrogen synthetase, in the granulosa cells stimulated by FSH [188,189].

As estrogen concentrations rise due to the developing follicle, a concentration-dependent estrogen receptor induces positive feedback on GnRH secretion, resulting in a surge in both LH and FSH secretion [190]. This spike of LH concentration induces ovulation and the formation of the corpus luteum (remnant of the developing follicle). The corpus luteum secretes estrogen and progesterone, inhibiting kisspeptin, GnRH, FSH, and LH secretion. Progesterone induces endometrium secretory and vascular activity in preparation of embryo implantation. It also increases the thermostat slightly (approximately 1°C) [191]. Once the corpus luteum dies at 14 days, the progesterone levels plummet, resulting in endometrial sloughing (menstruation), and allow for the initiation of the next follicle-stimulating cycle. Circulating estrogen levels are also necessary for the development of secondary sexual features during puberty, protein synthesis, and lipid cycling, coagulation, and libido (in conjunction with androgens) [192].

Essentially all molecules of the gonadal axes can be pharmacologically replaced. There are numerous formulations of testosterone (i.e., injectable, topical cream, gel, or patch), estrogen, and progesterone (pills or patch) [193]. Human gonadotropins can be replaced to help induce ovulation, though clomiphene, an estrogen receptor inhibitor, can be effective in inducing ovulation [194]. The GnRH replacement therapy (pulsatile) can be used for infertility in both men and women, particularly for GnRH-deficient patients [195]. Conversely, long-acting GnRH (leuprorelin) can be used to suppress endogenous gonadotropin secretion for the treatment of certain cancers, endometriosis, and uterine fibroids as well as an adjunct for in vitro fertilization [196].

5.1.5 Lactotroph Axis

The lactotroph axis is unique in that it lacks an obvious negative feedback loop. The lactotroph cell secretes prolactin, a peptide hormone that primarily induces lactation (milk production) in the mammary glands [197]. This is induced in the third trimester of pregnancy, as progesterone levels fall. It is also induced by the suckling reflex. Milk letdown, also induced by the suckling reflex, is stimulated by oxytocin discussed in the following section. Prolactin is thought to cause the sexual refractory period in opposition to dopamine, which induces sexual arousal [198,199].

Nonreproductive functions of prolactin include immune system mediation, osmoregulation, and angiogenesis [200–202]. Prolactin secretion is dependent on the circadian rhythm, with the highest concentrations found during sleep [203]. Prolactin has inhibitory effects on both FSH and LH secretion by the pituitary gland.

Prolactin is regulated by tonic hypothalamic suppression by dopamine (prolactin inhibitory factor [PIF]). Dopamine acts on D2 receptors to inhibit prolactin secretion [204]. Other PIFs include somatostatin and gamma-aminobutyric acid. To balance this inhibitory effect, a prolactin-releasing factor has been identified in TRH as well as oxytocin and neurotensin [205]. There are numerous physiological stimuli that can increase prolactin levels, including coitus, exercise, breast-feeding, pregnancy, epileptic seizures, and stress. Additionally, many medications can increase prolactin levels, including agents that have dopamine antagonist activity, such as neuroleptics, antipsychotics, antihistamines, and antihypertensives [206].

Given that there is a clinically relevant distinction in the degree of hyperprolactinemia to differentiate between prolactin-secreting tumors and "stalk effect" from disruption of prolactin inhibition, much attention has been given to the laboratory analysis of prolactin [207]. The immunometric prolactin assay is prone to develop a "hook effect," where the concentration reported is erroneously lower than the true concentration as a result of antibody saturation [208]. To account for this, serial dilutions are routinely performed. Prolactin levels as high as 280,000 ng/mL have been diagnosed with serial dilution (undiluted concentration 31 ng/mL) [209].

Another physiological variant that can interfere with true laboratory assessment is the presence of macroprolactin [210]. Prolactin is active in the monomeric state (23 kDa protein). However, prolactin does exist in dimeric (big-prolactin) and tetrameric (big-big-prolactin) forms. These are inactive but are still detected by immunometric assays with multiple signals [211]. Typically about 20% of circulating prolactin is macroprolactin. Patients with a significant percentage of macroprolactin (> 50%) are minimally symptomatic despite elevated immunometric assay levels [212]. Specific assays are available to measure monomeric prolactin, including gel filtration chromatography and polyethylene-glycol precipitation methods [213,214].

5.2 Posterior Pituitary Function

The hypothalamus directly controls neurohypophyseal hormone release via axonal communication. The cell bodies of these neurons comprise the magnocellular region of the paraventricular and supraoptic nuclei of the hypothalamus [45]. The two hormones released by the neurohypophysis are oxytocin and ADH (vasopressin). These are synthesized from the precursor proteins preprooxyphysin and preprovasophysin that are cleaved to the active hormone as well as neurophysin [215]. They are rapidly transported down the axons to the posterior pituitary gland.

The secretion of ADH is regulated by baroreceptor signals via the vagus nerve input into the tractus solitarious nucleus. When there is a decrease in blood pressure, this stimulates ADH secretion [216]. Concurrently, osmoreceptors in the organum vasculosum of the lamina terminalis as well as the subforniceal organ stimulate ADH release in the setting of increased serum osmolality. The ADH binds to V_2 receptors in the collecting ducts of the kidney, a cAMP-mediated signal transduction system that ultimately results in the insertion of aquaphorins into the cell membrane [217].

Oxytocin is similarly controlled by direct neuronal regulation. Stretch receptors in the cervix stimulate the magnocellular neurons of the paraventricular hypothalamic nuclei. Though the initiation of parturition is not mediated by cervical stretch, once begun, oxytocin facilitates its completion [218]. Similarly, the suckling reflex during breastfeeding also induces oxytocin secretion, stimulating the same neurons. Interestingly, milk letdown can also be stimulated by psychogenic stimuli, such as the sound of a crying infant [219].

Both oxytocin and vasopressin are available pharmacologically. Oxytocin is available parenterally and is used to induce uterine contractions. Vasopressin is available as an injectable agent, used primarily for hypotensive shock. The synthetic formulation of ADH, 1-desamino-8-D-arginine vasopressin (DDAVP or desmopressin), has a much longer half-life. It is available in parenteric and enteric formulations. Its primary use is to treat hypernatremia from diabetes insipidus [220].

5.3 Intermediate Gland Function

The melanotrophs secrete MSH, which regulates melanin deposition in skin melanocytes. Melanocyte-stimulating hormone has three subtypes, each of which is derived from variable splicing of POMC. The regulation of this hormone is poorly understood, however, there may be an interaction with CRH [221]. Interestingly, there may be a correlation between MSH and body-weight regulation [222].

6 HOMEOSTASIS

The hypothalamus in conjunction with the pituitary gland and its feedback loops regulate the homeostasis of systemic organ systems. This is mediated through homeostatic mechanisms (e.g., hunger, thirst, libido, and circadian rhythm), endocrine control (via the pituitary gland and intermediary glands), autonomic control, and limbic mechanisms. For example, thermoregulation is governed by the anterior and posterior hypothalamic nuclei and mediated via thyroid hormone release as well as a balance of sympathetic and parasympathetic tone [223].

Many of the hormones secreted by the pituitary gland and their downstream glands rely on circadian rhythm generated by the interaction of the suprachiasmatic hypothalamic nuclei, pineal gland, and visual stimuli. Systemic energy homeostasis involves multiple pituitary axes systems (i.e., thyroid, adrenal, and growth hormone) and a balance between the hunger and satiety centers of the hypothalamus. This is tied to the limbic reward systems, affecting behavior [224]. Similarly, reproduction is modulated by hypothalamic regulation of behavior and libido (via the limbic system), endocrine-mediated control of libido (testosterone/prolactin), and endocrine-mediated regulation of gametogenesis and pregnancy [225].

7 HYPOPITUITARISM

Pituitary dysfunction can occur as a result of a multitude of etiologies, including tumors, trauma, vascular injury, inflammatory conditions, adverse medication effects, congenital causes, and infections. Each of these can affect the different HPAs differentially. Intrinsic pituitary tumors, such as pituitary adenomas, have a somewhat predictable sequence of dysfunction, starting with hypogonadism and hyposomatism, followed by hypothyroidism and ultimately hypocortisolism [226]. These patients rarely present with diabetes insipidus. Conversely, patients with the autoimmune condition, lymphocytic hypophysitis, initially present with hypocortisolism, and a number of patients also develop diabetes insipidus [227].

The pituitary is a very resilient gland and can tolerate significant compromise before demonstrating dysfunction. As with other endocrine organs, the gland can tolerate partial resection without developing significant new endocrinopathy [64]. Patients who present with hypopituitarism can experience improvement of their dysfunction. This is dependent on the etiology of the hypopituitarism, number of axes involved, and the duration of symptoms. Hypopituitary patients with pituitary tumors and inflammatory conditions have a higher chance of improvement than those who sustained traumatic brain injury or subarachnoid hemorrhage [228–230].

When assessing patients with hormone-secreting pituitary tumors (e.g., Cushing's disease, acromegaly, or prolactinomas), one should not only address the primary disease diagnosis but should also assess the remaining pituitary axes for pituitary dysfunction. This is particularly relevant in patients with secretory macroadenomas, causing pituitary gland compression (more commonly in acromegaly and prolactinomas compared to Cushing's disease) [231,232]. Given the interaction of the hormone systems as previously delineated, the clinician should be aware of the consequences of replenishing one hormone group in the setting of hypopituitarism. For example, patients with severe central hypocortisolism and diabetes insipidus may not present with polyurea and hypernatremia until the cortisol is replaced [233,234]. Similarly, patients with severe central hypothyroidism and hypocortisolism can develop an Addisonian crisis if thyroid hormone is replaced before cortisol replacement (as a result of the sudden increase in metabolism) [235,236].

8 CONCLUSIONS

The pituitary gland has numerous regulatory and homeostatic roles as the master gland of the body. Its unique location and intimate relation with the hypothalamus allows it to be the primary communication between the CNS and the other organ systems. Understanding normal pituitary physiology, including the feedback loop system of each HPA and their cross-reactivity, is necessary to help diagnose and treat patients with pituitary tumors and disorders.

References

[1] Starling E. The chemical correlation of the functions of the body. Croonian lecture II. Lancet 1905;2:423–5.

[2] De Groot L, Beck-Peccoz P, Chrousos G, et al. Functional anatomy of the hypothalamus and pituitary. Endotext. [Internet]. South Dartmouth, MA: MDText.com, 2000.

[3] Hyrtl J. Onomatologia Anatomica: Geschichte und Kritik der Anatomischen Sprache der Gegenwart, mit Besonderer Berücksichtigung ihrer Barbarismen, Widersinnigkeiten, Tropen, und Grammatikalischen Fehler. Wien: Wilhem Braumüller; 1880.

[4] Schreger C, Schreger H, Schreger T. Synonymia Anatomica. Furth: Bureau par Literatur; 1803.

[5] Rathke M. Über die entstehung der glandula pituitaria. Arch Anat Physiol Wiss Med 1838;5:482–5.

[6] Swedenborg E. The Brain, Considered Anatomically, Physiologically and Philosophically. London: James Speirs; 1882.

[7] Luschka H. Der Hirnanhang und die Striessdruse des Menschen. Berlin: Reimer; 1860.

[8] Hutchinson J. A case of acromegaly. Arch Surg II. 1889;141:148.

[9] Cushing H. The Pituitary Body and Its Disorders. Philadelphia and London: Lippincott; 1912.

[10] Cushing H. The basophil adenomas of the pituitary body and their clinical manifestations (pituitary basophilism). Obes Res 1994;2(5):486–508.

[11] Frank E. Ueber beziehungen der hypophyse zum diabetes insipidus. Berliner klin Wschr 1912;49:393–7.

[12] Riddle O, Bates RW, Dykshorn SW. The preparation, identification and assay of prolactin—a hormone of the anterior pituitary. Am J Physiol (Legacy Content) 1933;105(1):191–216.

[13] Steelman SL, Segaloff A, Andersen RN. Purification of human pituitary follicle-stimulating (FSH) and luteinizing (LH) hormones. Exp Biol Med 1959;101(3):452–4.

[14] Li CH, Simpson ME, Evans HM. Isolation of adrenocorticotropic hormone from sheep pituitaries. Science 1942;96(2498):450.

[15] Schloffer H. Erfolgreiche operation eines hypophysentumors auf nasalem wege. Wien Clin Wochenschr 1907;20:621–4.

[16] Cushing H. Intracranial Tumors. Baltimore: Charles C Thomas; 1932. p. 150.

[17] Hardy J, Wigser SM. Trans-sphenoidal surgery of pituitary fossa tumors with televised radiofluoroscopic control. J Neurosurg 1965;23(6):612–9.

[18] Hardy J. Trans-sphenoidal microsurgical removal of pituitary micro-adenoma. In: Krayenbuhl H, et al. editor. Progress in neurological surgery, vol. 6. Basel: Karger; 1975. p. 200–16.

[19] Liu JK, Das K, Weiss MH, et al. The history and evolution of transsphenoidal surgery. J Neurosurg 2001;95(6):1083–96.

[20] Cappabianca P, Cavallo LM, de Divitiis E. Endoscopic endonasal transsphenoidal surgery. Neurosurgery 2004;55(4):933–41.

[21] Jho H-D, Carrau RL. Endoscopic endonasal transsphenoidal surgery: experience with 50 patients. J Neurosurg 1997;87(1):44–51.

[22] Haddad G, Bassagasteguy L, Carrau R. A novel reconstructive technique after endoscopic expanded endonasal approaches: vascular pedicled nasoseptal flap. Laryngoscope 2006;116:1882–6.

[23] Kassam AB, Carrau RL, Snyderman CH, et al. Endoscopic reconstruction of the cranial base using a pedicled nasoseptal flap. Neurosurgery 2008;63(1):ons44–53.

[24] Dubois PM, Eiamraoui A. Embryology of the pituitary gland. Trends Endocrinol Metab 1995;6(1):1–7.

[25] Takuma N, Sheng HZ, Furuta Y, et al. Formation of Rathke's pouch requires dual induction from the diencephalon. Development 1998;125(23):4835–40.

[26] Sheng HZ, Westphal H. Early steps in pituitary organogenesis. Trends Genet 1999;15(6):236–40.

[27] Dubois PM, Hemming FJ. Fetal development and regulation of pituitary cell types. J Electron Microsc Tech 1991;19(1):2–20.

[28] Dubois PM, El Amraoui A, Heritier AG. Development and differentiation of pituitary cells. Microsc Res Tech 1997;39(2):98–113.

[29] Simeone A, Acampora D, Gulisano M, et al. Nested expression domains of four homeobox genes in developing rostral brain. Nature 1992;358(6388):687–90.

[30] Figdor MC, Stern CD. Segmental organization of embryonic diencephalon. Nature 1993;363(6430):630–4.

[31] Begeot M, Dubois M, Dubois P. Growth hormone and ACTH in the pituitary of normal and anencephalic human fetuses: immunocytochemical evidence for hypothalamic influences during development. Neuroendocrinology 1977;24(3-4):208–20.

[32] Begeot M, Dubois M, Dubois P. Evolution of lactotropes in normal and anencephalic human fetuses. J Clin Endocr Metab 1984;58(4):726–30.

[33] Simmons D, Voss J, Ingraham H, et al. Pituitary cell phenotypes involve cell-specific Pit-1 mRNA translation and synergistic interactions with other classes of transcription factors. Genes Dev 1990;4(5):695–711.

[34] Harris FS, Rhoton AL Jr. Anatomy of the cavernous sinus: a microsurgical study. J Neurosurg 1976;45(2):169–80.

[35] Renn WH, Rhoton AL Jr. Microsurgical anatomy of the sellar region. J Neurosurg 1975;43(3):288–98.

[36] Rhoton AL Jr. The sellar region. Neurosurgery 2002;51(4):S335–74.

[37] Yamamoto I, Rhoton AL Jr, Peace DA. Microsurgery of the third ventricle: part 1: microsurgical anatomy. Neurosurgery 1981;8(3):334–56.

[38] Holmes RL, Ball JN. The pituitary gland: a comparative account. Oakland: University of California Press; 1974.

[39] Horvath E, Kovacs K. Pituitary gland. Pathol Res Pract 1988;183(2):129–42.

[40] Passolli H, Torres A, Aoki A. The mammosomatotroph: a transitional cell between growth hormone and prolactin producing cells? An immunocytochemical study. Histochemistry 1994;102(4):287–96.

[41] Coates P, Doniach I, Wells C, et al. Peptides related to α-melanocyte-stimulating hormone are commonly produced by human pituitary corticotroph adenomas: no relationship with pars intermedia origin. J Endocrinol 1989;120(3):531.

[42] Takeuchi M. The mammalian pars intermedia-structure and function. Zoolog Sci 2001;18(2):133–44.

[43] Kobayashi Y. Quantitative and electron microscopic studies on the pars intermedia of the hypophysis. Cell Tissue Res 1974;154(3):321–7.

[44] Bergland RM, Ray BS, Torack RM. Anatomical variations in the pituitary gland and adjacent structures in 225 human autopsy cases. J Neurosurg 1968;28(2):93–9.

[45] Brownstein MJ, Russell JT, Gainer H. Synthesis, transport, and release of posterior pituitary hormones. Science 1980;207(4429):373–8.

[46] Swaab D, Hofman M, Mirmiran M, et al. Anatomy of the human hypothalamus (chiasmatic and tuberal region). Hum Hypothal Health Dis 1992;93:3.

[47] Gibo H, Lenkey C, Rhoton AL Jr. Microsurgical anatomy of the supraclinoid portion of the internal carotid artery. J Neurosurg 1981;55(4):560–74.

[48] Popa G, Fielding U. A portal circulation from the pituitary to the hypothalamic region. J Anat 1930;65(Pt 1):88.

[49] Bergland RM, Page RB. Pituitary-brain vascular relations: a new paradigm. Science 1979;204(4388):18–24.

[50] Griffiths CF, Cutler AR, Duong HT, et al. Avoidance of postoperative epistaxis and anosmia in endonasal endoscopic skull base surgery: a technical note. Acta Neurochir 2014;156(7):1393–401.

[51] Voegels RL, Thomé DC, Iturralde PPV, et al. Endoscopic ligature of the sphenopalatine artery for severe posterior epistaxis. Otolaryngol Head Neck Surg 2001;124(4):464–7.

[52] Rumboldt Z, Castillo M, Smith JK. The palatovaginal canal: can it be identified on routine CT and MR imaging? Am J Roentgenol 2002;179(1):267–72.

[53] Pinheiro-Neto CD, Fernandez-Miranda JC, Rivera-Serrano CM, et al. Endoscopic anatomy of the palatovaginal canal (palatosphenoidal canal). Laryngoscope 2012;122(1):6–12.

[54] Fernandez-Miranda JC, Prevedello DM, Madhok R, et al. Sphenoid septations and their relationship with internal carotid arteries: anatomical and radiological study. Laryngoscope 2009;119(10):1893–6.

[55] Wang J, Bidari S, Inoue K, et al. Extensions of the sphenoid sinus: a new classification. Neurosurgery 2010;66(4):797–816.

[56] Güldner C, Pistorius SM, Diogo I, et al. Analysis of pneumatization and neurovascular structures of the sphenoid sinus, using cone-beam tomography (CBT). Acta Radiol 2012;53(2):214–9.

[57] Fujii K, Chambers SM, Rhoton AL Jr. Neurovascular relationships of the sphenoid sinus: a microsurgical study. J Neurosurg 1979;50(1):31–9.

[58] Rhoton AL Jr. Operative techniques and instrumentation for neurosurgery. Neurosurgery 2003;53(4):907–34.

[59] Unlu A, Meco C, Ugur H, et al. Endoscopic anatomy of sphenoid sinus for pituitary surgery. Clin Anat 2008;21(7):627–32.

[60] Jittapiromsak P, Sabuncuoglu H, Deshmukh P, et al. Greater superficial petrosal nerve dissection: back to front or front to back? Neurosurgery 2009;64(5):253–9.

[61] Lin P-Y, Cheng C-Y, Wu C-C, et al. Bilateral neurotrophic keratopathy complicating Vidian neurectomy. Am J Ophthalmol 2001;132(1):106–8.

[62] Dusick JR, Esposito F, Malkasian D, et al. Avoidance of carotid artiery in injuries in transsphenoidal surgery with the Doppler probe and micro-hook blades. Neurosurgery 2007;60(4):322–9.

[63] Cho CH, Barkhoudarian G, Hsu L, et al. Magnetic resonance imaging validation of pituitary gland compression and distortion by typical sellar pathology: clinical article. J Neurosurg 2013;119(6):1461–6.

[64] Barkhoudarian G, Cutler AR, Yost S, et al. Impact of selective pituitary gland incision or resection on hormonal function after adenoma or cyst resection. Pituitary 2015;18(6):868–75.

[65] Goto T, Tanaka Y, Kodama K, et al. Loss of visual evoked potential following temporary occlusion of the superior hypophyseal artery during aneurysm clip placement surgery. J Neurosurg 2007;107(4):865–7.

[66] Kassam AB, Prevedello DM, Thomas A, et al. Endoscopic endonasal pituitary transposition for a transdorsum sellae approach to the interpeduncular cistern. Neurosurgery 2008;62(3):57–74.

[67] Taussky P, Kalra R, Coppens J, et al. Endocrinological outcome after pituitary transposition (hypophysopexy) and adjuvant radiotherapy for tumors involving the cavernous sinus: clinical article. J Neurosurg 2011;115(1):55–62.

[68] Mikhael MA, Mattar AG. Intracranial pearly tumors: the roles of computed tomography, angiography, and pneumoencephalography. J Comput Assist Tomogr 1978;2(4):421–9.

[69] Davidoff LM, Epstein BS. The abnormal pneumoencephalogram. J Neuropathol Exp Neurol 1952;11(3):340.

[70] Powell DF, Baker HL Jr, Laws ER Jr. The primary angiographic findings in pituitary adenomas. Radiology 1974;110(3):589–96.

[71] Romero ADCB, Barkhoudarian G, Silva CE, et al. As variações na anatomia do seio esfenoidal e assoalho selar para realização de endoscopia transesfenoidal em adultos: revisão de literatura. J Bras Neurocir 2012;23(1):11–7.

[72] Elster AD. High-resolution, dynamic pituitary MR imaging: standard of care or academic pastime? Am J Roentgenol 1994;163(3):680–2.

[73] Tien R, Kucharczyk J, Kucharczyk W. MR imaging of the brain in patients with diabetes insipidus. Am J Neuroradiol 1991;12(3):533–42.

[74] Loh JA, Verbalis JG. Diabetes insipidus as a complication after pituitary surgery. Nature Clin Pract Endocrinol Metab 2007;3(6):489–94.

[75] Teramoto A, Hirakawa K, Sanno N, et al. Incidental pituitary lesions in 1,000 unselected autopsy specimens. Radiology 1994;193(1):161–4.

[76] Kucharczyk W, Bishop J, Plewes D, et al. Detection of pituitary microadenomas: comparison of dynamic keyhole fast spin-echo, unenhanced, and conventional contrast-enhanced MR imaging. Am J Roentgenol 1994;163(3):671–9.

[77] Melmed S, Kleinberg D, Ho K. Pituitary physiology and diagnostic evaluation. In: Melmed S, editor. Williams Textbook of Endocrinology. 12th ed. Philadelphia: Saunders Elsevier; 2011. p. 176–231.

[78] Szkudlinski MW, Fremont V, Ronin C, et al. Thyroid-stimulating hormone and thyroid-stimulating hormone receptor structure-function relationships. Physiol Rev 2002;82(2):473–502.

[79] Matzuk M, Kornmeier C, Whitfield GK, et al. The glycoprotein α-subunit is critical for secretion and stability of the human thyrotropin β-subunit. Mol Endocrinol 1988;2(2):95–100.

[80] Canteras NS. The medial hypothalamic defensive system: hodological organization and functional implications. Pharmacol Biochem Behav 2002;71(3):481–91.

[81] Skultety FM. Stimulation of periaqueductal gray and hypothalamus. Arch Neurol 1963;8(6):608–20.

[82] Parent A, Steriade M. Afferents from the periaqueductal gray, medial hypothalamus and medial thalamus to the midbrain reticular core. Brain Res Bull 1981;7(4):411–8.

[83] Elmquist JK, Bjørbæk C, Ahima RS, et al. Distributions of leptin receptor mRNA isoforms in the rat brain. J Compar Neurol 1998;395(4):535–47.

[84] Elias CF, Aschkenasi C, Lee C, et al. Leptin differentially regulates NPY and POMC neurons projecting to the lateral hypothalamic area. Neuron 1999;23(4):775–86.

[85] Harris GC, Wimmer M, Aston-Jones G. A role for lateral hypothalamic orexin neurons in reward seeking. Nature 2005;437(7058):556–9.

[86] Teitelbaum P, Epstein AN. The lateral hypothalamic syndrome: recovery of feeding and drinking after lateral hypothalamic lesions. Psychol Rev 1962;69(2):74.

[87] Anand BK, Brobeck JR. Hypothalamic control of food intake in rats and cats. Yale J Biol Med 1951;24(2):123.

[88] Goldman JK, Schnatz JD, Bernardis LL, et al. Adipose tissue metabolism of weanling rats after destruction of ventromedial hypothalamic nuclei: effect of hypophysectomy and growth hormone. Metabolism 1970;19(11):995–1005.

[89] Shimazu T, Takahashi A. Stimulation of hypothalamic nuclei has differential effects on lipid synthesis in brown and white adipose tissue. Nature 1980;284(5751):62–3.

[90] Halpern CH, Wolf JA, Bale TL, et al. Deep brain stimulation in the treatment of obesity. J Neurosurg 2008;109(4):625–34.

[91] Laćan G, De Salles AA, Gorgulho AA, et al. Modulation of food intake following deep brain stimulation of the ventromedial hypothalamus in the vervet monkey. J Neurosurg 2008;108(2):336–42.

[92] Sani S, Jobe K, Smith A, et al. Deep brain stimulation for treatment of obesity in rats. J Neurosurg 2007;117(1):809–13.

[93] Parmeggiani P, Azzaroni A, Lenzi P. On the functional significance of the circuit of Papez. Brain Res 1971;30(2):357–74.

[94] Kapur N, Crewes H, Wise R, et al. Mammillary body damage results in memory impairment but not amnesia. Neurocase 1998;4(6):509–17.

[95] Papez JW. A proposed mechanism of emotion. Arch Neurol Psychiatry 1937;38(4):725.

[96] Heilman KM, Sypert GW. Korsakoff's syndrome resulting from bilateral fornix lesions. Neurology 1977;27(5):490.

[97] Beglinger LJ, Haut MW, Parsons MW. The role of the mammillary bodies in memory: a case of amnesia following bilateral resection. Eur J Psychiatry 2006;20(2):88–95.

[98] Dalgleish T. The emotional brain. Nature Rev Neurosci 2004;5(7):583–9.

[99] Pessoa L. On the relationship between emotion and cognition. Nature Rev Neurosci 2008;9(2):148–58.

[100] Nishino H, Koizumi K, Brooks CM. The role of suprachiasmatic nuclei of the hypothalamus in the production of circadian rhythm. Brain Res 1976;112(1):45–59.

[101] Watts AG, Swanson LW, Sanchez-Watts G. Efferent projections of the suprachiasmatic nucleus. I. Studies using anterograde transport of *Phaseolus vulgaris* leucoagglutinin in the rat. J Compar Neurol 1987;258(2):204–29.

[102] Gillette MU, McArthur AJ. Circadian actions of melatonin at the suprachiasmatic nucleus. Behav Brain Res 1995;73(1):135–9.

[103] Moore RY. Neural control of the pineal gland. Behav Brain Res 1995;73(1):125–30.

[104] Klein D, Smoot R, Weller J, et al. Lesions of the paraventricular nucleus area of the hypothalamus disrupt the suprachiasmatic → spinal cord circuit in the melatonin rhythm generating system. Brain Res Bull 1983;10(5):647–52.

[105] Gudelsky GA, Porter JC. Release of dopamine from tuberoinfundibular neurons into pituitary stalk blood after prolactin or haloperidol administration. Endocrinology 1980;106(2):526–9.

[106] Lookingland K, Jarry H, Moore K. The metabolism of dopamine in the median eminence reflects the activity of tuberoinfundibular neurons. Brain Res 1987;419(1):303–10.

[107] Ferguson AV, Bains JS. Electrophysiology of the circumventricular organs. Front Neuroendocrinol 1996;17(4):440–75.

[108] Kawano H, Masuko S. Region-specific projections from the subfornical organ to the paraventricular hypothalamic nucleus in the rat. Neuroscience 2010;169(3):1227–34.

[109] Keil L, Summy-Long J, Severs W. Release of vasopressin by angiotensin II. Endocrinology 1975;96(4):1063–5.

[110] Mendelsohn FA, Aguilera G, Saavedra JM, et al. Characteristics and regulation of angiotensin II receptors in pituitary, circumventricular organs and kidney. Clin Expl Hypertens Part A: Theory Prac 1983;5(7-8):1081–97.

[111] Gaillard R, Grossman A, Gillies G, Angiotensin II, et al. stimulates the release of ACTH from dispersed rat anterior pituitary cells. Clin Endocrinol 1981;15(6):573–8.

[112] Sumitomo T, Suda T, Nakano Y, et al. Angiotensin II increases the corticotropin-releasing factor messenger ribonucleic acid level in the rat hypothalamus. Endocrinology 1991;128(5):2248–52.

[113] Irvine C, Alexander S. Factors affecting the circadian rhythm in plasma cortisol concentrations in the horse. Domes Animal Endocrinol 1994;11(2):227–38.

[114] Sherman B, Wysham W, Pfoh B. Age-related changes in the circadian rhythm of plasma cortisol in man. J Clin Endocrinol Metab 1985;61(3):439–43.

[115] Egana M, Sancho M, Macarulla J. An early effect of cortisol, previous to its glycogenogenic action. Horm Metabol Res 1981;13(11):609–11.

[116] Lecavalier L, Bolli G, Gerich J. Glucagon-cortisol interactions on glucose turnover and lactate gluconeogenesis in normal humans. Am J Physiol Endocrinol Metab 1990;258(4):E569–75.

[117] Rizza RA, Mandarino LJ, Gerich JE. Cortisol-induced insulin resistance in man: impaired suppression of glucose production and stimulation of glucose utilization due to a postreceptor defect of insulin action. J Clin Endocrinol Metab 1982;54(1):131–8.

[118] Djurhuus C, Gravholt CH, Nielsen S, et al. Effects of cortisol on lipolysis and regional interstitial glycerol levels in humans. Am J Physiol Endocrinol Metab 2002;283(1):E172–7.

[119] Simmons PS, Miles JM, Gerich J, et al. Increased proteolysis. An effect of increases in plasma cortisol within the physiologic range. J Clin Invest 1984;73(2):412.

[120] Walker BR, Connacher AA, Webb DJ, et al. Glucocorticoids and blood pressure: a role for the cortisol/cortisone shuttle in the control of vascular tone in man. Clin Sci 1992;83(2):171–8.

[121] Coderre L, Srivastava AK, Chiasson J-L. Role of glucocorticoid in the regulation of glycogen metabolism in skeletal muscle. Am J Physiol Endocrinol Metab 1991;260(6):E927–32.

[122] Young EA, Breslau N. Cortisol and catecholamines in posttraumatic stress disorder: an epidemiologic community study. Arch Gen Psychiatry 2004;61(4):394–401.

[123] Morgan CA III, Wang S, Rasmusson A, et al. Relationship among plasma cortisol, catecholamines, neuropeptide Y, and human performance during exposure to uncontrollable stress. Psychosom Med 2001;63(3):412–22.

[124] Udelsman R, Goldstein DS, Loriaux DL, et al. Catecholamine-glucocorticoid interactions during surgical stress. J Surg Res 1987;43(6):539–45.

[125] Cavallo R, Sartori M, Gatti G, et al. Cortisol and immune interferon can interact in the modulation of human natural killer cell activity. Experientia 1986;42(2):177–9.

[126] Elenkov IJ. Glucocorticoids and the Th1/Th2 balance. Ann NY Acad Sci 2004;1024(1):138–46.

[127] Mavoungou E, Bouyou-Akotet M, Kremsner P. Effects of prolactin and cortisol on natural killer (NK) cell surface expression and function of human natural cytotoxicity receptors (NKp46, NKp44 and NKp30). Clin Exp Immunol 2005;139(2):287–96.

[128] Nelson D, Ruhmann-Wennhold A. Corticosteroids increase superoxide anion production by rat liver microsomes. J Clin Invest 1975;56(4):1062.

[129] Sandle G, Keir M, Record C. The effect of hydrocortisone on the transport of water, sodium, and glucose in the jejunum: perfusion studies in normal subjects and patients with coeliac disease. Scand J Gastroenterol 1981;16(5):667–71.

[130] Lemann J Jr, Piering W, Lennon E. Studies of the acute effects of aldosterone and cortisol on the interrelationship between renal sodium, calcium and magnesium excretion in normal man. Nephron 1970;7(2):117–30.

[131] Ghaffar A, McGowan B, Tharakan G, et al. Unmasking of diabetes insipidus with steroid treatment. Endocrine Abstracts 2008;15:P227.

[132] Steven K. Adrenal cortical steroids. Drug facts and comparisons. 5th ed. St. Louis: Facts and Comparisons, Inc; 1997. pp. 122–128.

[133] Shibusawa N, Hollenberg AN, Wondisford FE. Thyroid hormone receptor DNA binding is required for both positive and negative gene regulation. J Biol Chem 2003;278(2):732–8.

[134] Phan TQ, Jow MM, Privalsky ML. DNA recognition by thyroid hormone and retinoic acid receptors: 3, 4, 5 rule modified. Mol Cell Endocrinol 2010;319(1):88–98.

[135] Visser WE, Friesema EC, Visser TJ. Minireview: thyroid hormone transporters: the knowns and the unknowns. Mol Endocrinol 2011;25(1):1–14.

[136] Dumitrescu AM, Liao X-H, Abdullah MS, et al. Mutations in SECISBP2 result in abnormal thyroid hormone metabolism. Nat Genet 2005;37(11):1247–52.

[137] Galo M, Unates L, Farias R. Effect of membrane fatty acid composition on the action of thyroid hormones on (Ca2 + + Mg2 +)-adenosine triphosphatase from rat erythrocyte. J Biol Chem 1981;256(14):7113–4.

[138] Toni R, Lechan R. Neuroendocrine regulation of thyrotropin-releasing hormone (TRH) in the tuberoinfundibular system. J Endocrinol Invest 1993;16(9):715–53.

[139] Shimon I, Taylor J, Dong J, et al. Somatostatin receptor subtype specificity in human fetal pituitary cultures. Differential role of SSTR2 and SSTR5 for growth hormone, thyroid-stimulating hormone, and prolactin regulation. J Clin Invest 1997;99(4):789.

[140] Critchlow V, Abe K, Urman S, et al. Effects of lesions in the periventricular nucleus of the preoptic-anterior hypothalamus on growth hormone and thyrotropin secretion and brain somatostatin. Brain Res 1981;222(2):267–76.

[141] Arancibia S, Rage F, Astier H, et al. Neuroendocrine and autonomous mechanisms underlying thermoregulation in cold environment. Neuroendocrinology 1996;64(4):257–67.

[142] Björklund A, Lindvall O. Catecholaminergic brainstem regulatory systems. Comprehensive Physiology. New York: John Wiley; 1984.

[143] Van Haasteren G, Linkels E, Klootwijk W, et al. Starvation-induced changes in the hypothalamic content of prothyrotrophin-releasing hormone (proTRH) mRNA and the hypothalamic release of proTRH-derived peptides: role of the adrenal gland. J Endocrinol 1995;145(1):143–53.

[144] Chan JL, Heist K, DePaoli AM, et al. The role of falling leptin levels in the neuroendocrine and metabolic adaptation to short-term starvation in healthy men. J Clin Invest 2003;111(9):1409–21.

[145] Sanchez VC, Goldstein J, Stuart RC, et al. Regulation of hypothalamic prohormone convertases 1 and 2 and effects on processing of prothyrotropin-releasing hormone. J Clin Invest 2004;114(3):357–69.

[146] Kim B. Thyroid hormone as a determinant of energy expenditure and the basal metabolic rate. Thyroid 2008;18(2):141–4.

[147] Cheng S-Y, Leonard JL, Davis PJ. Molecular aspects of thyroid hormone actions. Endo Rev 2010;31(2):139–70.

[148] Ribeiro MO, Carvalho SD, Schultz JJ, et al. Thyroid hormone–sympathetic interaction and adaptive thermogenesis are thyroid hormone receptor isoform–specific. J Clin Invest 2001;108(1):97–105.

[149] Liu Y-Y, Schultz JJ, Brent GA. A thyroid hormone receptor α gene mutation (P398H) is associated with visceral adiposity and impaired catecholamine-stimulated lipolysis in mice. J Biol Chem 2003;278(40):38913–20.

[150] Brand M. The efficiency and plasticity of mitochondrial energy transduction. Biochem Soc Trans 2005;33(5):897–904.

[151] Epstein FH, Klein I, Ojamaa K. Thyroid hormone and the cardiovascular system. New Engl J Med 2001;344(7):501–9.

[152] Dodd J, Jessell TM. Axon guidance and the patterning of neuronal projections in vertebrates. Science 1988;242(4879):692–9.

[153] Tessier-Lavigne M, Goodman CS. The molecular biology of axon guidance. Science 1996;274(5290):1123.

[154] Gelfand RA, Hutchinson-Williams KA, Bonde AA, et al. Catabolic effects of thyroid hormone excess: the contribution of adrenergic activity to hypermetabolism and protein breakdown. Metabolism 1987;36(6):562–9.

[155] Tannenbaum G. Somatostatin as a physiological regulator of pulsatile growth hormone secretion. Horm Res Paediatr 1988;29(2-3):70–4.

[156] Tannenbaum GS, Painson J-C, Lapointe M, et al. Interplay of somatostatin and growth hormone-releasing hormone in genesis of episodic growth hormone secretion. Metabolism 1990;39(9):35–9.

[157] Gabriel S, Roncancio J, Ruiz N. Growth hormone pulsatility and the endocrine milieu during sexual maturation in male and female rats. Neuroendocrinology 1992;56(5):619–28.

[158] Pal B, Matthews D, Edge J, et al. The frequency and amplitude of growth hormone secretory episodes as determined by deconvolution analysis are increased in adolescents with insulin-dependent diabetes mellitus and are unaffected by short-term euglycaemia. Clin Endocrinol 1993;38(1):93–100.

[159] Somatostatin (SRIF) resistance in the hypersecretion of growth hormon (GH) in insulin-dependent diabetes mellitus (IDDM) in man. In: Cohen R, Frohman L, editors. Clinical Research. Thorofare, NJ: Slack Inc; 1988.

[160] Finkelstein JW, Roffwarg HP, Boyar RM, et al. Age-related change in the twenty-four hour spontaneous secretion of growth hormone. J Clin Endocrinol Metab 1972;35(5):665–70.

[161] Isaksson OG, Lindahl A, Nilsson A, et al. Mechanism of the stimulatory effect of growth hormone on longitudinal bone growth. Endo Rev 1987;8(4):426–38.

[162] Schlechter NL, Russell SM, Spencer EM, et al. Evidence suggesting that the direct growth-promoting effect of growth hormone on cartilage in vivo is mediated by local production of somatomedin. Proc Nat Acad Sci 1986;83(20):7932–4.

[163] Chang HR, Kim HJ, Xu X, et al. Macrophage and adipocyte IGF1 maintain adipose tissue homeostasis during metabolic stresses. Obesity 2016;24(1):172–83.

[164] Rosenbaum M, Gertner JM, Leibel RL. Effects of systemic growth hormone (GH) administration on regional adipose tissue distribution and metabolism in GH-deficient children. J Clin Endocrinol Metab 1989;69(6):1274–81.

[165] Juul A, Main K, Blum WF, et al. The ratio between serum levels of insulin-like growth factor– (IGF-) I and the IGF binding proteins (IGFBP-1, 2 and 3) decreases with age in healthy adults and is increased in acromegalic patients. Clin Endocrinol 1994;41(1):85–93.

[166] Tillmann V, Patel L, Gill M, et al. Monitoring serum insulin-like growth factor-I (IGF-I), IGF binding protein-3 (IGFBP-3), IGF-I/IGFBP-3 molar ratio and leptin during growth hormone treatment for disordered growth. Clin Endocrinol Oxf 2000;53(3):329–36.

[167] Chomczynski P, Downs TR, Frohman LA. Feedback regulation of growth hormone (GH)-releasing hormone gene expression by GH in rat hypothalamus. Mol Endocrinol 1988;2(3):236–41.

[168] Chihara K, Minamitani N, Kaji H, et al. Intraventricularly injected growth hormone stimulates somatostatin release into rat hypophysial portal blood. Endocrinology 1981;109(6):2279–81.

[169] Robbins RJ, Leidy J Jr, Landon R. The effects of growth hormone, prolactin, corticotropin, and thyrotropin on the production and secretion of somatostatin by hypothalamic cells in vitro. Endocrinology 1985;117(2):538–43.

[170] Sakata I, Sakai T. Ghrelin cells in the gastrointestinal tract. Int J Peptides 2010;2010:7.

[171] Hataya Y, Akamizu T, Takaya K, et al. A low dose of ghrelin stimulates growth hormone (GH) release synergistically with GH-releasing hormone in humans. J Clin Endocrinol Metab 2001;86(9):4552.

[172] De Zegher F, Van Den Berghe G, Devlieger H, et al. Dopamine inhibits growth hormone and prolactin secretion in the human newborn. Pediatr Res 1993;34(5):642–5.

[173] Boyd A III, Lebovitz HE, Pfeiffer JB. Stimulation of human growth-hormone secretion by L-dopa. New Engl J Med 1970;283(26):1425–9.

[174] Jiang H, Betancourt L, Smith RG. Ghrelin amplifies dopamine signaling by cross talk involving formation of growth hormone secretagogue receptor/dopamine receptor subtype 1 heterodimers. Mol Endocrinol 2006;20(8):1772–85.

[175] Reed ML, Merriam GR, Kargi AY. Adult growth hormone deficiency-benefits, side effects, and risks of growth hormone replacement. Front Endocrinol (Lausanne) 2013;4:64.

[176] Plewe G, Krause U, Beyer J, et al. Long-acting and selective suppression of growth hormone secretion by somatostatin analogue SMS 201-995 in acromegaly. Lancet 1984;324(8406):782–4.

[177] Shimon I, Yan X, Taylor JE, et al. Somatostatin receptor (SSTR) subtype-selective analogues differentially suppress in vitro growth hormone and prolactin in human pituitary adenomas. Novel potential therapy for functional pituitary tumors. J Clin Invest 1997;100(9):2386.

[178] McNeilly A, Crawford J, Taragnat C, et al. The differential secretion of FSH and LH: regulation through genes, feedback and packaging. Reprod Cambridge Suppl 2003;61:463–76.

[179] Schulz RW, Miura T. Spermatogenesis and its endocrine regulation. Fish Physiol Biochem 2002;26(1):43–56.

[180] Demura R, Ono M, Demura H, et al. Prolactin directly inhibits basal as well as gonadotropin-stimulated secretion of progesterone and 17β-estradiol in the human ovary. J Clin Endocrinol Metab 1982;54(6):1246–50.

[181] Mooradian AD, Morley JE, Korenman SG. Biological actions of androgens. Endocr Rev 1987;8(1):1–28.

[182] Weinstein Y, Berkovich Z. Testosterone effect on bone marrow, thymus, and suppressor T cells in the (NZB X NZW) F1 mice: its relevance to autoimmunity. J Immunol 1981;126(3):998–1002.

[183] Wilson JD, George FW, Griffin JE. The hormonal control of sexual development. Science 1981;211:1278–84.

[184] Chrivia JC, Kwok RP, Lamb N, et al. Phosphorylated CREB binds specifically to the nuclear protein CBP. Nature 1993;365(6449):855–9.

[185] Negro-Vilar A, Ojeda S, McCann S. Evidence for changes in sensitivity to testosterone negative feedback on gonadotropin release during sexual development in the male rat. Endocrinology 1973;93(3):729–35.

[186] Walker WH, Cheng J. FSH and testosterone signaling in Sertoli cells. Reproduction 2005;130(1):15–28.

[187] de Tassigny XdA, Colledge WH. The role of kisspeptin signaling in reproduction. Physiology 2010;25(4):207–17.

[188] Hsueh A, Erickson G. Glucocorticoid inhibition of FSH-induced estrogen production in cultured rat granulosa cells. Steroids 1978;32(5):639–48.

[189] Słomczyńska M, Duda M. The expression of androgen receptor, cytochrome P450 aromatase and FSH receptor mRNA in the porcine ovary. Folia Histochem Cytobiol 2000;39(1):9–13.

[190] Wintermantel TM, Campbell RE, Porteous R, et al. Definition of estrogen receptor pathway critical for estrogen positive feedback to gonadotropin-releasing hormone neurons and fertility. Neuron 2006;52(2):271–80.

[191] Horvath S, Drinkwater B. Thermoregulation and the menstrual cycle. Aviat Space Environ Med 1982;53(8):790–4.

[192] Warnock JK, Swanson SG, Borel RW, et al. Combined esterified estrogens and methyltestosterone versus esterified estrogens alone in the treatment of loss of sexual interest in surgically menopausal women. Menopause 2005;12(4):374–84.

[193] Turgeon JL, McDonnell DP, Martin KA, et al. Hormone therapy: physiological complexity belies therapeutic simplicity. Science 2004;304(5675):1269–73.

[194] Holtkamp DE, Greslin JG, Root CA, et al. Gonadotrophin inhibiting and anti-fecundity effects of chloramiphene. Exp Biol Med 1960;105(1):197–201.

[195] Seminara SB, Beranova M, Oliveira LM, et al. Successful use of pulsatile gonadotropin-releasing hormone (GnRH) for ovulation induction and pregnancy in a patient with GnRH receptor mutations 1. J Clin Endocrinol Metab 2000;85(2):556–62.

[196] Crosignani P, Luciano A, Ray A, et al. Subcutaneous depot medroxyprogesterone acetate versus leuprolide acetate in the treatment of endometriosis-associated pain. Hum Reprod 2006;21(1):248–56.

[197] Bole-Feysot C, Goffin V, Edery M, et al. Prolactin (PRL) and its receptor: actions, signal transduction pathways and phenotypes observed in PRL receptor knockout mice. Endocr Rev 1998;19(3):225–68.

[198] Kruger T, Haake P, Haverkamp J, et al. Effects of acute prolactin manipulation on sexual drive and function in males. J Endocrinol 2003;179(3):357–65.

[199] Levin R. Is prolactin the biological 'off switch' for human sexual arousal? Sex Relation Ther 2003;18(2):237–43.

[200] Goffin V, Bouchard B, Ormandy CJ, et al. Prolactin: a hormone at the crossroads of neuroimmunoendocrinology. Ann NY Acad Sci 1998;840(1):498–509.

[201] Shennan DB. Regulation of water and solute transport across mammalian plasma cell membranes by prolactin. J Dairy Res 1994;61(01):155–66.

[202] Clapp C, de la Escalera GM. Prolactins: novel regulators of angiogenesis. Physiology 1997;12(5):231–7.

[203] Parker DC, Rossman LG, Vanderlaan E. Relation of sleep-entrained human prolactin release to REM-nonREM cycles. J Clin Endocrinol Metab 1974;38(4):646–51.

[204] Kebabian JW, Calne DB. Multiple receptors for dopamine. Nature 1979;277(5692):93–6.

[205] Freeman ME, Kanyicska B, Lerant A, et al. Prolactin: structure, function, and regulation of secretion. Physiol Rev 2000;80(4):1523–5631.

[206] La Torre D, Falorni A. Pharmacological causes of hyperprolactinemia. Ther Clin Risk Manage 2007;3(5):929.

[207] Biller B, Luciano A, Crosignani P, et al. Guidelines for the diagnosis and treatment of hyperprolactinemia. J Reprod Med 1999;44(12 Suppl):1075–84.

[208] Smith TP, Kavanagh L, Healy M-L, et al. Technology insight: measuring prolactin in clinical samples. Nature Clin Pract Endocrinol Metab 2007;3(3):279–89.

[209] Barkan AL, Chandler WF. Giant pituitary prolactinoma with falsely low serum prolactin: the pitfall of the "high-dose hook effect": case report. Neurosurgery 1998;42(4):913–5.

[210] Sadideen H, Swaminathan R. Macroprolactin: what is it and what is its importance? Int J Clin Prac 2006;60(4):457–61.

[211] Vaishya R, Gupta R, Arora S. Macroprolactin: a frequent cause of misdiagnosed hyperprolactinemia in clinical practice. J Reprod Infertil 2010;11(3):161.

[212] Taghavi M, Sedigheh F. Macroprolactinemia in patients presenting with hyperandrogenic symptoms and hyperprolactinemia. Int J Endocrinol Metab 2008;3(Summer):140–3.

[213] Vallette-Kasic S, Morange-Ramos I, Selim A, et al. Macroprolactinemia revisited: a study on 106 patients. J Clin Endocrinol Metab 2002;87(2):581–8.

[214] Leslie H, Courtney C, Bell P, et al. Laboratory and clinical experience in 55 patients with macroprolactinemia identified by a simple polyethylene glycol precipitation method. J Clin Endocrinol Metab 2001;86(6):2743–6.

[215] Chrétien M, Benjannet S, Lazure C, et al. Biosynthesis of hormonal and neural peptides. Trans Am Clin Climatol Assoc 1984;95:19.

[216] Robertson GL. Physiology of ADH secretion. Kidney Int Suppl 1987;21:S20.

[217] Berliner RW, Levinsky NG, Davidson DG, et al. Dilution and concentration of the urine and the action of antidiuretic hormone. Am J Med 1958;24(5):730–44.

[218] Blanks AM, Thornton S. The role of oxytocin in parturition. Int J Obstet Gynaecol 2003;110(Suppl. 20):S46–51.

[219] Riem MM, Bakermans-Kranenburg MJ, Pieper S, et al. Oxytocin modulates amygdala, insula, and inferior frontal gyrus responses to infant crying: a randomized controlled trial. Biol Psychiatry 2011;70(3):291–7.

[220] Robinson AG. DDAVP in the treatment of central diabetes insipidus. New Engl J Med 1976;294(10):507–11.

[221] Lu X-Y, Barsh GS, Akil H, et al. Interaction between α-melanocyte-stimulating hormone and corticotropin-releasing hormone in the regulation of feeding and hypothalamo-pituitary-adrenal responses. J Neurosci 2003;23(21):7863–72.

[222] Biebermann H, Castañeda TR, van Landeghem F, et al. A role for β-melanocyte-stimulating hormone in human body-weight regulation. Cell Metab 2006;3(2):141–6.

[223] Boulant JA. Role of the preoptic-anterior hypothalamus in thermoregulation and fever. Clin Infect Dis 2000;31(Suppl. 5):S157–61.

[224] Nieuwenhuizen AG, Rutters F. The hypothalamic-pituitary-adrenal-axis in the regulation of energy balance. Physiol Behav 2008;94(2):169–77.

[225] Zieba D, Amstalden M, Williams G. Regulatory roles of leptin in reproduction and metabolism: a comparative review. Domes Animal Endocrinol 2005;29(1):166–85.

[226] Arafah BM, Prunty D, Ybarra J, et al. The dominant role of increased intrasellar pressure in the pathogenesis of hypopituitarism, hyperprolactinemia, and headaches in patients with pituitary adenomas. J Clin Endocrinol Metab 2000;85(5):1789–93.

[227] Bellastella A, Bizzaro A, Coronella C, et al. Lymphocytic hypophysitis: a rare or underestimated disease? Eur J Endocrinol 2003;149(5):363–76.

[228] Fatemi N, Dusick JR, Mattozo C, et al. Pituitary hormonal loss and recovery after transsphenoidal adenoma removal. Neurosurgery 2008;63(4):709–19.

[229] Kelly DF, Chaloner C, Evans D, et al. Prevalence of pituitary hormone dysfunction, metabolic syndrome, and impaired quality of life in retired professional football players: a prospective study. J Neurotrauma 2014;31(13):1161–71.

[230] Kelly DF, Gaw Gonzalo IT, Cohan P, et al. Hypopituitarism following traumatic brain injury and aneurysmal subarachnoid hemorrhage: a preliminary report. J Neurosurg 2000;93(5):743–52.

[231] Molitch M. Clinical manifestations of acromegaly. Endocrinol Metab Clin North Am 1992;21(3):597–614.

[232] Tritos NA, Biller BM, Swearingen B. Management of Cushing disease. Nature Rev Endocrinol 2011;7(5):279–89.

[233] Linas SL, Berl T, Robertson GL, et al. Role of vasopressin in the impaired water excretion of glucocorticoid deficiency. Kidney Int 1980;18(1):58–67.

[234] Raff H. Glucocorticoid inhibition of neurohypophysial vasopressin secretion. Am J Physiol Regul Integr Comp Physiol 1987;252(4):R635–44.

[235] Graves L III, Klein RM, Walling AD. Addisonian crisis precipitated by thyroxine therapy: a complication of type 2 autoimmune polyglandular syndrome. South Med J 2003;96(8):824–8.

[236] Murray JS, Jayarajasingh R, Perros P. Deterioration of symptoms after start of thyroid hormone replacement. Br Med J 2001;323(7308):332.

CHAPTER

2

Epidemiology and Etiology of Cushing's Disease

N.A. Tritos, MD, DSc*,**, B.M.K. Biller, MD*,†

*Harvard Medical School, Boston, MA, United States; **Neuroscience Unit,
Massachusetts General Hospital, Boston, MA, United States; †Neuroendocrine Unit,
Massachusetts General Hospital, Boston, MA, United States

OUTLINE

1 INTRODUCTION

Cushing's disease is caused by a pituitary adenoma (or, rarely, carcinoma) secreting adrenocorticotropic hormone (ACTH), also known as corticotropin, autonomously, which leads to excess cortisol production by the adrenals [1,2]. This condition accounts for the majority (70%) of cases of endogenous Cushing's syndrome in adults; other underlying pathologies include ectopic ACTH secretion (10%) and adrenal masses (20%) [3,4]. Published data suggest that Cushing's disease is quite uncommon in the general population but is nevertheless associated with substantial morbidity and mortality [1–3]. Recent advances have begun to shed light on the molecular genetics of Cushing's disease.

The aims of the present chapter include a review of published epidemiologic data on the incidence and prevalence of Cushing's disease and a discussion of the Cushing's disease–associated morbidity and mortality. Subsequently, exciting recent data that have furthered our understanding of genetic abnormalities underlying Cushing's disease are reviewed here.

2 EPIDEMIOLOGY OF CUSHING'S DISEASE

2.1 Incidence and Prevalence

2.1.1 Population-Based Data

The incidence and prevalence of Cushing's disease were examined in a study of patients living in a region of Spain between 1975 and 1992 [5]. The crude incidence rate of Cushing's disease was estimated to be 2.4 new cases per million population per year. In the same study, the prevalence of Cushing's disease in 1992 was 39.1 patients per million population. There was a strong female predilection noted among patients with Cushing's disease, as evidenced by a 15:1 ratio between women and men [5].

More recently, another study reported on the incidence of Cushing's disease in Denmark during an 11-year period (1985–1995) [6]. The crude incidence rate of Cushing's disease was estimated to range between 1.2 and 1.7 new cases per million population per year, owing to uncertainties in establishing the location of the underlying tumor in some patients with endogenous Cushing's disease. In the same study, Cushing's disease accounted for approximately 70% of all cases of endogenous Cushing's syndrome, whose crude incidence rate was estimated to be 2.3 cases per million per year [6].

A study from Iceland found that the prevalence of Cushing's disease was 62.1 patients per million population, including 52.8 women per million and 9.3 men per million in 2012 [7]. These data are consistent with previous observations, indicating that Cushing's disease is much more common in women than men.

In the United States, a recent study examined the incidence of hypercortisolism, using data from a commercial claims database, and found an incidence of 6.2–7.6 new cases (Cushing's disease) per million population per year [8]. If confirmed in subsequent studies, these data would suggest that the incidence of Cushing's disease is higher than previously thought.

2.1.2 Hypercortisolism in Patients with Incidentally Found Pituitary Masses

Both autopsy and radiographic studies suggest that clinically unsuspected (incidental) pituitary lesions are common in the general population [9]. A meta-analysis of data on 18,631 autopsies found that 10.6% of pituitary glands contained incidental sellar lesions at autopsy [9]. Of note, most of these lesions were smaller than 10 mm in greatest diameter and were classified as microadenomas; only seven lesions exceeded this cut-point and were thought to represent macroadenomas [9]. These findings are corroborated by modern imaging data, suggesting that 10–38% of individuals in the general population have incidental sellar lesions on magnetic resonance imaging (MRI), which represent microadenomas or small cysts in most cases [10,11].

In a recent study of individuals with incidentally found pituitary lesions, the prevalence of ACTH-dependent hypercortisolism was 7.3% (5 out of 68 patients), including 2 patients with macroadenomas and 3 patients with microadenomas, none of whom had clinically evident hypercortisolism [12]. In the same study, 4.4% (3 out of 68) of patients underwent pituitary surgery and were all found to have pituitary adenomas on histologic examination, which were positive for ACTH on immunohistochemistry. These patients also developed hypoadrenalism for several months postoperatively, suggesting that their pituitary tumors were likely functioning [12]. Certainly, larger studies are needed to examine the diagnostic test performance and yield as well as the possible benefits and harms of widespread screening for hypercortisolism in patients with incidentally found sellar masses. At a minimum, sensitive case finding appears to be prudent in this patient population.

2.1.3 "Occult" Cushing's Disease in Patients with Diabetes Mellitus, Hypertension, Polycystic Ovary Syndrome, Obesity, and Osteoporosis

Several studies have examined the prevalence of Cushing's disease in adult patients with comorbidities associated with (or mimicking) hypercortisolism, including diabetes mellitus, hypertension, polycystic ovary syndrome (PCOS), obesity, and osteoporosis. The populations examined in many of these studies did not have specific features of pathological hypercortisolism (e.g., disproportionate supraclavicular adiposity; wide, pigmented striae; proximal myopathy; unexplained hypokalemia). Although prevalence estimates for Cushing's disease vary substantially among publications, it may be noted that the prevalence of Cushing's disease was reported to be higher than in the general population in some of these studies.

In a study of 200 overweight patients with poorly controlled type 2 diabetes mellitus, 26% failed the 1-mg dexamethasone suppression test (DST). Multiple additional endocrine and imaging tests were subsequently performed and excluded hypercortisolism in most study subjects. Of note, 3 patients (1.5%) were eventually confirmed to have Cushing's disease and underwent pituitary surgery, radiation therapy, or ketoconazole therapy [13]. In another study of 294 hospitalized patients (> 30 years old) with poorly controlled type 2 diabetes mellitus, there were 4 patients (1.4%) with documented hypercortisolism thought to be of pituitary origin (presumed Cushing's disease) [14]. However, only one of them underwent pituitary surgery. This patient was found to have an ACTH-positive pituitary microadenoma on immunohistochemical testing [14]. In contrast, two other studies that screened patients with type 2 diabetes mellitus found no patients with pathological hypercortisolism, including one study of 154 men (veterans) and another study of 201 patients who met at least two out of three criteria (i.e., overweight, hypertension, and poorly controlled diabetes mellitus) [15,16]. Differences in patient populations and methodology are likely to explain the discrepant findings among the previously mentioned studies.

The prevalence of Cushing's disease has been reported in two large studies investigating secondary causes of hypertension. In a study of 1020 patients in Japan, there were 5 (0.49%) individuals who were diagnosed with Cushing's disease (confirmed histologically) [17]. In a study of 4429 patients in the United States, there were 24 (0.5%) with Cushing's disease (details of the underlying pathology were not provided) [18]. Patients had presented with hypertension in these two studies. However, no details of the phenotype of patients with

Cushing's disease/Cushing's syndrome were reported. Consequently, it is not entirely clear if Cushing's disease was truly "occult" in these study populations.

Several clinical features of PCOS overlap with those of Cushing's disease, including obesity, oligomenorrhea, hirsutism, acne, and insulin resistance [19]. One study from Denmark examined the prevalence of underlying endocrinopathies in 340 women who had presented for evaluation of hirsutism [20]. Out of these, there was a single patient with Cushing's disease (0.3%), who had clinical evidence of hypercortisolism. However, it is unclear if patients with "occult" Cushing's disease might have been present in this population, since patients were tested for Cushing's disease only in the presence of clinical suspicion [20].

Obesity is a very common manifestation of hypercortisolism [3]. However, the management of patients with Cushing's disease/Cushing's syndrome is very different from that of patients with "simple" (idiopathic) obesity. Accordingly, evaluating the prevalence of hypercortisolism in obese populations is a clinically relevant issue. Several studies have attempted to answer this question, albeit with divergent findings. In one study, 3 out of 86 obese patients (half of whom had diabetes mellitus or hypertension) screened for hypercortisolism were diagnosed with Cushing's disease and underwent confirmatory pituitary surgery, yielding a prevalence of Cushing's disease of 3.5% [21]. Another study from Turkey found that 9 out of 150 obese patients (6%) had "occult" Cushing's disease [22]. In contrast, a study (in the United States) of 369 individuals, who were obese or overweight reported that none of the screened patients had pathological hypercortisolism [23]. On the other hand, there have been reports of patients who were diagnosed with Cushing's disease after undergoing bariatric surgical procedures to treat severe obesity, suggesting that careful case finding is important in the evaluation of this population group [24].

The prevalence of Cushing's disease has also been examined in a study of 219 patients who had no specific features of hypercortisolism and were referred for evaluation of bone health, wherein the diagnosis of Cushing's disease was made in 1 patient (0.4%) [25]. This individual had low bone mineral density and previous fractures [25]. However, if the subgroup of patients with low bone mineral density, previous fractures, or both was considered ($n = 147$), then the estimated prevalence of Cushing's disease was higher (0.7%) in this study [25].

It may be noted that the aforementioned studies were performed in tertiary referral centers, where more severely ill patients tend to be referred. In addition, false-positive test results on preliminary testing for hypercortisolism are not uncommon [23]. Accordingly, sensitive case finding, but not widespread screening, for hypercortisolism seems prudent in patients with type 2 diabetes mellitus, hypertension, presumed PCOS, obesity, or osteoporosis.

2.2 Mortality

Hypercortisolism is associated with excess mortality as a consequence of cardiovascular disease, stroke, and infection [6]. The reported 5-year survival rate was 50% in Harvey Cushing's era [1]. Similar findings were reported in the early 1950s [26]. With the advent of bilateral adrenalectomy, 5-year survival exceeded 85% in the 1980s [27]. More recent studies from pituitary centers have reported even higher survival rates in patients with Cushing's disease undergoing transsphenoidal pituitary surgery [28–30]. Indeed, the 5-year survival rate was reported as 99% in a more recent study [29].

However, overall mortality in Cushing's disease remains significantly higher than in the general population [6]. In a meta-analysis of seven studies, the standardized mortality ratio (SMR) was 2.22 (confidence interval [CI]: 1.45–3.41) [31]. More encouragingly, the SMR (CI) was not elevated above the general population in the subgroup of patients with Cushing's disease who were in remission postoperatively, albeit with substantial heterogeneity among individual reports (1.2 [0.45–3.18]) [31]. It may be noted that the diagnostic criteria used to establish remission varied among individual studies. As a corollary, it is possible that some of the patients reported to be in remission may have had subtle, recurrent hypercortisolism, thereby raising their mortality risk. Another possible source of increased mortality among some patients in remission may have been supraphysiologic glucocorticoid replacement. In the same meta-analysis, patients with persistent Cushing's disease experienced significantly higher mortality (SMR [CI]: 5.5 [2.7–11.3]) [31]. These findings underscore the importance of prompt diagnosis and effective management in patients with Cushing's disease in order to mitigate the adverse consequences of hypercortisolism on survival.

2.3 Long-Term Morbidity and Quality of Life

Several studies suggest that many of the comorbidities associated with Cushing's disease may persist in patients who are considered to be in remission. Indeed, a number of studies have reported that these patients may have an increased cardiovascular risk [32–34]. An increased prevalence of cardiovascular risk factors (i.e., central obesity, high blood pressure, dyslipidemia, and high glucose), carotid atherosclerosis, and a high risk of myocardial infarction have been found in patients with Cushing's disease in remission [33,32]. While cardiac hypertrophy improves with successful treatment of hypercortisolism, it may not completely resolve in some patients [34]. As a corollary, a thorough assessment and intense management of cardiovascular risk factors is important in patients with Cushing's disease, including those who are thought to be in remission, in an effort to improve their cardiovascular risk.

Low bone mass, premature osteoporosis, and increased fracture risk are well-known comorbidities in Cushing's disease [35]. Bone mineral density (BMD) generally improves after hypercortisolism resolves. However, it may take up to 9 years for BMD to normalize after sustained remission of Cushing's disease is achieved [36,37].

Psychiatric symptoms, which are also frequent in patients with active Cushing's disease, often improve in patients who enter remission [38,39]. However, it is important to be aware that there can be an acute deterioration in psychiatric symptoms postoperatively in a minority of patients. Of note, residual psychopathologic manifestations as well as impairments in self-reported quality of life and neurocognitive function appear to persist in some patients, despite remission of hypercortisolism [39–42]. Imaging studies have reported decreased brain volume, including hippocampal atrophy, in patients with active Cushing's disease, which is only partly reversible in patients in remission [43].

Not surprisingly, health-related expenses are high in patients with active Cushing's disease, about four times those in the general population and twice those in patients with nonfunctioning pituitary adenomas [44]. Based on 2010 claims data in the United States, the annual cost of care for each patient with Cushing's disease was estimated to be $35,000 per year [45]. Although health-related expenses declined after successful surgery, they remained higher than in controls, presumably in relation to the ongoing need for evaluation and management of residual comorbidities present in this population [44].

It is clear that some of the symptoms and conditions associated with hypercortisolism may persist for years after remission has been achieved. Nevertheless, the reasons underlying these observations have not been fully elucidated. It is possible, or even likely, that some patients with persistent mild hypercortisolism might have been misclassified as being in remission in published reports. In addition, it is possible that some of the associated comorbidities in Cushing's disease are either slowly reversible after long periods of time or perhaps not at all. Recent research findings have suggested an association between polymorphic variations of genes that have an important role in glucocorticoid physiology, including the glucocorticoid receptor (*GR*) gene or the 11β-hydroxysteroid dehydrogenase type 1 (*11β-HSD type 1*) gene and the risk of persistent neurocognitive symptoms in patients with Cushing's disease in remission [46]. These findings raise the possibility that variations in sensitivity to glucocorticoid tissue availability or action may be associated with long-lasting residual symptoms despite "cure" of hypercortisolism. In the same study, 43% of patients were on glucocorticoid replacement, raising the possibility that nonphysiologic replacement might be contributing to the persistence of residual symptoms in some patients thought to be in remission [46]. Regardless of the underlying mechanisms, all patients with Cushing's disease in remission require regular follow-up, evaluation, and management of associated comorbidities to optimize their recovery [47].

3 ETIOLOGY OF CUSHING'S DISEASE

An ACTH-secreting pituitary adenoma is the underlying pathology in most patients with Cushing's disease; pituitary carcinomas are truly rare. The genetic abnormalities underlying tumorigenesis in the pituitary have been incompletely elucidated. However, recent studies have significantly improved our understanding of the molecular mechanisms involved in the pathogenesis of corticotropinomas.

3.1 Mutations in the Deubiquitinase Gene (*USP8*)

Using whole exome sequencing, parallel studies from two different groups have found that activating, heterozygous somatic mutations in the deubiquitinase [ubiquitin-specific peptidase 8 (*USP8*)] gene are common in ACTH-secreting pituitary adenomas [48,49]. In one study, 35% of 17 corticotropinomas had such a mutation, which was not present in other pituitary tumors (i.e., nonfunctioning or prolactin- and growth hormone–secreting) [48]. These findings were confirmed in a large multicenter study, which found that 36% of 134 ACTH-secreting adenomas carried such a mutation [50]. A study from a second group found that 62% of 108 corticotropinomas had an activating somatic mutation in the *USP8* gene, which was again specific to corticotropin-secreting pituitary adenomas [49]. Such mutations have been found more often in tumors from women than men [49,48].

In all published studies, the identified mutations disrupt 14-3-3 protein binding to the USP8 deubiquitinase [48,49]. Since 14-3-3 protein binding normally serves to decrease the enzymatic activity of the deubiquitinase, the mutant USP8 protein has constitutively increased enzymatic activity. This leads to enhanced protein target deubiquitination and, consequently, decreased degradation of several signaling molecules, including the erb-b2 receptor, the epidermal growth factor receptor (EGFR), and possibly, the receptors for corticotropin-releasing hormone (CRH) or arginine vasopressin (AVP), among others. It has been postulated that these events may culminate in corticotroph cell proliferation and increased ACTH secretion [51]. These exciting findings open new areas for research into the pathogenesis of ACTH-secreting pituitary adenomas and may ultimately translate into the development of new effective tumor-targeted therapies for Cushing's disease.

3.2 Multiple Endocrine Neoplasia 1 Syndrome

Cardinal features of the multiple endocrine neoplasia 1 (MEN 1) syndrome include pituitary adenomas (30% of patients), primary hyperparathyroidism (90% of patients, occurring as a consequence of multiple parathyroid gland hyperplasia or metachronous adenomas), and enteropancreatic neuroendocrine tumors (in 30–80% of patients, depending on the series) [52]. Germline mutations in the *MEN1* gene, which encodes menin, have been identified in most patients with the MEN 1 syndrome and result in autosomal dominant transmission of the disease with high penetrance [52].

Germline *MEN1* gene mutations have been reported in small numbers of patients with Cushing's disease, wherein hypercortisolism is the presenting manifestation of MEN 1 [53,54]. However, such mutations appear to be quite uncommon among patients with sporadic Cushing's disease. Indeed, in a study of 74 patients (including both children and adolescents) with sporadic Cushing's disease, there were no germline *MEN1* mutations identified [55]. In the same study, 2 out of 4 patients with Cushing's disease in the setting of a suspected or known familial syndrome were found to have *MEN1* gene mutations [55]. Based on available data, the possibility that a patient may have MEN 1 syndrome needs to be considered in individuals with at least two cardinal manifestations or those with a positive family history. However, *MEN1* gene mutations appear unlikely to account for a substantial fraction of ACTH-secreting pituitary adenomas.

3.3 Mutations in the Aryl-hydrocarbon Receptor Interacting Protein (AIP) Gene

Familial isolated pituitary adenomas (FIPAs), defined as pituitary tumors occurring in several family members without evidence of syndromes, such as MEN 1 or the Carney complex, are uncommon and account for only 2% of all pituitary adenomas [56]. In 20% of FIPA patients, germline mutations of the gene encoding the aryl-hydrocarbon receptor interacting protein (AIP) are present and thought to confer a predisposition to pituitary tumorigenesis with variable penetrance [56,57]. Most of the pituitary adenomas in patients with *AIP* gene mutations are growth hormone– or prolactin-secreting; however, ACTH-secreting pituitary adenomas may occur in a small number of patients [56,57].

Of note, *AIP* gene mutations appear to be uncommon in patients with sporadic Cushing's disease [55,58]. In a study of 74 young patients with sporadic Cushing's disease, there was only 1 patient who was found to have a germline *AIP* gene mutation [55]. Therefore, *AIP* gene mutations may explain only a small portion of the burden of Cushing's disease.

3.4 Other Gene Mutations

A variety of germline and somatic gene mutations have been identified in very small numbers of patients with Cushing's disease. These include mutations in the following genes: *DICER1*, *CDKN1B*, *GR*, and *p53*.

3.4.1 Mutations in the DICER1 (Ribonuclease Type III) Gene

The *DICER1* gene encodes a ribonuclease (type III) that cleaves specific RNA molecules into microRNA (miRNA), which binds to complementary mRNA sequences and inhibits transcription [59–61]. Germline, heterozygous mutations in the *DICER1* gene lead to impaired transcription regulation and confer pleiotropic tumor predisposition, including an increased risk of pleuropulmonary blastoma, cystic nephroma, Wilms tumor, ovarian Sertoli–Leydig tumor, medulloblastoma, germ cell tumor, medulloepithelioma, multinodular goiter, and pituitary blastoma [59,60,62].

A recent report identified the case of a patient with Cushing's disease with onset in infancy, who was found to have both a germline and a somatic *DICER1* mutation in tumor tissue [63]. However, the DICER1 syndrome is rare and is unlikely to account for a substantial fraction of Cushing's disease cases.

3.4.2 Mutations in Cyclin-Dependent Kinase Inhibitor Subtype 1B Gene

The cyclin-dependent kinase inhibitor subtype 1B (*CDKN1B*) gene encodes a protein (p27/Kip1) that functions as a cell-cycle regulator [64]. Germline, inactivating mutations of the *CDKN1B* gene have been described in patients with pituitary and parathyroid tumors who lack mutations of the *MEN1* gene, a syndrome termed MEN 4 [64]. One study reported that a single patient with MEN 4 developed Cushing's disease [65].

3.4.3 Mutations in the GR Gene

The *GR* gene plays a pivotal role in mediating glucocorticoid action, including the negative feedback regulation of ACTH secretion by endogenous cortisol [66]. Corticotropinomas have blunted regulation of ACTH secretion in response to exogenous glucocorticoid administration but nevertheless maintain some degree of feedback inhibition by dexamethasone administered in high doses [66].

There are limited data involving *GR* gene mutations in patients with Nelson's syndrome (NS) [67]. Nelson's syndrome occurs as a consequence of corticotroph tumor progression and a concurrent increase in ACTH secretion in some patients with Cushing's disease after bilateral adrenalectomy [68,69]. Corticotroph pituitary adenomas may become locally aggressive in these patients, leading to substantial mass effect [70]. These patients often develop skin hyperpigmentation as a result of ACTH excess [68]. A somatic frameshift mutation of the *GR* gene was detected in the tumor tissue of 1 out of 4 patients with NS and might have a role in tumor progression in this patient by interfering with negative feedback regulation mechanisms in tumorous corticotrophs [67].

3.4.4 Mutations in the p53 Gene

The tumor suppressor p53 protein plays an important role in cell-cycle regulation, and its inactivating mutations are pivotal to tumorigenesis in many human malignancies [71].

TABLE 2.1 Gene Mutations in Cushing's Disease

Gene name	Role and function of the gene product (known or putative)
USP8	Protein deubiquitinase
MEN1	Transcription regulation; cell-cycle regulation
AIP	Tumor suppressor
DICER1	Type III ribonuclease
CDKN1B	Cell-cycle regulation
GR	Glucocorticoid action
p53	Cell-cycle regulation; tumor suppressor

AIP, aryl-hydrocarbon receptor interacting protein; *CDKN1B*, cyclin-dependent kinase inhibitor subtype 1B; *GR*, glucocorticoid receptor; *MEN1*, multiple endocrine neoplasia 1; and *USP8*, ubiquitin-specific peptidase 8.

There are two reports of somatic *p53* gene mutations in patients with ACTH-secreting tumors, including one patient with Cushing's disease caused by an atypical pituitary adenoma and another patient with NS caused by an aggressive tumor [72,73]. Of note, a *p53* gene mutation was only detected after the patient with NS received radiation therapy to the sella, raising the possibility that the mutation might have been induced by previous radiotherapy [73]. In both patients, it is conceivable that p53 inactivation may have contributed to tumor aggressiveness. A summary of gene mutations in Cushing's disease is shown in Table 2.1 [48,49,53–59,63–67,72,73].

3.5 Gene and Protein Expression Abnormalities in Corticotropinomas

Many alterations in gene and protein expression have been described in studies examining tissue specimens from ACTH-secreting tumors, using a variety of methods, including Northern blotting, reverse transcriptase–polymerase chain reaction, Western blotting, and immunohistochemistry [74–77].

These abnormalities may involve genes/proteins that have a known or putative role in cell-cycle regulation (cyclin D1, cyclin E, EGFR, kisseptin 1 and its receptor, p16, p27/Kip1, pituitary tumor transforming [*PTTG*] gene) [74–76,78–82], transcription regulation (*brahma-related gene 1* [*Brg1*], *histone deacetylase 2* [*HDAC2*]), *miR-493, NeuroD1, testicular orphan receptor 4* [*TR4*]) [77,83–85], protein folding (heat shock protein 90 [*HSP90*]) [86], intracellular signaling (*Akt1, Akt2*) [87], or corticotroph cell function/signaling (ACTH receptor, AVP receptor, CRH receptor, GR, 11β-HSD type 1, 11β-HSD type 2, proopiomelanocortin [*POMC*]) [88–93]. A summary of overexpressed and underexpressed proteins in corticotropinomas is shown in Table 2.2.

The functional significance of these alterations in protein expression has not been fully established and requires further study. It is possible that some of these molecules might turn out to be important drug targets and lead to the development of efficacious pharmacologic agents in Cushing's disease [90].

TABLE 2.2 Abnormalities in Gene and Protein Expression in Cushing's Disease

Name	Role and function (known or putative)	Expression in Cushing's disease
Cyclin D1	Cell-cycle regulation	Increased
Cyclin E	Cell-cycle regulation	Increased
EGFR	Downregulation of p27/Kip1	Increased
Kisspeptin 1 and its receptor	Cell apoptosis (possibly)	Decreased
p16	Cell-cycle regulation	Decreased
p27/Kip1	Cell-cycle regulation	Decreased
PTTG	Cell-cycle regulation	Increased
Brg1	Transcription regulation	Decreased
HDAC2	Transcription regulation	Decreased
miR-493	Transcription regulation	Decreased
NeuroD1	Transcription regulation	Increased
TR4	Transcription regulation	Increased
HSP90	Protein folding (chaperone)	Increased
Akt1 and Akt2	Intracellular signaling	Increased
ACTH receptor	ACTH signaling	Decreased
AVP receptor	ACTH secretion	Increased
CRH receptor	ACTH secretion	Increased
GR	Feedback inhibition of ACTH secretion	Variable (increased or decreased)
11β-HSD type 1	Cortisone to cortisol interconversion	Decreased
11β-HSD type 2	Cortisol inactivation	Increased
POMC	ACTH precursor	Increased

ACTH, adrenocorticotropic hormone; AVP, arginine vasopressin; Brg1, brahma-related gene 1; CRH, corticotropin-releasing hormone; EGFR, epidermal growth factor receptor; GR, glucocorticoid receptor; HDAC2, histone deacetylase 2; HSD, hydroxysteroid dehydrogenase; HSP90, heat shock protein 90; POMC, pro-opiomelanocortin; PTTG, pituitary tumor transforming gene; and TR4, testicular orphan receptor.

4 CONCLUSIONS

Cushing's disease is very uncommon in the general population and is associated with substantial morbidity and mortality, which can be mitigated by early diagnosis and effective therapy. Sensitive case finding aimed at detecting Cushing's disease is advisable in the evaluation of patients belonging to groups wherein Cushing's disease appears to be more common, including patients with incidentally found pituitary adenomas, type 2 diabetes mellitus, hypertension, PCOS, obesity, and osteoporosis. Recent advances in molecular genetics, including the identification of mutations in the USP8 gene in a substantial fraction of corticotropinomas as well as the detection of a host of abnormalities in gene and protein expression in these tumors, have begun to unravel the pathogenesis of Cushing's disease and offer renewed hope that novel therapeutic developments will soon follow.

Disclosures

BMKB has received research grants (to MGH) from Cortendo and Novartis, and has consulted for Cortendo, HRA Pharma, Ipsen, and Novartis. NAT has received research grants (to MGH) from Ipsen, Novartis, Novo Nordisk, and Pfizer.

References

[1] Cushing H. The basophil adenomas of the pituitary body and their clinical manifestations (pituitary basophilism). Bull Johns Hopkins Hosp 1932;50:137–95.

[2] Cushing H. The basophil adenomas of the pituitary body. Ann R Coll Surg Engl 1969;44(4):180–1.

[3] Newell-Price J, Bertagna X, Grossman AB, et al. Cushing's syndrome. Lancet 2006;367(9522):1605–17.

[4] Nieman LK, Biller BM, Findling JW, et al. The diagnosis of Cushing's syndrome: an Endocrine Society Clinical Practice Guideline. J Clin Endocrinol Metab 2008;93(5):1526–40.

[5] Etxabe J, Vazquez JA. Morbidity and mortality in Cushing's disease: an epidemiological approach. Clin Endocrinol (Oxf) 1994;40(4):479–84.

[6] Lindholm J, Juul S, Jorgensen JO, et al. Incidence and late prognosis of Cushing's syndrome: a population-based study. J Clin Endocrinol Metab 2001;86(1):117–23.

[7] Agustsson TT, Baldvinsdottir T, Jonasson JG, et al. The epidemiology of pituitary adenomas in Iceland, 1955–2012: a nationwide population-based study. Eur J Endocrinol 2015;173(5):655–64.

[8] Broder MS, Neary MP, Chang E, et al. Incidence of Cushing's syndrome and Cushing's disease in commercially insured patients < 65 years old in the United States. Pituitary 2015;18(3):283–9.

[9] Molitch ME. Nonfunctioning pituitary tumors and pituitary incidentalomas. Endocrinol Metab Clin North Am 2008;37(1):151–71.

[10] Hall WA, Luciano MG, Doppman JL, et al. Pituitary magnetic resonance imaging in normal human volunteers: occult adenomas in the general population. Ann Intern Med 1994;120(10):817–20.

[11] Chong BW, Kucharczyk W, Singer W, et al. Pituitary gland MRI: a comparative study of healthy volunteers and patients with microadenomas. Am J Neuroradiol 1994;15(4):675–9.

[12] Toini A, Dolci A, Ferrante E, et al. Screening for ACTH-dependent hypercortisolism in patients affected with pituitary incidentaloma. Eur J Endocrinol 2015;172(4):363–9.

[13] Catargi B, Rigalleau V, Poussin A, et al. Occult Cushing's syndrome in type-2 diabetes. J Clin Endocrinol Metab 2003;88(12):5808–13.

[14] Chiodini I, Torlontano M, Scillitani A, et al. Association of subclinical hypercortisolism with type 2 diabetes mellitus: a case-control study in hospitalized patients. Eur J Endocrinol 2005;153(6):837–44.

[15] Liu H, Bravata DM, Cabaccan J, et al. Elevated late-night salivary cortisol levels in elderly male type 2 diabetic veterans. Clin Endocrinol (Oxf) 2005;63(6):642–9.

[16] Mullan K, Black N, Thiraviaraj A, et al. Is there value in routine screening for Cushing's syndrome in patients with diabetes? J Clin Endocrinol Metab 2010;95(5):2262–5.

[17] Omura M, Saito J, Yamaguchi K, et al. Prospective study on the prevalence of secondary hypertension among hypertensive patients visiting a general outpatient clinic in Japan. Hypertens Res 2004;27(3):193–202.

[18] Anderson GH Jr, Blakeman N, Streeten DH. The effect of age on prevalence of secondary forms of hypertension in 4429 consecutively referred patients. J Hypertens 1994;12(5):609–15.

[19] Azziz R. Diagnostic criteria for polycystic ovary syndrome: a reappraisal. Fertil Steril 2005;83(5):1343–6.

[20] Glintborg D, Henriksen JE, Andersen M. Prevalence of endocrine diseases and abnormal glucose tolerance tests in 340 Caucasian premenopausal women with hirsutism as the referral diagnosis. Fertil Steril 2004;82(6):1570–9.

[21] Ness-Abramof R, Nabriski D, Apovian CM, et al. Overnight dexamethasone suppression test: a reliable screen for Cushing's syndrome in the obese. Obes Res 2002;10(12):1217–21.

[22] Tiryakioglu O, Ugurlu S, Yalin S, et al. Screening for Cushing's syndrome in obese patients. Clinics (Sao Paulo) 2010;65(1):9–13.

[23] Baid SK, Rubino D, Sinaii N, et al. Specificity of screening tests for Cushing's syndrome in an overweight and obese population. J Clin Endocrinol Metab 2009;94(10):3857–64.

[24] Javorsky BR, Carroll TB, Tritos NA, et al. Discovery of Cushing's syndrome after bariatric surgery: multicenter series of 16 patients. Obes Surg 2015;25(12):2306–13.

[25] Chiodini I, Mascia ML, Muscarella S, et al. Subclinical hypercortisolism among outpatients referred for osteo-porosis. Ann Intern Med 2007;147(8):541–8.

[26] Plotz CM, Knowlton AI, Ragan C. The natural history of Cushing's syndrome. Am J Med 1952;13(5):597–614.

[27] O'Riordain DS, Farley DR, Young WF Jr, et al. Long-term outcome of bilateral adrenalectomy in patients with Cushing's syndrome. Surgery 1994;116(6):1088–93. discussion 1093–1084.

[28] Swearingen B, Barker FG II, Zervas NT. The management of pituitary adenomas: the MGH experience. Clin Neurosurg 1999;45:48–56.

[29] Swearingen B, Biller BM, Barker FG 2nd. Long-term mortality after transsphenoidal surgery for Cushing disease. Ann Intern Med 1999;130(10):821–4.

[30] Laws ER Jr. The evolution of Cushing's surgical treatment of pituitary lesions. World Neurosurg 2013;79(2):290–1.

[31] Clayton RN, Raskauskiene D, Reulen RC. Mortality and morbidity in Cushing's disease over 50 years in Stoke-on-Trent, UK: audit and meta-analysis of literature. J Clin Endocrinol Metab 2011;96(3):632–42.

[32] Colao A, Pivonello R, Spiezia S. Persistence of increased cardiovascular risk in patients with Cushing's disease after five years of successful cure. J Clin Endocrinol Metab 1999;84(8):2664–72.

[33] Dekkers OM, Horvath-Puho E, Jorgensen JO, et al. Multisystem morbidity and mortality in Cushing's syndrome: a cohort study. J Clin Endocrinol Metab 2013;98(6):2277–84.

[34] Toja PM, Branzi G, Ciambellotti F, et al. Clinical relevance of cardiac structure and function abnormalities in patients with Cushing's syndrome before and after cure. Clin Endocrinol (Oxf) 2012;76(3):332–8.

[35] Valassi E, Santos A, Yaneva M, et al. The European Registry on Cushing's syndrome: 2-year experience. Baseline demographic and clinical characteristics. Eur J Endocrinol 2011;165(3):383–92.

[36] Manning PJ, Evans MC, Reid IR. Normal bone mineral density following cure of Cushing's syndrome. Clin Endocrinol (Oxf) 1992;36(3):229–34.

[37] Kristo C, Jemtland R, Ueland T, et al. Restoration of the coupling process and normalization of bone mass following successful treatment of endogenous Cushing's syndrome: a prospective, long-term study. Eur J Endocrinol 2006;154(1):109–18.

[38] Dorn LD, Burgess ES, Dubbert B, et al. Psychopathology in patients with endogenous Cushing's syndrome: 'atypical' or melancholic features. Clin Endocrinol (Oxf) 1995;43(4):433–42.

[39] Dorn LD, Burgess ES, Friedman TC, et al. The longitudinal course of psychopathology in Cushing's syndrome after correction of hypercortisolism. J Clin Endocrinol Metab 1997;82(3):912–9.

[40] Lindsay JR, Nansel T, Baid S, et al. Long-term impaired quality of life in Cushing's syndrome despite initial improvement after surgical remission. J Clin Endocrinol Metab 2006;91(2):447–53.

[41] Andela CD, Scharloo M, Pereira AM, et al. Quality of life (QoL) impairments in patients with a pituitary adenoma: a systematic review of QoL studies. Pituitary 2015;18(5):752–76.

[42] Ragnarsson O, Berglund P, Eder DN, et al. Long-term cognitive impairments and attentional deficits in patients with Cushing's disease and cortisol-producing adrenal adenoma in remission. J Clin Endocrinol Metab 2012;97(9):E1640–8.

[43] Andela CD, van Haalen FM, Ragnarsson O, et al. Mechanisms in endocrinology: Cushing's syndrome causes irreversible effects on the human brain: a systematic review of structural and functional magnetic resonance imaging studies. Eur J Endocrinol 2015;173(1):R1–R14.

[44] Swearingen B, Wu N, Chen SY, et al. Health care resource use and costs among patients with Cushing disease. Endocr Pract 2011;17(5):681–90.

[45] Broder MS, Neary MP, Chang E, et al. Burden of illness, annual healthcare utilization, and costs associated with commercially insured patients with Cushing disease in the United States. Endocr Pract 2015;21(1):77–86.

[46] Ragnarsson O, Glad CA, Berglund P, et al. Common genetic variants in the glucocorticoid receptor and the 11beta-hydroxysteroid dehydrogenase type 1 genes influence long-term cognitive impairments in patients with Cushing's syndrome in remission. J Clin Endocrinol Metab 2014;99(9):E1803–7.

[47] Nieman LK, Biller BM, Findling JW, et al. Treatment of Cushing's syndrome: an Endocrine Society Clinical Practice Guideline. J Clin Endocrinol Metab 2015;100(8):2807–31.

[48] Reincke M, Sbiera S, Hayakawa A, et al. Mutations in the deubiquitinase gene *USP8* cause Cushing's disease. Nat Genet 2015;47(1):31–8.

[49] Ma ZY, Song ZJ, Chen JH, et al. Recurrent gain-of-function *USP8* mutations in Cushing's disease. Cell Res 2015;25(3):306–17.

[50] Perez-Rivas LG, Theodoropoulou M, Ferrau F, et al. The gene of the ubiquitin-specific protease 8 is frequently mutated in adenomas causing Cushing's disease. J Clin Endocrinol Metab 2015;100(7):E997–E1004.

[51] Perez-Rivas LG, Reincke M. Genetics of Cushing's disease: an update. J Endocrinol Invest 2016;39(1):29–35.

[52] Thakker RV, Newey PJ, Walls GV, et al. Clinical practice guidelines for multiple endocrine neoplasia type 1 (MEN1). J Clin Endocrinol Metab 2012;97(9):2990–3011.

[53] Matsuzaki LN, Canto-Costa MH, Hauache OM. Cushing's disease as the first clinical manifestation of multiple endocrine neoplasia type 1 (MEN1) associated with an R460X mutation of the MEN1 gene. Clin Endocrinol (Oxf) 2004;60(1):142–3.

[54] Rix M, Hertel NT, Nielsen FC, et al. Cushing's disease in childhood as the first manifestation of multiple endocrine neoplasia syndrome type 1. Eur J Endocrinol 2004;151(6):709–15.

[55] Stratakis CA, Tichomirowa MA, Boikos S, et al. The role of germline *AIP, MEN1, PRKAR1A, CDKN1B* and *CDKN2C* mutations in causing pituitary adenomas in a large cohort of children, adolescents, and patients with genetic syndromes. Clin Genet 2010;78(5):457–63.

[56] Beckers A, Aaltonen LA, Daly AF. Familial isolated pituitary adenomas (FIPA) and the pituitary adenoma predisposition due to mutations in the aryl hydrocarbon receptor interacting protein (*AIP*) gene. Endocr Rev 2013;34(2):239–77.

[57] Daly AF, Tichomirowa MA, Petrossians P, et al. Clinical characteristics and therapeutic responses in patients with germ-line AIP mutations and pituitary adenomas: an international collaborative study. J Clin Endocrinol Metab 2010;95(11):E373–83.

[58] Dinesen PT, Dal J, Gabrovska P, et al. An unusual case of an ACTH-secreting macroadenoma with a germline variant in the aryl hydrocarbon receptor-interacting protein (AIP) gene. Endocrinol Diab Metab Case Rep 2015;2015:140105.

[59] Foulkes WD, Bahubeshi A, Hamel N, et al. Extending the phenotypes associated with *DICER1* mutations. Hum Mutat 2011;32(12):1381–4.

[60] Rio Frio T, Bahubeshi A, Kanellopoulou C, et al. *DICER1* mutations in familial multinodular goiter with and without ovarian Sertoli–Leydig cell tumors. JAMA 2011;305(1):68–77.

[61] Carthew RW, Sontheimer EJ. Origins and mechanisms of miRNAs and siRNAs. Cell 2009;136(4):642–55.

[62] Slade I, Bacchelli C, Davies H, et al. DICER1 syndrome: clarifying the diagnosis, clinical features and management implications of a pleiotropic tumour predisposition syndrome. J Med Genet 2011;48(4):273–8.

[63] Sahakitrungruang T, Srichomthong C, Pornkunwilai S, et al. Germline and somatic *DICER1* mutations in a pituitary blastoma causing infantile-onset Cushing's disease. J Clin Endocrinol Metab 2014;99(8):E1487–92.

[64] Pellegata NS, Quintanilla-Martinez L, Siggelkow H, et al. Germ-line mutations in p27Kip1 cause a multiple endocrine neoplasia syndrome in rats and humans. Proc Natl Acad Sci USA 2006;103(42):15558–63.

[65] Georgitsi M, Raitila A, Karhu A, et al. Germline *CDKN1B/p27Kip1* mutation in multiple endocrine neoplasia. J Clin Endocrinol Metab 2007;92(8):3321–5.

[66] Briassoulis G, Damjanovic S, Xekouki P, et al. The glucocorticoid receptor and its expression in the anterior pituitary and the adrenal cortex: a source of variation in hypothalamic-pituitary-adrenal axis function; implications for pituitary and adrenal tumors. Endocr Pract 2011;17(6):941–8.

[67] Karl M, Von Wichert G, Kempter E, et al. Nelson's syndrome associated with a somatic frame shift mutation in the glucocorticoid receptor gene. J Clin Endocrinol Metab 1996;81(1):124–9.

[68] Nelson DH, Meakin JW, Dealy JB Jr, et al. ACTH-producing tumor of the pituitary gland. N Engl J Med 1958;259(4):161–4.

[69] Assie G, Bahurel H, Coste J, et al. Corticotroph tumor progression after adrenalectomy in Cushing's disease: a reappraisal of Nelson's syndrome. J Clin Endocrinol Metab 2007;92(1):172–9.

[70] Tritos NA, Schaefer PW, Stein TD. Case records of the Massachusetts General Hospital. Case 40-2011. A 52-year-old man with weakness, infections, and enlarged adrenal glands. N Engl J Med 2011;365(26):2520–30.

[71] Cadwell C, Zambetti GP. The effects of wild-type p53 tumor suppressor activity and mutant *p53* gain-of-function on cell growth. Gene 2001;277(1–2):15–30.

[72] Kawashima ST, Usui T, Sano T, et al. P53 gene mutation in an atypical corticotroph adenoma with Cushing's disease. Clin Endocrinol (Oxf) 2009;70(4):656–7.

[73] Pinto EM, Siqueira SA, Cukier P, et al. Possible role of a radiation-induced p53 mutation in a Nelson's syndrome patient with a fatal outcome. Pituitary 2011;14(4):400–4.

[74] Lee EH, Kim KH, Kwon JH, et al. Results of immunohistochemical staining of cell-cycle regulators: the prediction of recurrence of functioning pituitary adenoma. World Neurosurg 2014;81(3–4):563–75.

[75] Jordan S, Lidhar K, Korbonits M, et al. Cyclin D and cyclin E expression in normal and adenomatous pituitary. Eur J Endocrinol 2000;143(1):R1–6.

[76] Theodoropoulou M, Arzberger T, Gruebler Y, et al. Expression of epidermal growth factor receptor in neoplastic pituitary cells: evidence for a role in corticotropinoma cells. J Endocrinol 2004;183(2):385–94.

[77] Oyama K, Sanno N, Teramoto A, et al. Expression of neuro D1 in human normal pituitaries and pituitary adenomas. Mod Pathol 2001;14(9):892–9.

[78] Turner HE, Nagy Z, Sullivan N, et al. Expression analysis of cyclins in pituitary adenomas and the normal pituitary gland. Clin Endocrinol (Oxf) 2000;53(3):337–44.

[79] Martinez-Fuentes AJ, Molina M, Vazquez-Martinez R, et al. Expression of functional KISS1 and KISS1R system is altered in human pituitary adenomas: evidence for apoptotic action of kisspeptin-10. Eur J Endocrinol 2011;164(3):355–62.

[80] Seemann N, Kuhn D, Wrocklage C, et al. CDKN2A/p16 inactivation is related to pituitary adenoma type and size. J Pathol 2001;193(4):491–7.

[81] Lidhar K, Korbonits M, Jordan S, et al. Low expression of the cell cycle inhibitor p27Kip1 in normal corticotroph cells, corticotroph tumors, and malignant pituitary tumors. J Clin Endocrinol Metab 1999;84(10):3823–30.

[82] Filippella M, Galland F, Kujas M, et al. Pituitary tumour transforming gene (PTTG) expression correlates with the proliferative activity and recurrence status of pituitary adenomas: a clinical and immunohistochemical study. Clin Endocrinol (Oxf) 2006;65(4):536–43.

[83] Bilodeau S, Vallette-Kasic S, Gauthier Y, et al. Role of Brg1 and HDAC2 in GR trans-repression of the pituitary POMC gene and misexpression in Cushing disease. Genes Dev 2006;20(20):2871–86.

[84] Stilling G, Sun Z, Zhang S, et al. MicroRNA expression in ACTH-producing pituitary tumors: up-regulation of microRNA-122 and -493 in pituitary carcinomas. Endocrine 2010;38(1):67–75.

[85] Du L, Bergsneider M, Mirsadraei L, et al. Evidence for orphan nuclear receptor TR4 in the etiology of Cushing disease. Proc Natl Acad Sci USA 2013;110(21):8555–60.

[86] Riebold M, Kozany C, Freiburger L, et al. A C-terminal HSP90 inhibitor restores glucocorticoid sensitivity and relieves a mouse allograft model of Cushing disease. Nat Med 2015;21(3):276–80.

[87] Musat M, Korbonits M, Kola B, et al. Enhanced protein kinase B/Akt signalling in pituitary tumours. Endocr Relat Cancer 2005;12(2):423–33.

[88] Morris DG, Kola B, Borboli N, et al. Identification of adrenocorticotropin receptor messenger ribonucleic acid in the human pituitary and its loss of expression in pituitary adenomas. J Clin Endocrinol Metab 2003;88(12):6080–7.

[89] Dahia PL, Ahmed-Shuaib A, Jacobs RA, et al. Vasopressin receptor expression and mutation analysis in corticotropin-secreting tumors. J Clin Endocrinol Metab 1996;81(5):1768–71.

[90] Luque RM, Ibanez-Costa A, Lopez-Sanchez LM, et al. A cellular and molecular basis for the selective desmopressin-induced ACTH release in Cushing disease patients: key role of AVPR1b receptor and potential therapeutic implications. J Clin Endocrinol Metab 2013;98(10):4160–9.

[91] Tateno T, Izumiyama H, Doi M, et al. Differential gene expression in ACTH-secreting and non-functioning pituitary tumors. Eur J Endocrinol 2007;157(6):717–24.

[92] Korbonits M, Bujalska I, Shimojo M, et al. Expression of 11 beta-hydroxysteroid dehydrogenase isoenzymes in the human pituitary: induction of the type 2 enzyme in corticotropinomas and other pituitary tumors. J Clin Endocrinol Metab 2001;86(6):2728–33.

[93] Raverot G, Wierinckx A, Jouanneau E, et al. Clinical, hormonal and molecular characterization of pituitary ACTH adenomas without (silent corticotroph adenomas) and with Cushing's disease. Eur J Endocrinol 2010;163(1):35–43.

Physical Presentation of Cushing's Syndrome: Typical and Atypical Presentations

M.L. Vance, MD

Departments of Medicine and Neurological Surgery, Division of Endocrinology and Metabolism,
University of Virginia Health System, Charlottesville, VA, United States

O U T L I N E

Cushing's Disease. http://dx.doi.org/10.1016/B978-0-12-804340-0.00003-6

1 INTRODUCTION

The most common cause of Cushing's syndrome is "iatrogenic," that is, the administration of oral, intramuscular, or intraarticular steroids to treat a variety of medical problems, such as arthritis, asthma, chronic obstructive pulmonary disease, joint pain, rheumatoid arthritis, spinal stenosis, and spinal disc disease. When suspicious about Cushing's syndrome, the first question a physician must ask is about exposure to exogenous steroid treatment. Any patient who has been treated at an orthopedic or pain clinic likely received multiple injections of a potent and long-acting depot steroid (most commonly triamcinolone, the most potent, long-acting synthetic steroid available). Repeated injections or frequent oral steroid treatment causes clinical features of Cushing's syndrome.

There is no one "typical" presentation of patients with Cushing's syndrome, regardless of the cause [e.g., a pituitary adenoma, an adrenal adenoma or carcinoma, or ectopic adrenocorticotropic hormone (ACTH) production]. The clinical features vary and depend on both the duration and severity of excessive cortisol production and the individual patient's response to excessive cortisol. Weight gain, new onset diabetes mellitus, and hypertension or worsening of control of diabetes and hypertension are probably the most common features of Cushing's. In most patients, medications are adjusted to control these disorders without consideration of the reason behind them. New bone fractures without an obvious cause should raise concern, regarding excessive cortisol production. Depression and mood changes are a prominent part of Cushing's but are usually treated with antidepressant medications, without consideration of possible Cushing's. This is the reality. In our pituitary clinic, we conducted a survey of 245 patients with Cushing's (almost all had pituitary Cushing's) and asked the following questions: How long did you have symptoms? How many physicians did you see before a definitive diagnosis of Cushing's syndrome? The average time from onset of symptoms to diagnosis was 3.5–5 years, and the number of physicians consulted ranged from 2 to over 12.

2 SYMPTOMS OF CUSHING'S DISEASE

2.1 Subjective Symptoms

Patient-reported symptoms are highly variable and may be nonspecific. The more commonly reported psychological symptoms are changes in mood, including depression, irritability, and crying spells for no particular reason; difficulty sleeping with frequent awakening during the night, sometimes described as feeling "wired"; difficulty concentrating; and memory problems. The emotional and memory issues are often attributed to depression, and the patient is given antidepressant or antianxiety medication with a variable and often a suboptimal response. Weight gain is usual, even in overweight or obese patients, but may not occur in patients who exercise rigorously. An increase in appetite is often reported, or weight gain occurs despite no change in diet, activity, or even with an attempt to restrict calories. A prominent feature is overwhelming fatigue and feeling generally warm or hot most of the time (not the typical features of "hot flashes" in menopausal women). Muscle weakness is usually associated with either severe Cushing's or long-standing unrecognized disease (e.g., difficulty walking up a flight of stairs). Many patients also report a change in facial features

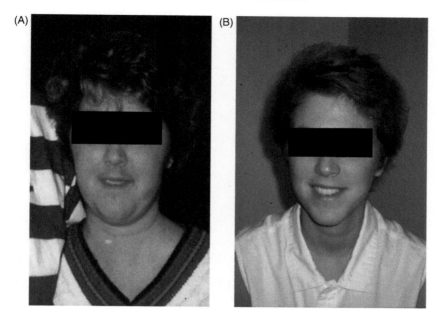

FIGURE 3.1   Cushing's patient shown pretreatment (A) and 6 months after treatment (B).

and body shape, which should be assessed by asking to see previous photos, a driver's license, or an identification card.

Women often report new onset or worsening acne, development of dark facial and body hair, development of lanugo hair over the cheeks and sideburn area, and thinning of scalp hair, typically in the frontal area. Premenopausal women often report changes in their menstrual cycles, most commonly irregular menses and infertility. Many premenopausal women have been diagnosed previously with polycystic ovary syndrome (PCOS) long before the diagnosis of Cushing's syndrome is entertained because symptoms and signs of both of these disorders overlap.

Men often report a decrease in libido and erectile dysfunction. They also often report a loss of muscle strength, a decrease in exercise tolerance, and fatigue. Diminished libido and erectile dysfunction are common presenting features.

2.2 Objective Symptoms

The recent onset of hypertension, glucose intolerance, or diabetes mellitus, which have usually been treated before the patient is evaluated for possible Cushing's syndrome, are typical presenting symptoms. More indicative is worsening control of preexisting hypertension, requiring additional medications, or worsening control of preexisting diabetes mellitus, also requiring additional medications. The important feature is the need for a *change* in medications to control these conditions. Changes in facial features are common, requiring a review by the physician of earlier photos to mark any change, such as facial rounding and facial plethora (Fig. 3.1A–B). Hirsutism and thinning of frontal hair should be assessed, and

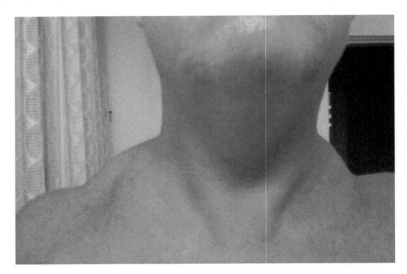

FIGURE 3.2   **A patient with Cushing's syndrome exhibits supraclavicular fat pads, which are characteristic of this disease.** Thus, examination of the neck is an important part of the physical examination.

the patient should be asked about any recent hair removal, especially on the face. Examination of the neck is vital. Also, it should be determined if the clavicles are visible and if there are supraclavicular fat pads (Fig. 3.2). Palpation of the supraclavicular area is a key part of the physical examination. A posterior cervical fat pad is less indicative of Cushing's syndrome because this is often present in obese patients (Fig. 3.3). Muscle strength should be assessed with a very simple test: patients are asked to cross their arms and then rise from a seated position. When patients have to lean forward to accomplish this or push up with their hands, this test suggests proximal muscle weakness. Another test is to ask patients to squat and rise without using their arms to push upward. These are very simple tests and require no "high-tech" studies. Examination of the skin may determine the presence of violaceous striae, which are diagnostic but present in only 50% of patients with Cushing's; thus, the absence of violaceous striae does not exclude Cushing's (Fig. 3.4). Thinning of the skin and bruising (or ecchymoses) suggest a steroid effect, presuming the patient is not taking an anticoagulation medication, aspirin, or vitamin E. Hyperpigmentation of the knuckles or elbows may be present in ACTH-dependent Cushing's. Another dermatologic finding is the superficial fungal infection, tinea corporis, most commonly over the anterior chest. Since high-cortisol levels are immunosuppressive, patients may also have frequent urinary tract infections, sepsis, and in women, recurrent vaginal infections. Hypokalemia occurs in patients with severe Cushing's and raises the concern about ectopic ACTH syndrome as very high cortisol production may cause hypokalemia. Peripheral edema may also occur (Table 3.1).

2.3 Atypical Symptoms

Patients who are dedicated to regular and strenuous exercise may not present with the typical weight gain of Cushing's disease. However, these patients often report a decrease in

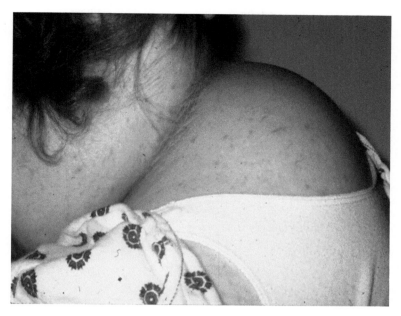

FIGURE 3.3   **A patient with Cushing's syndrome exhibits posterior cervical fat pads and acanthosis nigricans.** These fat pads are less indicative of Cushing's syndrome than supraclavicular fat pads and are also seen in patients with diabetes, obesity, polycystic ovary syndrome, and metabolic syndrome.

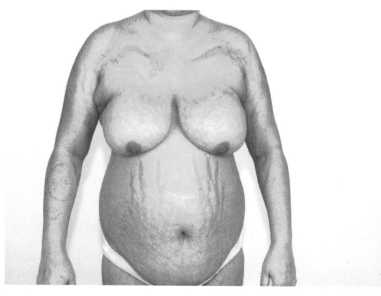

FIGURE 3.4   **A patient is shown with violaceous striae, which appears in approximately 50% of Cushing's patients.**

TABLE 3.1   Clinical Features of Cushing's Disease

- Obesity (central or generalized)
- Facial rounding (moon-face)
- Glucose intolerance and diabetes
- Hypertension
- Psychological changes (e.g., depression; anxiety disorders; psychosis, which is rare; mood disorders, especially bipolar disorder; substance abuse; and cognitive impairment, especially memory problems)
- Weakness, proximal myopathy, and hypokalemia
- Easy bruisability and skin pigmentation
- Oligo-amenorrhea and infertility
- Impotence
- Acne (new onset or worsening)
- Hirsutism but loss of scalp hair
- Striae (50% of patients)
- Peripheral edema
- Osteoporosis and fractures (also spontaneous rupture of the Achilles tendon)
- Polydipsia/polyuria
- Renal calculi
- Recurrent infections
- Supraclavicular fat pads
- Glaucoma and cataracts

exercise endurance, muscle strength, and fatigue. The presentation of symptoms of psychosis, including suicidal ideation, while atypical and uncommon, may occur. Cushing's patients are also prone to opportunistic infections that may be masked by the hypercortisolism and, therefore, may be potentially life-threatening.

3   SIGNS OF CUSHING'S DISEASE

Physicians should be alert to changes in body habitus in their patients, including an increase in abdominal girth, which may also occur in their obese patients; new thickening around the neck, such as supraclavicular fat pads and posterior cervical fat pads; skin changes, including easy bruising, ecchymosis, hyperpigmentation of the knuckles and elbows (ACTH-dependent Cushing's), and acathosis nigricans; and changes in hair in women, including frontal hair loss and new onset hirsutism or lanugo hair of the cheeks and sideburn area. New onset or worsening acne is also common in women and children.

4   COMORBIDITIES ASSOCIATED WITH CUSHING'S SYNDROME

Untreated Cushing's syndrome increases the risk of premature mortality; the 5-year survival was reported as only 50% in 1952 with the most common causes of death being myocardial infarction or stroke. More recent data indicate that the risk of premature mortality is twice that of the normal population with an increased risk of venous thromboembolism, myocardial infarction, peptic ulcer disease, fractures, and infections.

4.1 Diabetes Mellitus

Diabetes mellitus type 2 is most common in patients with Cushing's syndrome, but patients with type 1 diabetes may also develop Cushing's. This is either new onset or worsening control of preexisting diabetes. Approximately 75% of patients with Cushing's have insulin resistance or glucose intolerance; the prevalence of diabetes ranges from 20 to 47% of patients.

4.2 Hypertension

Hypertension is common in the general population and in patients with obesity and diabetes. However, new onset hypertension or worsening control of treated hypertension should raise a question as to why this has occurred. This occurrence in conjunction with other features should prompt additional evaluation.

4.3 Sleep Disturbances

Frequent awakening, difficulty falling asleep (feeling "wired"), and sleep apnea are all common features of Cushing's syndrome. The sleep apnea may be a direct result of weight gain and obesity.

4.4 Osteoporosis and Bone Fractures

Bone loss (decreased bone formation and increased bone resorption) occurs with both exogenous and endogenous exposure to high levels of glucocorticoid. Osteopenia, osteoporosis, and nontraumatic bone fractures occur commonly in patients with Cushing's syndrome. These may be unrecognized unless a bone density study is obtained.

4.5 Depression and Psychosis

Depression is very common; it has been estimated that at some time in life approximately 25–30% of the population has depression; the prevalence is more common in women than in men. Additionally, studies conducted at the National Institutes of Health demonstrated that patients with severe depression do have overactive hypothalamic-pituitary-adrenal function. The challenge is to consider the totality of the patient's symptoms and signs before concluding that a patient has only depression. The precise occurrence of depression in patients with Cushing's is not known, but from clinical experience and reported studies, this occurs in approximately 50% or more of Cushing's syndrome patients. Psychosis is an uncommon feature of Cushing's syndrome, but it does occur. The prevalence of psychosis in Cushing's syndrome is not precisely known.

4.6 Memory and Cognitive Function

Chronically high cortisol levels have been shown to affect brain anatomy with a decrease in brain volume in patients with Cushing's compared with normal subjects and patients with other types of pituitary adenomas. Many patients with Cushing's report difficulty with memory and cognitive function (e.g., no longer able to perform in high level work, such as accounting or banking). The memory dysfunction is not that of patients with Alzheimer's disease, but it has some similarities, including forgetfulness (Chapter 4).

5 CYCLICAL CUSHING'S SYNDROME

Cyclical Cushing's syndrome is a controversial subject. It is known that patients with proven Cushing's syndrome may have variable production of cortisol (normal and abnormal) over time when numerous studies are obtained. In some patients the symptoms can also be sporadic. The length of the varying cycles has been reported to be weeks to months. Additionally, normal subjects have variable amounts of cortisol production. The screening tests for Cushing's disease, such as 24-h urinary free cortisol (UFC), late-night salivary cortisol, and 1-mg overnight dexamethasone suppression test, are equally reliable and approximately 92% accurate. Thus, 8% of these screening tests yield either false-positive or false-negative results (most commonly false-positive results). A particular caveat regarding the 24-h UFC test is excessive fluid ingestion with large urinary volume, which falsely increases the 24-h UFC result.

While endocrine tumors (pituitary, adrenal, ectopic) are autonomous, there are still varying amounts of hormone production with each tumor type. There are well-documented case reports of "cyclic" Cushing's; however, this syndrome is considered very uncommon. In the event that this diagnosis is entertained, "time" is the best course to document cortisol production as it may take several months to establish a firm diagnosis of *consistent* overproduction of cortisol. With the common use of the Internet, including websites and blogs, there is a subset of patients who actually seek the diagnosis of Cushing's to explain symptoms, and when most of the studies are normal, the question of "cyclic" Cushing's is raised. Again, "time" and repeated appropriate tests are needed to establish the consistent overproduction of cortisol.

6 CUSHING'S SYNDROME IN ATHLETES

This is an uninvestigated entity. Anyone can develop Cushing's disease. The most common presentation among athletes is the patient who exercises regularly and vigorously in whom exercise tolerance and muscle strength have decreased. There may also be complaints of fatigue. Again, the important issue is *change* in a patients' ability to continue his or her regular exercise regimen. Vigorous exercise increases cortisol production transiently but not sufficiently to cause symptoms or signs of Cushing's syndrome.

7 PSEUDO-CUSHING'S DISEASE

The description of pseudo-Cushing's is based on the clinical features of Cushing's in patients who do not have consistent biochemical evidence of excessive cortisol production. This can also be attributed to excessive alcohol consumption, resulting in physical findings suggestive of Cushing's syndrome related to decreased hepatic metabolism of cortisol. If alcohol is a factor, the patient should refrain from alcohol for at least a month to be evaluated properly

TABLE 3.2   Clinical Features of Cushing's Syndrome in Children and Adolescents

- Growth retardation (delayed bone age)
- Weight gain and obesity
- Virilism and hirsutism
- Hypertension
- Striae, easy bruising, and hyperpigmentation
- Acne (new onset or worsening)
- Delay of secondary sexual development
- Mental changes (but fewer psychiatric changes than in adults)
- Sleep difficulties
- Muscle weakness

for Cushing's. Alcoholics can and do develop Cushing's, but unless there is abstinence from alcohol, the evaluation is compromised. Laboratory studies in patients with pseudo-Cushing's may be abnormal if they have a problem with alcohol, emphasizing the need to evaluate these patients when they have been free of alcohol, preferably for a month. The diagnosis of pseudo-Cushing's could also be applied to obese women who have PCOS because there is so much overlap in the clinical features of both disorders.

8 CUSHING'S SYNDROME IN CHILDREN AND ADOLESCENTS

The incidence of Cushing's in prepubertal children is equal between girls and boys. The most common presentation in children is a decline in growth velocity with a resultant decline in the percentile of growth for age; thus, it is important to review the child's growth chart. Signs of virilism and hypertension are also common presenting symptoms. This is usually accompanied by an increase in weight and an increase in percentile of weight for age. Delay in pubertal development also occurs in adolescents. Table 3.2 shows the typical signs and symptoms seen in children and adolescents; see also Chapter 11.

9 CONCLUSIONS

Unfortunately, unlike an X-ray that shows a bone fracture, there are no specific clinical features of Cushing's and no one test that is diagnostic in most patients. Thus, it is essential for physicians to pay close attention to the patient's symptoms and signs. The diagnosis of Cushing's syndrome is dependent on the awareness of many nonspecific symptoms and signs that prompt the physician to consider the disease and to obtain the appropriate tests. A firm diagnosis is usually best made by referring the patient to an endocrinologist who has experience with patients with Cushing's. This remains a challenge for nonendocrinologists who care for most of these patients but do not recognize the disease. The delay in diagnosis remains a problem for these patients, but hopefully, this will improve with more awareness by all physicians.

4

The Cognitive, Psychological, and Emotional Presentation of Cushing's Disease

L. Katznelson, MD

Pituitary Center, Stanford School of Medicine, Stanford, CA, United States

OUTLINE

1 INTRODUCTION

Cushing's syndrome refers to the presence of pathologic hypercortisolism, and Cushing's disease refers to the presence of an adrenocorticotropic– (ACTH-) secreting pituitary adenoma, leading to hypercortisolism. Cushing's disease is associated with a number of medical comorbidities (e.g., diabetes mellitus, hypertension, osteoporosis, and obesity) as a result of

Cushing's Disease. http://dx.doi.org/10.1016/B978-0-12-804340-0.00004-8

the hypercortisolism. Patients with Cushing's disease are also confronted with psychological and cognitive limitations. This chapter describes the psychological and cognitive deficits associated with Cushing's disease and reviews the anatomic and metabolic findings that may underlie the clinical presentations. Of note, patients with Cushing's disease may have hypopituitarism, particularly with pituitary macroadenomas. Hypopituitarism may affect psychological and cognitive health as well. This chapter focuses on the impact of hypercortisolism, although hypopituitarism may also have a role in a subset of patients.

2 COGNITIVE AND EMOTIONAL ASPECTS OF CUSHING'S DISEASE

2.1 Clinical Presentations

2.1.1 Effects on Psychological Health

Psychiatric disorders are common with Cushing's disease and may be the presenting symptoms [1]. In particular, mood disorders, especially depression, are common in patients with Cushing's disease. In a study of 209 subjects with Cushing's syndrome, there was a history of significant psychiatric illness, usually depression, which preceded the onset of signs and symptoms of Cushing's syndrome in up to 12% of subjects [1]. In this study, significant psychiatric illness, usually depression, was present or had been a feature of the Cushing's syndrome at diagnosis in 57% of subjects. Overall, depression may be found in over 60% of patients [2]. In a study of 29 subjects with Cushing's syndrome, 24% were found to have mild depression and 62% were found to have moderate-to-severe depression [3]. In these studies, serum cortisol levels correlated with the degree of mood disturbance. Other psychiatric disturbances linked with excess glucocorticoids include anxiety, excitability, hypomania, and psychosis [4]. Of note, these psychological concerns may occur at presentation or may exacerbate in the period following therapy.

2.1.2 Effects on Sleep

Sleep disorders including insomnia, are associated with hypercortisolism. In a study of patients with Cushing's syndrome, 50% of subjects had evidence of mild-to-moderate OSA [5]. In a recent study, Cushing's syndrome subjects had higher fragmented sleep and nocturnal motor activity as compared to controls [6]. No correlation was found between sleep alterations and urinary free cortisol (UFC) in patients. Insomnia is an early symptom of Cushing's disease and may also be seen with pharmacologic use of glucocorticoids. In a study by Born and coworkers, infusion of either cortisol or corticotrophin resulted in reduced rapid eye movement sleep as well as increased time awake [7]. Insomnia in these populations is thought to be caused by high serum cortisol concentrations during sleep due to the absence of normal diurnal variation in cortisol secretion [7]. Sleep disturbances may contribute to the worsening of quality of life as well as the metabolic comorbidities associated with Cushing's syndrome.

2.1.3 Effects on Cognitive Function

Hypercortisolism impacts cognitive function in several ways, including verbal intellectual skills, learning, and memory. These cognitive deficits may correlate with cortisol levels [8].

In this study by Starkman and coworkers, the largest decline in cognitive function occurred in measures of the verbal intelligence quotient, verbal learning, and recall [8]. These impairments are consistent with complaints of cognitive deficits reported by patients with Cushing's disease [9]. Attention span and memory (largely short-term memory) are impaired in patients with hypercortisolism [10]. In contrast to increased vulnerability across visuospatial measures found in dementia and delirium, verbal functions are most prominently affected in Cushing's disease. The deficits in verbal intellectual skills suggest involvement of the neocortex, whereas impairments in verbal learning and recall are consistent with the increasingly accepted view that the hippocampus is especially vulnerable to the effects of glucocorticoids [8,11–13]. Depression may contribute to the loss of attention and memory skills, but a direct impact of glucocorticoid excess is likely a strong contributing factor.

3 EFFECTS OF GLUCOCORTICOID EXCESS ON BRAIN STRUCTURES

3.1 Hippocampal Size and Atrophy

3.1.1 Animal Models

In rodent and primate animal models, hypercortisolism has consistently been shown to reduce hippocampal volume [14]. For example, in a study by Sapolsky and coworkers, using stereotactically implanted glucocorticoid and control pellets in the hippocampi of vervet monkeys, both hippocampal damage and volume loss were detected after 1 year [11]. Of note, exposure to excess glucocorticoids does not kill or reduce the number of pyramidal or glial cells in the hippocampus [15]. Several early studies showed cell-layer irregularities, some shrinkage, and condensation of the pyramidal cells after excess glucocorticoid administration [11,16]. More recent studies, however, have not shown decreases in pyramidal cell diameter, condensation, or cell-layer irregularities [17,18].

3.1.2 Clinical Studies

Brain and hippocampal atrophy have been demonstrated, using imaging studies in patients receiving glucocorticoid therapy for a variety of indications, including asthma, rheumatic diseases, and multiple sclerosis [11–22]. In addition, there are several pathological conditions resulting in elevated cortisol levels, including Cushing's disease, major depression, and post-traumatic stress disorder (PTSD). These disorders also share cognitive impairments, such as memory deficits. Since the hippocampus is critical in memory processing, it is possible that excess glucocorticoids (endogenous or exogenous) are responsible for changes in the hippocampus and, consequently, for the hippocampal-dependent memory impairment. Magnetic resonance imaging studies have documented a decrease in the hippocampal volume of patients with excess glucocorticoids and have shown correlations between this decrease and the presence of cognitive deficits [20,23,24].

3.2 Neurons: Mechanism of Changes in Hippocampal and Cortical Size

The mechanisms underlying the reduction in hippocampal volume are unclear. Exposure to excess glucocorticoids appears to alter the dendritic shape of the hippocampal pyramidal neurons [13,16]. The apical dendrites in the CA3 region of the hippocampus decrease in length and show decreased branching. This decrease in apical dendritic neuropil volume (dendritic atrophy) appears to be responsible for the hippocampal volume loss. Decreases in mitochondrial volume have also been reported and may contribute to hippocampal volume loss [17]. In addition, glucocorticoids may cause a profound loss of synapses in the CA3 region of the hippocampus, independent of the volume loss [18]. This suggests that volume measures may significantly underestimate the effects of glucocorticoids on the brain.

Glucocorticoid receptors are distributed throughout the brain, and the highest density of glucocorticoid receptors in the central nervous system is in the hippocampus [25]. Coburn-Litvak and coworkers have demonstrated that chronic glucocorticoid exposure not only decreases hippocampal volume but also reduces total brain weight [17]. Therefore, glucocorticoids may cause atrophy in the prefrontal cortex and other cortical areas, in addition to that of the hippocampus [19,26].

3.3 Impact of Duration of Excess Glucocorticoid Exposure on Brain Atrophy

Primate studies using exogenous glucocorticoids show that hippocampal changes are present within 1 year of glucocorticoid exposure. There are scant data in humans linking exposure to glucocorticoids and brain atrophy given the often insidious onset of symptoms in Cushing's disease. Cerebral atrophy may be seen within 2–6 months in subjects receiving exogenous glucocorticoid therapy [15,20], suggesting that glucocorticoids may impact cerebral volume in a relatively short time period.

4 EFFECTS OF GLUCOCORTICOID EXCESS ON BRAIN METABOLISM

There are limited data available regarding the impact of hypercortisolism on cerebral metabolism, using functional magnetic resonance imaging (fMRI). In one study with fMRI, adults with Cushing's syndrome demonstrated less activation in the left anterior superior temporal gyrus and higher activation in the frontal, medial, and subcortical regions during the identification of emotional faces. These findings indicated alterations in brain activity in regions used for perception, processing, and regulation of emotion [27]. Furthermore, a study in adolescents with active Cushing's syndrome showed increased activation in the left amygdala and right anterior hippocampus during the performance of an emotional facial memory task [28]. These results point toward alterations in brain activity that impact mood (related to depressive symptoms) and emotional memory.

5 REVERSIBILITY OF COGNITIVE AND PSYCHOLOGICAL EFFECTS WITH TREATMENT OF CUSHING'S DISEASE

5.1 Clinical Presentation

Following biochemical remission of the Cushing's disease, there is improvement in the psychiatric symptoms; however, resolution is variable. In one study of 33 patients with

Cushing's syndrome, important psychopathology (predominantly atypical depression) was present in 55% of subjects with active Cushing's syndrome [29]. Following remission for 1 year, 24% of subjects had persistent psychopathology with a significant improvement in overall mood score; however, important psychopathology, including an increase in the frequency of suicidal ideation and panic was found. The slight increase in the incidence of panic after correction of hypercortisolism might be due to a decreased glucocorticoid restraint at the central arousal/sympathetic catecholaminergic system. In a study of 36 subjects, Hamilton scores for depression improved from 9.2 to 2.4 (controls were 2.0) following biochemical remission for 14 months [2]. This study shows that biochemical control reduced scores well within the depression range into that of controls [2]. In another cross-sectional study involving 15 patients in surgical remission for Cushing's disease, psychological well-being and psychosocial adjustment were significantly impaired in patients with Cushing's disease when compared with all other types of pituitary tumors, where scores were similar [30]. Subjects with Cushing's disease had impaired psychosocial functioning compared with other groups (e.g., nonfunctioning adenomas, macroprolactinomas, and acromegaly). This study did not include data, such as preoperative quality of life data, time since successful surgery, nor prevalence of hypopituitarism in the other tumor groups, all of which would have been useful to explain these findings. This study, however, did indicate that patients with Cushing's disease in biochemical remission had significantly worse scores on measures of psychosocial well-being and psychosocial functioning compared to patients with other types of pituitary tumors. Nevertheless, Cushing's disease appears to be associated with long-term adverse effects on mood and social functioning, even when patients are in biochemical remission. Therefore, despite an overall improvement but with an incomplete reversal in mood disorders, there may be persistent reductions in quality of life. Close monitoring for mood disorders should continue even after successful biochemical remission of Cushing's disease.

Similarly, attainment of biochemical remission is associated with an improvement in cognitive function, though function may not return to baseline. In a study of 24 patients studied before and after biochemical remission, some, but not all, had an improvement in cognitive and memory function [31]. There was an increase in hippocampal formation volume in these patients; however, there were no significant associations between improvement in paragraph or paired-word learning or memory tasks and an increase in hippocampal formation volume [30]. In contrast, the structural volumetric increase in hypothalamic formation volume was associated with functional improvement in learning of unrelated words. Therefore, some measures of cognitive function may show greater responses than others. In another study that compared 74 subjects after successful treatment of Cushing's disease to controls and patients with nonfunctioning pituitary adenomas, cognitive function, specifically memory and executive functions, was impaired despite long-term remission of the hypercortisolism [32]. Of note, age has been identified as a significant factor that influences the speed of recovery [33]. Younger patients regain and sustain their improvement in cognitive functioning more quickly than older subjects. These data suggest that biochemical remission is associated with an improvement in cognitive function but that dysfunction may, in part, be irreversible especially in older patients. Moreover, the improvement in hippocampal size does not necessarily correlate with cognitive improvements.

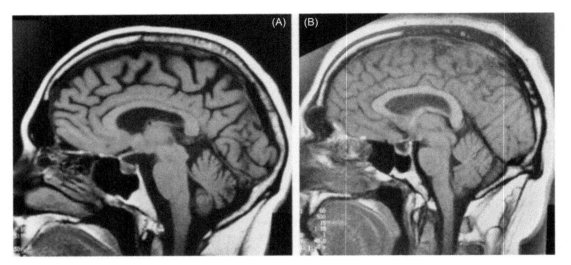

FIGURE 4.1   (A) T1-weighted sagittal MRIs of a 32-year-old patient with Cushing's disease and (B) an age- and sex-matched control. Note the significant cerebral atrophy (A), evidenced by the widened sulci. *MRI*, Magnetic resonance imaging. *Source: Reproduced with permission from Simmons NE, Do HM, Lipper MH, et al. Cerebral atrophy in Cushing's disease. Surg Neurol 2000; 53(1): 72–76.*

5.2 Brain Structures and Function

5.2.1 Brain Atrophy

Cerebral atrophy has been shown to be at least partially reversible in patients with Cushing's disease (Fig. 4.1) [34]. Following normalization of cortisol levels, brain volume increases but does not always return to normal [35]. In a study of 38 subjects with Cushing's syndrome, there was a notable increase in third ventricle and bicaudate diameters (measures of hydrocephalus ex vacuo) compared to controls: this suggests the presence of cerebral atrophy. In 22 subjects followed after biochemical remission, there was an improvement in the imaging parameters, although these did not reach that of control values. These data suggest that the atrophy does not normalize following therapy. In other studies, biochemical remission has been associated with an increase in hippocampal volume by as much as 10% [24]. The increase in hippocampal volume correlates with the magnitude of decrease in UFC excretion. In addition, improvements in memory correlate with decreases in cortisol levels as well as with increases in hippocampal volume [33]. These findings suggest that at least some of the deleterious effects of prolonged hypercortisolism on hippocampal volume are reversible.

5.2.2 Cerebral Metabolism

Studies using fMRI have shown improvement but persistent alterations in metabolism following recovery from Cushing's syndrome. In one study comparing Cushing's disease subjects in long-term remission with controls, there was hypoactivation of the ventromedial prefrontal cortex (vmPFC) during processing of facial expressions (vs. scrambled faces), without alterations in amygdala activation [36]. These findings suggest that patients with long-term remission of Cushing's disease have persistent abnormalities in cerebral metabolism, as well as functional connectivity at rest. This may, in part, explain the persistent psychological morbidity found in patients with Cushing's disease in biochemical remission. These results contrast with earlier findings in patients with active Cushing's disease that showed higher activation levels in frontal, medial, and subcortical regions during the identification of emotional faces [27].

The vmPFC has a role in fear learning and fear extinction and is functionally and structurally connected to the amygdala. Hence, the vmPFC is implicated in the pathogenesis of anxiety and mood disorders, including phobia, panic disorders, and PTSD [37]. The present results, however, are in striking contrast with earlier findings in patients with active Cushing's disease, since patients with active disease demonstrated higher activation levels in frontal, medial, and subcortical regions during the identification of emotional faces [27]. These findings tentatively suggest that correction of hypercortisolism may induce a switch in vmPFC activation levels from hyperactivation to hypoactivation in response to emotional stimuli. This finding may play a role in the persistent psychological deficits following successful treatment of Cushing's disease.

6 CONCLUSIONS

Cushing's disease is associated with a number of psychological and cognitive impairments. These impairments improve with biochemical control of the hypercortisolism but may persist despite endocrine control. These clinical findings are associated with changes in anatomic (including cerebral and hippocampal atrophy) and in site-specific cerebral metabolism that may, in part, explain these clinical findings. Further research is important to define the structural and clinical manifestations associated with glucocorticoid excess as well as the interventions that may improve these findings.

References

[1] Kelly WF. Psychiatric aspects of Cushing's syndrome. QJM 1996;89(7):543–51.
[2] Kelly WF, Kelly MJ, Faragher B. A prospective study of psychiatric and psychological aspects of Cushing's syndrome. Clin Endocrinol 1996;45(6):715–20.
[3] Cohen SI. Cushing's syndrome: a psychiatric study of 29 patients. Brit J Psychiatry 1980;136:120–4.
[4] Haskett RF. Diagnostic categorization of psychiatric disturbance in Cushing's syndrome. Am J Psychiatry 1985;142(8):911–6.
[5] Shipley JE, Schteingart DE, Tandon R, et al. Sleep architecture and sleep apnea in patients with Cushing's disease. Sleep 1992;15(6):514–88.
[6] D'Angelo V, Beccuti G, Berardelli R, et al. Cushing's syndrome is associated with sleep alterations detected by wrist actigraphy. Pituitary 2015;18(6):893–7.
[7] Born J, Spath-Schwalbe E, Schwakenhofer H, et al. Influences of corticotropin-releasing hormone, adrenocorticotropin, and cortisol on sleep in normal man. J Clin Endocrinol Metab 1989;68(5):904–11.
[8] Starkman MN, Giordani B, Berent S, et al. Elevated cortisol levels in Cushing's disease are associated with cognitive decrements. Psychosom Med 2001;63(6):985–93.
[9] Starkman MN, Schteingart DE. Neuropsychiatric manifestations of patients with Cushing's syndrome. Relationship to cortisol and adrenocorticotropic hormone levels. Arch Intern Med 1981;141(2):215–9.
[10] Forget H, Lacroix A, Somma M, et al. Cognitive decline in patients with Cushing's syndrome. J Int Neuropsychol Soc 2000;6(1):20–9.
[11] Sapolsky RM, Uno H, Rebert CS, et al. Hippocampal damage associated with prolonged glucocorticoid exposure in primates. J Neurosci 1990;10(9):2897–902.

[12] Uno H, Tarara R, Else JG, et al. Hippocampal damage associated with prolonged and fatal stress in primates. J Neurosci 1989;9(5):1705–11.

[13] Watanabe Y, Gould E, Cameron HA, et al. Phenytoin prevents stress- and corticosterone-induced atrophy of CA3 pyramidal neurons. Hippocampus 1992;2(4):431–5.

[14] Sousa N, Madeira MD, Paula-Barbosa MM. Effects of corticosterone treatment and rehabilitation on the hippocampal formation of neonatal and adult rats. An unbiased stereological study. Brain Res 1998;794(2):199–210.

[15] Spiegel W, McGeady SJ, Mansmann HC Jr. Cerebral cortical atrophy and central nervous system (CNS) symptoms in a steroid-treated child with asthma. J Allergy Clin Immunol 1992;89(4):918–9.

[16] Woolley CS, Gould E, McEwen BS. Exposure to excess glucocorticoids alters dendritic morphology of adult hippocampal pyramidal neurons. Brain Res 1990;531(1–2):225–31.

[17] Coburn-Litvak PS, Tata DA, Gorby HE, et al. Chronic corticosterone affects brain weight, and mitochondrial, but not glial volume fraction in hippocampal area CA3. Neuroscience 2004;124(2):429–38.

[18] Tata DA, Marciano VA, Anderson BJ. Synapse loss from chronically elevated glucocorticoids: relationship to neuropil volume and cell number in hippocampal area CA3. J Comp Neurol 2006;498(3):363–74.

[19] Bentson J, Reza M, Winter J, et al. Steroids and apparent cerebral atrophy on computed tomography scans. J Comput Assist Tomogr 1978;2(1):16–23.

[20] Brown ES, J Woolston D, Frol A, et al. Hippocampal volume, spectroscopy, cognition, and mood in patients receiving corticosteroid therapy. Biol Psychiatry 2004;55(5):538–45.

[21] Chapman C, Tubridy N, Cook MJ, et al. Short-term effects of methylprednisolone on cerebral volume in multiple sclerosis relapses. J Clin Neurosci (Australasia) 2006;13(6):636–8.

[22] Momose KJ, Kjellberg RN, Kliman B. High incidence of cortical atrophy of the cerebral and cerebellar hemispheres in Cushing's disease. Radiology 1971;99(2):341–8.

[23] Sheline YI. Hippocampal atrophy in major depression: a result of depression-induced neurotoxicity? Mol Psychiatry 1996;1(4):298–9.

[24] Starkman MN, Giordani B, Gebarski SS, et al. Decrease in cortisol reverses human hippocampal atrophy following treatment of Cushing's disease. Biol Psychiatry 1999;46(12):1595–602.

[25] Cereseto M, Reines A, Ferrero A, et al. Chronic treatment with high doses of corticosterone decreases cytoskeletal proteins in the rat hippocampus. Euro J Neurosci 2006;24(12):3354–64.

[26] McEwen BS. Glucocorticoids, depression, and mood disorders: structural remodeling in the brain. Metabolism 2005;54(5 Suppl. 1):20–3.

[27] Langenecker SA, Weisenbach SL, Giordani B, et al. Impact of chronic hypercortisolemia on affective processing. Neuropharmacology 2012;62(1):217–25.

[28] Maheu FS, Mazzone L, Merke DP, et al. Altered amygdala and hippocampus function in adolescents with hypercortisolemia: a functional magnetic resonance imaging study of Cushing syndrome. Dev Psychopathol 2008;20(4):1177–89.

[29] Dorn LD, Burgess ES, Friedman TC, et al. The longitudinal course of psychopathology in Cushing's syndrome after correction of hypercortisolism. J Clin Endocrinol Metab 1997;82(3):912–9.

[30] Heald AH, Ghosh S, Bray S, et al. Long-term negative impact on quality of life in patients with successfully treated Cushing's disease. Clin Endocrinol 2004;61(4):458–65.

[31] Starkman MN, Giordani B, Gebarski SS, et al. Improvement in learning associated with increase in hippocampal formation volume. Biol Psychiatry 2003;53(3):233–8.

[32] Tiemensma J, Kokshoorn NE, Biermasz NR, et al. Subtle cognitive impairments in patients with long-term cure of Cushing's disease. J Clin Endocrinol Metab 2010;95(6):2699–714.

[33] Hook JN, Giordani B, Schteingart DE, et al. Patterns of cognitive change over time and relationship to age following successful treatment of Cushing's disease. J Int Neuropsychol Soc 2007;13(1):21–9.

[34] Heinz ER, Martinez J, Haenggeli A. Reversibility of cerebral atrophy in anorexia nervosa and Cushing's syndrome. J Comput Assist Tomogr 1977;1(4):415–8.

[35] Bourdeau I, Bard C, Noel B, et al. Loss of brain volume in endogenous Cushing's syndrome and its reversibility after correction of hypercortisolism. J Clin Endocrinol Metab 2002;87(5):1949–54.

[36] van der Werff SJ, Pannekoek JN, Andela CD, et al. Resting-state functional connectivity in patients with long-term remission of Cushing's disease. Neuropsychopharmacology 2015;40(8):1888–98.

[37] Kim MJ, Loucks RA, Palmer AL, et al. The structural and functional connectivity of the amygdala: from normal emotion to pathological anxiety. Behav Brain Res 2011;223(2):403–10.

Making the Diagnosis: Laboratory Testing and Imaging Studies

L. Nieman, MD, FACP

Diabetes, Endocrine, and Obesity Branch, The National Institute of Diabetes and Digestive and Kidney Diseases, Bethesda, MD, United States; Endocrinology Consultation Service, National Institutes of Health, Bethesda, MD, United States

OUTLINE

1 MAKING THE DIAGNOSIS OF CUSHING'S SYNDROME

1.1 History and Physical Examination

Cushing's syndrome is a rare disorder characterized by a variety of clinical signs and symptoms that reflect chronic exposure to hypercortisolism, including obesity, hypertension, glucose intolerance, infections, psychiatric disturbance, impaired cognition, and

Cushing's Disease. http://dx.doi.org/10.1016/B978-0-12-804340-0.00005-X
2017 Published by Elsevier Inc.

hypercoagulability (Table 5.1) [1–4]. It is important to screen for this treatable disorder so as to prevent its associated morbidity and mortality.

As implied by its designation as a syndrome, Cushing's syndrome may present in different ways. Table 5.1 lists signs and symptoms of the disorder and, when possible, shows the positive and negative predictive value of the clinical feature. It is readily apparent that no one feature confidently establishes the diagnosis; rather, the number of features and their accumulation and worsening over time best predict the diagnosis. When a patient presents with one or more features of Cushing's syndrome, it is important to ask about all other features, when they occurred, and whether they are worsening.

A number of the characteristic presentations "map" to various medical specialties. Hence, patients may be seen by gynecologists for menstrual abnormalities, infertility, and hirsutism; psychiatrists for depression, anxiety, and suicidality; neurologists for headache, back pain, and proximal muscle weakness; infectious disease physicians for typical community acquired and unusual infections associated with an immunocompromised state; endocrinologists for diabetes; rheumatologists and orthopedists for osteoporosis and fractures; general internists for fatigue and weight gain; urologists for decreased libido (among male patients); cardiologists for myocardial infarction and hypertension; and dermatologists for ruddy skin and striae. Unfortunately, Cushing's syndrome may not be recognized because of the focus on a specialty-specific differential diagnosis that does not consider this disorder.

The clinical features of Cushing's syndrome tend to reflect the severity and duration of hypercortisolism; thus, the pretest probability is high when there are many features or if they have worsened and increased in number over time. Conversely, the clinical presentation may be subtle in a patient with mild or cyclic hypercortisolism. In all patients, but particularly those in whom the disorder is mild, it is important to ask about changes over time related to the patient's own baseline state. For example, a male patient may report a current ability to bench press 150 lbs; this would be an important piece of diagnostic import if he had previously been able to bench press 250 lbs. Similarly, amenorrhea of 6-months duration is more concerning in a 32-year old woman with previously regular menses than in a woman with oligomenorrhea since menarche.

Although not all patients with Cushing's syndrome have all of the associated clinical features, nearly all have gained weight and have difficulty losing weight. Overweight [body mass index (BMI) > 25.0] and obesity (BMI > 30.0) are common in the general population. Recent National Health and Nutrition Examination Survey data [5] indicate that weight gain affects as much as 70% of the adult population. Other features of Cushing's syndrome also are common in the general population, including hypertension (after age 40), glucose intolerance, depression, irregular menses, and hirsutism. By contrast, features most specific to Cushing's syndrome, such as wide purple striae (>1 cm) and proximal muscle weakness, are uncommon both in the general population and in the Cushing's syndrome population, where they are found most often in the context of an unmistakable clinical syndrome with very high urinary free cortisol (UFC) excretion.

Many overweight individuals may have at least one other feature of Cushing's syndrome. This presents physicians with the dilemma of deciding when to screen for the disorder. As the prevalence of Cushing's syndrome in individuals with multiple features of the syndrome is unknown, there are few data to inform this decision. Nugent and colleagues developed an equation to calculate the probability of Cushing's syndrome, using weighted clinical and

TABLE 5.1   Clinical Features of Cushing's Syndrome

Clinical features	Sensitivity specificity (%)	Likelihood ratio		References and notes
		Positive result	Negative result	
Increased fatigue	100			[3]
Decreased libido	33–100			
Weight gain	79–97			
Irritability, emotional lability	40–86			
Insomnia	69			[3]
Decreased concentration	66			[3]
Impaired short-term memory	83			[3]
Changes in appetite	54			[3]
Lethargy, depression	40–67			[3,4]
Menstrual changes	35–86	49	0.68–1.68	1.3–0.29
Osteopenia or recent fracture	48–83	94	8–13.8	0.55–0.18
Headache	47–58	63	1.27–1.57	0.67–0.84
Backache	39–83			
Glucose intolerance				
Recurrent infections	14–25			
Generalized obesity or weight gain	51–90	71	1.75–3.10	0.14–0.69
Truncal obesity	3–97	38	0.05–1.56	0.08–2.6
Plethora	78–94	69	2.51–3.03	0.09–0.32
Round face	88–92			
Hirsutism	64–84	61	2.21–2.90	0.26–0.59
Hypertension	74–90	83	4.35–5.29	0.12–0.31
Ecchymoses	60–68	94	10–11.3	0.34–0.43
Striae wider than 1 cm and purple in color	50–64	78	2.72–2.91	0.46–0.64
Weakness	56–90	93	8–12.6	0.11–0.69	Proximal muscle weakness is most specific
Abnormal fat distribution: centripetal, dorso-cervical, supraclavicular, and temporal	34–67			
Edema	48–66	83	2.82–3.88	0.41–0.63
Thinness and fragility of skin	84			
Abdominal pain	21			
Acne	21–82	76	0.88–3.42	0.24–1.01
Female balding	13–51			

biochemical features, such as obesity, osteoporosis, weakness, plethora, elevated white blood cell count, acne, striae, hypertension, edema, and hirsutism [2]. When applied to 111 patients suspected of having Cushing's syndrome, the diagnosis could be confirmed or excluded with a high degree of confidence in about 50%. The study, reported in 1964, was not followed by any confirmatory studies that included large numbers of patients suspected of having Cushing's syndrome. Also, compared to 1964, some clinical features (e.g., weight gain) are now more common in the general population, and the question of Cushing's syndrome may be raised more often in individuals without the syndrome; thus, the current utility of this strategy is unknown.

1.2 Screening Biochemical Tests for the Diagnosis of Cushing's Syndrome

As clinical features do not reliably identify patients with Cushing's syndrome, screening tests must be used to establish the diagnosis. Guidelines for the diagnosis of Cushing's syndrome recommend that two of three tests be used for this purpose: 24-h UFC, late-night salivary cortisol, the 1-mg dexamethasone suppression test (DST), or the 2-mg, 2-day DST [6]. In some situations, other tests are useful, such as plasma adrenocorticotropic hormone (ACTH) and the dehydroepiandrosterone sulfate (DHEAS) levels.

There are a number of caveats for all tests, which relate to technical assay issues and cyclic hypercortisolism. Each of the tests requires a reliable assay with appropriately developed reference ranges. Additionally, the DST requires use of a cortisol assay with a low functional limit of detection. Patients with cyclic Cushing's syndrome may have normal responses to any of the tests during a nonactive eucortisolemic period and may require persistent testing over a long period of time to establish the diagnosis. The choice of tests should be individualized so as to minimize potential false-negative and false-positive results, as shown in Tables 5.2 and 5.3.

1.2.1 Urinary Free Cortisol

The UFC reflects the integrated production of cortisol over a 24-h period and for many years was the mainstay of diagnosis. When circulating cortisol levels exceed the capacity of corticosteroid-binding globulin (CBG) to bind cortisol (around 27 μg/dL), the excess free cortisol is excreted. Thus, patients with sustained daily elevations in cortisol should have increased UFC.

Historically, assays that measured excess glucocorticoid production evolved from the measurement of urine 17-hydroxysteroids, using the Porter–Silber reaction; to measurement of urinary "cortisol," using immunoassays with antibodies that cross-react with cortisol and to some extent with other precursors and metabolites of cortisol; and finally to current structurally based assays [e.g., liquid chromatography (LC) or LC combined with tandem mass spectrometry (LC-MS/MS)]. As the structurally based assays only measure cortisol, the upper limit of normal (ULN) has decreased. When reviewing the literature, it is important to keep these assay differences in mind, as they are likely to influence diagnostic accuracy.

Concomitantly, an increasing number of patients with proven Cushing's syndrome have normal UFC, using structurally based assays, probably because other glucocorticoids are not measured [7] and because patients with mild hypercortisolism may not consistently increase CBG-binding capacity.

TABLE 5.2 Screening Tests for the Diagnosis of Cushing's Syndrome: Caveats and Cautions

Test	Cautions	When not to use	When best used	Assay issues
UFC	Must obtain complete collection; check with volume and creatinine; inconvenient; must obtain two or more measurements; physiologic (nonpathologic) causes of increased UFC	If GFR < 60 mL/min	Women taking oral contraceptives with elevated CBG	False-positive result when volume is >5 L
Late-night salivary cortisol	Requires consistent sleep–wake pattern; may be abnormal in older patient with comorbidities	Shift workers unless shift is consistent 24/7 and sample is obtained at bedtime; users of licorice, chewing tobacco, cigarettes	Patients <60 years old; when Cushing's syndrome is suspected but UFC by structural assays is normal or only mildly elevated; in women taking oral contraceptives	Immunoassay and MS/MS have very different reference ranges; immunoassay may cross-react with cortisone.
DST	False-positive (abnormal) results may occur with increased CBG after oral estrogen. Metabolized via CYP3A4; medications may alter metabolism.	Use with caution in patients on many medications; consider obtaining a level.	For evaluation of adrenal mass	Cortisol assay should be robust at 1–2 µg/dL range.

CBG, Corticosteroid-binding globulin; CYP3A4, cytochrome P450 3A4; DST, dexamethasone suppression test; GFR, glomerular filtration rate; MS/MS, tandem mass spectrometry; and UFC, urinary free cortisol.

TABLE 5.3 Suggested Tests for Various Patient Characteristics

Patient group	Outcome of test in each patient group[a]			
	1-mg DST	UFC	Dex-CRH	Late-night serum/salivary cortisol
Obesity	FP	FP	LR	LR
Psychiatric	FP	FP	?	FP
Alcohol	FP	FP	?	FP
Acute illness	FP	FP	?	?
Exercise	?	FP	FP	?
Shift work/time zone changes	LR	?	?	FP
Estrogen (increased CBG)	FP	LR	FP	LR
Increased CYP3A4	FP	LR	FP	LR
Periodic/cyclic hypercortisolism	FN	FN	?	?
Abnormal dexamethasone clearance	FN	LR	FN	LR

CBG, Corticosteroid-binding globulin; CRH, corticotropin-releasing hormone; CYP3A4, cytochrome P450 3A4; DEX-CRH, dexamethasone–corticotropin–releasing hormone test; and DST, dexamethasone suppression test; and UFC, urinary free cortisol test.
[a]FN, False-negative results may occur; FP, false-positive results may occur; and LR, low risk of false results.

Urinary cortisol excretion is a good reflection of cortisol production but may be elevated in a variety of conditions, apart from Cushing's syndrome. These include psychiatric disorders, chronic pain, severe exercise, diabetes, and morbid obesity (see later) [4,8–10]. It is thought that central brain mechanisms stimulate corticotropin-releasing hormone (CRH) release in these so-called pseudo-Cushing states and that CRH stimulates activation of the entire hypothalamic-pituitary-adrenal axis [11]. Negative feedback inhibition by cortisol on CRH and pituitary ACTH release restrains the resulting "hypercortisoluria" to less than fourfold normal; thus, if UFC levels above the ULN are considered to indicate Cushing's syndrome, many patients with pseudo-Cushing states would be falsely diagnosed with Cushing's syndrome [10]. Conversely, patients with Cushing's syndrome may have normal UFC levels when measured by immunoassay, either because of intermittent hypercortisolism or because of altered renal metabolism of cortisol [4,12].

The UFC level is increased when the 24-h urine volume is more than 5 L [13] (although 17-hydroxysteroid and creatinine excretion are not affected) and decreases as the glomerular filtration rate falls below 60 mL/min [14].

1.2.2 Late-Night Salivary Cortisol

Salivary cortisol levels are in equilibrium with free cortisol levels in the blood; as such salivary cortisol is not affected by CBG abnormalities and follows the circadian rhythm of circulating cortisol. Like in the blood, the nadir of salivary cortisol is entrained to sleep so that the lowest daily values occur within 1 h of sleep onset [15]. Hence, a late night (i.e., bedtime) salivary cortisol is increased in patients with Cushing's syndrome, who lose the diurnal variation in cortisol [16,17]. Some studies tested the utility of measurement at a specific time (2300 or 2400); because of the physiologic entrainment, falsely abnormal values are probably less likely if the sample is obtained just before going to bed. Advantages to using salivary cortisol include the convenience of obtaining saliva at home and the thermal stability of salivary cortisol so that samples can be mailed to the laboratory [18].

As shift workers who alternate sleep schedules lack a normal cortisol nadir, measurement of late-night salivary cortisol is not a good screening test for these individuals. For shift workers with a consistent daily sleep time who do not sleep at night, measurement of salivary cortisol just before bedtime (regardless of the clock hour) may be a good alternative. However, as this has not been studied formally, one might accept a normal (low) value but have some skepticism regarding a slightly abnormal result.

The salivary glands convert cortisol to cortisone via 11β-hydroxysteroid dehydrogenase type 2 (11β-HSD 2); as a result, patients using or ingesting inhibitors of that enzyme (e.g., chewing tobacco, licorice) may have falsely abnormal results. Individuals who smoke cigarettes also have elevated values [19].

Immunoassays whose antibodies cross-react with noncortisol glucocorticoids may have superior sensitivity compared to the structurally based assays [20]. However, immunoassays may give false-positive results if other steroids are present because of exogenous contamination of the pledget used to collect the sample. This can be evaluated by measurement of cortisol and cortisone, using a structurally based assay; in cases of endogenous hypercortisolism both the cortisol and cortisone values are elevated, while cortisone is normal in cases of contamination [21].

Liu et al. showed an association between comorbidities (e.g., age, hypertension, diabetes mellitus) and elevated late-night salivary cortisol levels in male veterans [22], suggesting that the test should be interpreted with caution, or not used, in these settings. Measurement of midnight plasma cortisol has a high diagnostic accuracy, but it is not practical because of the requirement for clinic or hospital collection [23].

1.2.3 Dexamethasone Suppression Tests

The overnight DST evaluates whether glucocorticoid negative feedback is normal. This test evaluates whether the potent glucocorticoid dexamethasone, at a 1-mg dose, reduces pituitary ACTH secretion, and hence cortisol values, through negative inhibition. Dexamethasone, 1 mg, is taken orally between 2300 and 2400, and plasma cortisol is measured the next morning between 0800 and 0900. Cortisol levels suppress to less than 1.8 µg/dL after this dose in normal individuals and those with pseudo-Cushing states. Pituitary tumors that produce ACTH, which cause Cushing's disease, also decrease ACTH in response to negative feedback but have a higher set point and require a higher dose of dexamethasone to respond. Other causes of Cushing's syndrome, such as cortisol-producing tumors or ectopic ACTH-producing tumors, do not respond to glucocorticoid administration. Thus, in theory, all individuals without Cushing's syndrome should suppress cortisol, and all patients with Cushing's syndrome should fail to respond to dexamethasone at this dose.

In practice, up to 30% of normal individuals and those hospitalized with nonendocrine disorders do not suppress cortisol normally after 1 mg of dexamethasone [24]. These unexpected responses may reflect fast metabolic clearance of dexamethasone in "normal" individuals, who thus experience a less biologically active dose of dexamethasone. Conversely, the cortisol suppression seen in some patients with Cushing's disease may reflect slower metabolic clearance of dexamethasone, resulting in a more biologically active dose. Inter-individual dexamethasone clearance is variable [25]. Additionally, renal and liver diseases slow dexamethasone metabolism, and certain medications (e.g., phenytoin, dilantin, barbiturates) enhance its clearance through stimulation of the hepatic P450 enzymes. Patients taking multiple medications are less likely to have a normal response than those not taking medications [26].

The 2-day 2-mg DST (also known as the low-dose DST) is a variation of the more commonly used overnight test. It involves administration of dexamethasone, 500 µg, every 6 h for eight doses, and measurement of plasma cortisol 2 h after the last dose. Two studies showed a sensitivity of 90–100% and a specificity of 97–100% for discriminating Cushing's syndrome, using criteria of 1.4 or 2.2 µg/dL [10].

1.2.4 Other Useful Tests

The 2-day 2-mg DST followed by CRH stimulation may help to discriminate patients with a pseudo-Cushing state. The CRH (1 µg/kg body weight, intravenously) stimulation is given 6 h after the last dose of dexamethasone, and cortisol is measured 15 min later. This increased the sensitivity and specificity of the low-dose DST to 100% in a small study of 58 patients [10]. While this test has a very high diagnostic accuracy, it is costly and cumbersome and may not work properly if the patient does not take dexamethasone at the prescribed times.

Measurement of cortisol in scalp hair may be useful but requires careful designation of a reference range, as it appears elevated in other conditions, such as cardiovascular disease. Hair cortisol levels are increased by age and the presence of diabetes mellitus and are decreased as hair-washing frequency increases [27]. The test is not commercially available.

When evaluation is initiated because of the incidental recognition of an adrenal mass, measurement of ACTH and DHEAS may be helpful, if they are suppressed because of consistent hypercortisolism [28]. This strategy is more likely to be useful in younger patients because DHEAS decreases with age.

1.3 Other Conditions with Physiologic Increases in Cortisol

When a patient has an abnormal response to a screening test, a variety of additional approaches may exclude a pseudo-Cushing state. Continued observation over time may reveal progression of clinical features and biochemical abnormalities, suggesting Cushing's syndrome. Conversely, biochemical tests may normalize after treatment of pseudo-Cushing states, such as depression or pain.

1.3.1 Depression, Stress, and Other Psychiatric Conditions

Some, but not all, patients with major depression show increased basal cortisol values in urine, blood, and hair (the latter of which measures integrated values over many days) [29]. This appears to result from the increased amplitude of ACTH bursts [30]; ACTH half-life is shortened, however, so that the mean 24-h ACTH concentration is normal. The association between cardiovascular disease and depression may be mediated in part by this increase in cortisol, with consequent increased intraabdominal adiposity [31].

There are no reports of the responses of depressed individuals to other screening tests for Cushing's syndrome. Other psychiatric disorders (e.g., eating disorders, withdrawal from substance abuse, bipolar disease, undifferentiated somatoform disorder, adjustment disorder with mixed emotional features, and avoidant personality disorder) have been associated with hypercortisolism [10]. It is well established that stressful situations (e.g., the Trier test) are associated with increased salivary cortisol values, but in general UFC and DST have not been measured in these studies.

1.3.2 Polycystic Ovary Syndrome

Like obesity, hirsutism raises the question of possible Cushing's syndrome. Moran and colleagues found that 1 of 250 women with hirsutism had Cushing's syndrome, suggesting that this may be a useful marker [32]. However, Pecori-Geraldi and colleagues reported that the prevalence of polycystic ovary syndrome (PCOS) was lower (<10%) in women with Cushing's syndrome than in those in whom Cushing's syndrome was excluded (~42%) [33]. Putignano and colleagues evaluated the diagnostic performance of screening tests in women in whom Cushing's syndrome was excluded and did or did not have PCOS and compared it with the results in premenopausal women found to have Cushing's syndrome. They found that UFC levels were higher in women with PCOS, but only when compared to women without PCOS, and that the performance of the midnight salivary cortisol and 1-mg overnight DSTs were not affected by the presence of PCOS [34].

1.3.3 Diabetes Mellitus

As noted earlier, about 25% of diabetic men were reported to have elevated late-night salivary cortisol values [22]. In another study, 86% of 382 adults with type 2 diabetes had an abnormal late-night salivary result; only 20% had an abnormal response to dexamethasone [35]. The UFC level may also be increased [36]. While Cushing's syndrome has been reported in up to 3% of patients in a diabetes clinic [37], none of the previous studies found any cases of Cushing's syndrome. Another large screening study found that 37 out of 993 (3.7%) patients had an abnormal response ($\geq 1.8 \ \mu g/dL$) to the 1-mg overnight DST, but none was found to have Cushing's syndrome on further testing [38]. Thus, widespread screening for Cushing's syndrome is not warranted in diabetic patients without other features of the syndrome. If screening is needed, the late-night salivary cortisol test should be avoided, particularly in older patients.

2 THE DIFFERENTIAL DIAGNOSIS OF CUSHING'S SYNDROME

2.1 ACTH-Dependent and ACTH-Independent Causes of Cushing's Syndrome

The causes of endogenous Cushing's syndrome can be broadly characterized as ACTH-dependent or independent. The ACTH-dependent causes are most common (~80%) and represent tumors that secrete ACTH (or rarely CRH); they arise from pituitary corticotrope cells, termed Cushing's disease, or from other sites, termed ectopic ACTH syndrome or secretion. The excess ACTH stimulates cortisol production and is not normalized by endogenous negative feedback.

Adrenocorticotropic hormone–independent causes represent primary adrenal overproduction of cortisol. In this setting negative feedback suppresses ACTH secretion by the normal corticotropes, and plasma ACTH levels are low normal or suppressed.

2.1.1 ACTH-Dependent Forms

2.1.1.1 PITUITARY TUMOR PRODUCTION OF ACTH: CUSHING'S DISEASE

Nearly all (90%) of these benign tumors are microadenomas (<1-cm diameter), with an average diameter of 6 mm in surgical series. They are more frequent in adult women than men (3–5:1) and are diagnosed on average in the fourth decade of life. In children, the average age of diagnosis is around 13 years, and each gender is equally represented in prepubertal patients [39].

2.1.1.2 ECTOPIC TUMOR PRODUCTION OF ACTH

In 10–15% of patients, Cushing's syndrome results from ectopic production of ACTH and very rarely from ectopic CRH production. Small cell carcinoma of the lung, medullary thyroid cancer, pheochromocytoma, and foregut (pulmonary, pancreas) carcinoid tumors are the most common sources of ectopic ACTH production. The potential for malignancy varies, according to tumor type, but it should be kept in mind when searching for the source. The male:female ratio is different from Cushing's disease, from 1–2:1 [40], and the age of onset is about a decade later. However, while it has been said that a man with Cushing's syndrome should be considered to have ectopic ACTH secretion, this is not true because Cushing's disease is much more common. Hypokalemia is associated with ectopic ACTH secretion. It occurs because of inadequate renal conversion of cortisol to cortisone by 11β-HSD in patients with extremely high cortisol levels [41]. However, patients with Cushing's disease also may develop hypokalemia if the UFC levels are very high. Some ectopic ACTH-producing tumors are indolent and may be occult for some time, so that the clinical presentation is similar to that of patients with Cushing's disease. Others present with a more rapid course and severe features of hypercortisolism. Such a presentation is very suggestive of an ectopic ACTH-producing tumor.

2.1.2 ACTH-Independent Forms

2.1.2.1 ADRENAL ADENOMA

Adrenal adenomas are the most common cause of ACTH-independent Cushing's syndrome, comprising 10–20% of all patients with Cushing's syndrome [42]. These tumors frequently contain mutations of the beta-catenin signaling or cyclic adenosine monophosphate (cAMP)–dependent pathways. Once removed, they do not recur, unless the histologic diagnosis of a benign lesion was incorrect.

2.1.2.2 ADRENAL CARCINOMA

Adrenal carcinoma accounts for up to 7% of Cushing's syndrome patients, most commonly occurring in infancy and older individuals (5th–6th decade). These patients may present with hypercortisolism alone or in combination with hyperandrogenism. In general, steroidogenesis is inefficient, and the degree of hypercortisolism may be modest in relationship to the tumor burden.

2.1.2.3 BILATERAL MACRONODULAR ADRENAL DISEASE

Bilateral macronodular adrenal hyperplasia (BMAH) is rare and may be sporadic or familial. Inactivating mutations of armadillo repeat-containing 5 gene (*ARMC5*) have been identified in large families with BMAH and in about half of patients without a clear family history [43]. Although an assay for this gene is not yet commercially available, in the future, genetic screening may help to identify family members at risk for development of BMAH.

Bilateral macronodular adrenal hyperplasia is often associated with the aberrant expression of one or several nonmutated G-protein–coupled receptors, both with eutopic expression (AVPR1, LH/HCGR, and HT4R) or ectopic/illicit expression (glucose-dependent insulinotropic peptide (GIPR), β-adrenergic ligands, vasopressin (AVPR2/3), and serotonin (HT7R) [42].

2.1.2.4 MICRONODULAR ADRENAL DISEASE

Bilateral micronodular adrenal disease is a rare cause of Cushing's syndrome that presents in childhood and young adulthood. It may be associated with the Carney complex, which includes cardiac and skin myxomas, lentigenes, blue nevi, and growth hormone (GH) excess. These conditions are most often associated with mutations in the type 1α regulatory subunit of cAMP-dependent protein kinase A (PRKAR1) [42].

3 PREREQUISITES FOR DIFFERENTIAL DIAGNOSTIC TESTING

3.1 Consistent Hypercortisolism

The differential diagnostic testing in Cushing's syndrome requires exposure to persistent negative feedback that is sufficient to suppress normal corticotrope function. If this occurs, the test responses reflect only the underlying tumors. Corticotrope tumors have biochemical responses to diagnostic tests that are similar to those of healthy people, albeit sometimes exaggerated (e.g., after CRH) or attenuated (e.g., after 1-mg dexamethasone), while other causes of Cushing's syndrome tend not to respond. As a result, it is important to document persistent hypercortisolism before testing [44]. The duration and amount of hypercortisolism needed to suppress normal corticotropes are not known, however.

3.2 Testing Strategies for the Differential Diagnosis

3.2.1 ACTH Level

Due to the differences in pathophysiology, measurement of plasma ACTH is the first step in the differential diagnostic testing. Values below 10 pg/mL are almost always associated with ACTH-independent hypercortisolism, while values more than 20 pg/mL are usually associated with ACTH-dependent hypercortisolism. Values between 10 and 20 pg/mL are indeterminate; in this setting, measurement of DHEAS, if suppressed, points to a primary adrenal etiology, while a response to CRH tends to point to a pituitary etiology.

If the ACTH level indicates an adrenal etiology, imaging of the adrenal glands, generally with computed tomography (CT) with and without contrast, is the next step, to identify whether there is a unilateral adenoma or carcinoma, bilateral hyperplasia, or nodularity. No further biochemical testing is necessary except for patients in whom the ACTH value is intermediate, patients suspected of having adrenal cancer in whom other hormonal markers are sought, or for patients with suspected Carney complex, in whom cardiac myxomas and GH excess should be excluded.

3.2.2 CRH Stimulation Test

The CRH stimulation test was introduced in 1982 [45] to discriminate between the ACTH-dependent causes of Cushing's syndrome. Healthy individuals show an increase in ACTH and cortisol levels after intravenous administration of ovine or human CRH, 1 mg/kg or 100 mg. Patients with corticotrope tumors retain CRH receptors and can secrete ACTH in response, while patients with ectopic ACTH-secreting tumors do not have the machinery to respond. The criteria and timepoints for hormone measurement vary across studies of a given form of CRH. Human CRH is less potent than ovine CRH [46]; the latter analog is available in the United States, and the human analog is more readily available in Europe.

The two largest studies reported a sensitivity of 93% [47] and 70% [48] for the ACTH response to CRH, and both reported a specificity of 100%. For the cortisol response, sensitivity was 91 and 85%, and specificity was 88 and 100% to detect Cushing's disease.

3.2.3 High-Dose (8-mg) DST

The high-dose DST interrogates whether potent glucocorticoid negative feedback can reduce ACTH and hence cortisol levels. Corticotrope tumors retain this response but require larger amounts of glucocorticoid to suppress than do healthy individuals. This is reflected in the different doses of dexamethasone used in the overnight screening test (1 mg) versus the high-dose test (8 mg). In general, patients with ectopic ACTH secretion do not suppress, although suppression has been reported in patients with pulmonary carcinoid tumors [4,24]. Patients with primary adrenal causes of Cushing's syndrome do not respond to dexamethasone. The test is hampered by false-positive and false-negative results. This may be caused by endogenous variability in cortisol levels, a true ability of some ectopic ACTH-secreting tumors to respond to negative feedback, and variability in dexamethasone metabolism (e.g., a patient with a corticotrope adenoma and fast clearance of dexamethasone may not respond).

Using a criterion of 50% suppression of UFC or serum cortisol, Aron and colleagues reported 81% sensitivity and 67% specificity for the 8-mg DST for the diagnosis of pituitary-dependent Cushing's syndrome [49]. Their analysis also revealed a complete overlap in responses between patients with ectopic ACTH secretion and Cushing's disease. As a result, they do not recommend routine use of the test if inferior petrosal sinus sampling (IPSS) is available (see later).

3.2.4 Inferior Petrosal Sinus Sampling

To distinguish a pituitary from an ectopic source of ACTH, IPSS demonstrates higher ACTH concentrations in the petrosal sinus blood (representing venous drainage of a corticotropinoma) as compared to a peripheral vein [50]. Catheters are guided from the groin into the inferior petrosal sinus, and their position is confirmed with retrograde venography. Blood is obtained simultaneously from the IPSS and periphery before (two timepoints) and after (usually at 3, 5, and 10 min) administration of CRH (1 mg/kg or 100 mg). A central (i.e., petrosal) to peripheral ratio in ACTH of more than 2 before CRH or more than 3 after CRH is consistent with Cushing's disease; patients with ectopic ACTH secretion have lower values.

In general, IPSS is the "gold standard" for discrimination of the causes of ACTH-dependent Cushing's syndrome, with a sensitivity and specificity of 95–99% [39,51]. However, false-positive results may occur in patients with ectopic ACTH secretion whose normal pituitary corticotropes are not fully suppressed because of cyclic hypercortisolism or medical treatment to decrease cortisol levels [44]. False-negative results may occur in patients with Cushing's disease who have abnormal venous anatomy or when the radiologist is not able technically to catheterize the petrosal sinuses [51]. The latter point highlights the importance of choosing a center with extensive experience in performing the procedure, as the success of catheterization varies from about 65–99% [39].

Patients with Cushing's disease who have unsuccessful catheterizations almost always have low-peak ACTH levels in the petrosal sinus blood (<200 pg/mL before or <400 pg/mL after CRH administration) [52]. Prolactin can be used as an index of pituitary excretion, to normalize the petrosal sinus ACTH values in relation to the peripheral values; this approach is not necessary if the results show a clear central-to-peripheral step-up but can improve the diagnostic efficacy if there is a negative result [53,54].

If IPSS is not available, an alternative approach is to evaluate the response to the 8-mg DST and (separately) the CRH stimulation test. Patients who respond to both tests have a 98% probability of having Cushing's disease. Unfortunately, discordant or negative responses are not diagnostically useful [55].

3.3 Imaging

3.3.1 Pituitary Magnetic Resonance Imaging

Only about 50% of corticotrope tumors are detected on routine T1 spin-echo (T1SE) magnetic resonance imaging (MRI) protocols of the pituitary gland [56]. The T1SE imaging works best if the field of view is restricted (i.e., to the pituitary and not including the entire brain), and TR/TE is modulated [57]. Use of high-resolution, spoiled-gradient recalled (SPGR) acquisition MRI sequences improve detection of these tumors by up to 30%, with a slight increase in false-positive results [58].

3.3.2 Localization Studies for Ectopic ACTH-Producing Tumors

Anatomic (structural) imaging with CT and adjunctive use of MRI are the mainstays of efforts to localize an ectopic ACTH-secreting tumor. As most of these tumors are located in the thoracic cavity (pulmonary and thymic carcinoids) [40,59], initial imaging of the chest may have the greatest yield. However, as tumors may be located from the pharynx/neck to the pelvis, additional studies are often needed.

Functional imaging with somatostatin analogs can help verify that a finding on CT scan is consistent with a tumor. Many ACTH-secreting tumors express somatostatin receptors, and somatostatin-receptor scintigraphy, using [^{111}In-DTPA-D-Phe]-pentetreotide (octreoscan) at a 6 mCi dose, has been reported to have an approximate 50–90% sensitivity [60–62]. Other somatostatin analogs labeled with ^{68}Ga are available in Europe and may offer improved sensitivity. For example, ^{68}Ga-DOTATATE, a positron emission tomography (PET) radiopharmaceutical, has high affinity for SSTR2 and delivers a lower total body radiation dose than octreotide (0.48 vs. 1 rem). Kayani and colleagues demonstrated positive uptake in all 11 typical and 2 of 5 atypical tumors [63]. A second group also reported very high sensitivity (19/20 patients) [64]. Neither of these studies, however, included patients with ACTH-secreting tumors, and nearly all tumors were more than 1 cm in diameter and easily detected by conventional imaging. Many ACTH-secreting pulmonary neuroendocrine tumors have a diameter less than 1 cm. Additional research is needed to assess the diagnostic utility of the ^{68}Ga-labeled somatostatin analogs.

The ^{18}F-fluorodeoxyglucose (FDG) PET has been used for years for tumor localization, reflecting the increased glycolytic metabolic rate of lung, bone, and colorectal cancers compared to normal tissue [65]. We have found a sensitivity of approximately 50% for ^{18}F-FDG-PET [62,66]. However, ^{18}F-FDG-PET did not detect (or suggest) any tumors that were not identified by CT or MRI.

Neuroendocrine tumors, such as foregut carcinoids, have been classified as apudomas based on the demonstration of amine precursor uptake and decarboxylation. These tumors may take up and decarboxylate L-3,4-dihydroxyphenylalanine (L-DOPA). In a series of small studies, ^{18}F-DOPA PET or ^{11}C-DOPA PET had a 50–85% sensitivity to detect pancreatic neuroendocrine tumors, gastrointestinal carcinoids, other carcinoids, melanoma, small cell lung cancer, pheochromocytoma, glomus tumor, and medullary thyroid cancer [67].

References

[1] Plotz CM, Knowlton AI, Regan C. The natural history of Cushing's syndrome. Am J Med 1952;13:597–614.

[2] Nugent CA, Warner HR, Dunn JT, et al. Probability theory in the diagnosis of Cushing's syndrome. J Clin Endocrinol 1964;24:621–7.

[3] Starkman MN, Schteingart DE. Neuropsychiatric manifestations of patients with Cushing's syndrome. Relationship to cortisol and adrenocorticotropic hormone levels. Arch Intern Med 1981;141:215–9.

[4] Newell-Price J, Trainer P, Besser M, et al. The diagnosis and differential diagnosis of Cushing's syndrome and pseudo-Cushing's states. Endocr Rev 1998;19:647–72.

[5] National Center for Health Statistics. Health, United States, 2015: With Special Feature on Racial and Ethnic Health Disparities. Hyattsville, MD, 2016.

[6] Nieman LK, Biller BM, Findling JW, et al. The diagnosis of Cushing's syndrome: an Endocrine Society Clinical Practice Guideline. J Clin Endocrinol Metab 2008;93:1526–40.

[7] Wood L, Ducroq DH, Fraser HL, et al. Measurement of urinary free cortisol by tandem mass spectrometry and comparison with results obtained by gas chromatography-mass spectrometry and two commercial immunoassays. Ann Clin Biochem 2008;45:380–8.

[8] Rees LH, Besser GM, Jeffcoate WJ, et al. Alcohol-induced pseudo-Cushing's syndrome. Lancet 1977;1:726–8.

[9] Tsigos C, Young RJ, White A. Diabetic neuropathy is associated with increased activity of the hypothalamic-pituitary-adrenal axis. J Clin Endocrinol Metab 1993;76:554–8.

[10] Yanovski JA, Cutler GB Jr, Chrousos GP, et al. Corticotropin-releasing hormone stimulation following low-dose dexamethasone administration. A new test to distinguish Cushing's syndrome from pseudo-Cushing's states. JAMA 1993;269:2232–8.

[11] Gold PW, Loriaux DL, Roy A, et al. Responses to corticotropin-releasing hormone in the hypercortisolism of depression and Cushing's disease. Pathophysiologic and diagnostic implications. N Engl J Med 1986;314:1329–35.

[12] Voccia E, Saenger P, Peterson RE, et al. 6-beta-Hydroxycortisol excretion in hypercortisolemic states. J Clin Endocrinol Metab 1979;48:467–71.

[13] Mericq MV, Cutler GB Jr. High fluid intake increases urine free cortisol excretion in normal subjects. J Clin Endocrinol Metab 1998;83:682–4.

[14] Chan KC, Lit LC, Law EL, et al. Diminished urinary free cortisol excretion in patients with moderate and severe renal impairment. Clin Chem 2004;50:757–9.

[15] Krieger DT, Allen W, Rizzo F, et al. Characterization of the normal temporal pattern of plasma corticosteroid levels. J Clin Endocrinol Metab 1971;32:266–84.

[16] Raff H, Raff JL, Findling JW. Late-night salivary cortisol as a screening test for Cushing's syndrome. J Clin Endocrinol Metab 1998;83:2681–6.

[17] Raff H. Update on late-night salivary cortisol for the diagnosis of Cushing's syndrome: methodological considerations. Endocrine 2013;44:346–9.

[18] Graham UM, Hunter SJ, McDonnell M, et al. A comparison of the use of urinary cortisol to creatinine ratios and nocturnal salivary cortisol in the evaluation of cyclicity in patients with Cushing's syndrome. J Clin Endocrinol Metab 2013;98:E72–6.

[19] Steptoe A, Ussher M. Smoking, cortisol and nicotine. Int J Psychophysiol 2006;59:228–35.

[20] Erickson D, Singh RJ, Sathananthan A, et al. Late-night salivary cortisol for diagnosis of Cushing's syndrome by liquid chromatography/tandem mass spectrometry assay. Clin Endocrinol (Oxf) 2012;76:467–72.

[21] Raff H, Singh RJ. Measurement of late-night salivary cortisol and cortisone by LC-MS/MS to assess preanalytical sample contamination with topical hydrocortisone. Clin Chem 2012;58:947–8.

[22] Liu H, Bravata DM, Cabaccan J, et al. Elevated late-night salivary cortisol levels in elderly male type 2 diabetic veterans. Clin Endocrinol (Oxf) 2005;63:642–9.

[23] Papanicolaou DA, Yanovski JA, Cutler GB Jr, et al. A single midnight serum cortisol measurement accurately distinguishes Cushing syndrome from pseudo-Cushing states. J Clin Endocrinol Metab 1998;83:1163–7.

[24] Crapo L. The Cushing syndrome: a review of diagnostic tests. Metabolism 1979;28:955–77.

[25] Meikle AW. Dexamethasone suppression tests: usefulness of simultaneous measurement of plasma cortisol and dexamethasone. Clin Endocrinol (Oxf) 1982;16:401–8.

[26] Valassi E, Swearingen B, Lee H, et al. Concomitant medication use can confound interpretation of the combined dexamethasone-corticotropin releasing hormone test in Cushing's syndrome. J Clin Endocrinol Metab 2009;94:4851–9.

[27] Staufenbiel SM, Penninx BW, de Rijke YB, et al. Determinants of hair cortisol and hair cortisone concentrations in adults. Psychoneuroendocrinology 2015;60:182–94.

[28] Terzolo M, Stigliano A, Chiodini I, et al. Italian Association of Clinical Endocrinologists. AME position statement on adrenal incidentaloma. Eur J Endocrinol 2011;164:851–70.

[29] Dettenborn L, Muhtz C, Skoluda N, et al. Introducing a novel method to assess cumulative steroid concentrations: increased hair cortisol concentrations over 6 months in medicated patients with depression. Stress 2012;15:348–53.

[30] Carroll BJ, Cassidy F, Naftolowitz D, et al. Pathophysiology of hypercortisolism in depression. Acta Psychiatr Scand Suppl 2007;433:90–103.

[31] Weber-Hamann B, Hentschel F, Kniest A, et al. Hypercortisolemic depression is associated with increased intra-abdominal fat. Psychosom Med 2002;64:274–7.

[32] Moran C, Tapia MC, Hernandez E, et al. Etiological review of hirsutism in 250 patients. Arch Med Res 1994;25:311–4.

[33] Pecori Giraldi F, Pivonello R, Ambrogio AG, et al. The dexamethasone-suppressed corticotropin-releasing hormone test and the desmopressin test to distinguish Cushing's syndrome from pseudo-Cushing's states. Clin Endocrinol (Oxf) 2007;66:251–7.

[34] Putignano P, Bertolini M, Losa M, et al. Screening for Cushing's syndrome in obese women with and without polycystic ovary syndrome. J Endocrinol Invest 2003;26:539–44.

[35] Steffensen CH, Thomsen H, Dekkers OM, et al. Low positive predictive value of midnight salivary cortisol measurement to detect hypercortisolism in type 2 diabetes. Clin Endocrinol (Oxf) 2016;85(2):202–6.

[36] Roy MS, Roy A, Brown S. Increased urinary-free cortisol outputs in diabetic patients. J Diabetes Complications 1998;12:24–7.

[37] Catargi B, Rigalleau V, Poussin A, et al. Occult Cushing's syndrome in type-2 diabetes. J Clin Endocrinol Metab 2003;88:5808–13.

[38] Budyal S, Jadhav SS, Kasaliwal R, et al. Is it worthwhile to screen patients with type 2 diabetes mellitus for subclinical Cushing's syndrome? Endocr Connect 2015;4:242–8.

[39] Lonser RR, Nieman L, Oldfield EH. Cushing's disease: pathobiology, diagnosis, and management. J Neurosurg 2016;1–14. [Epub ahead of print].

[40] Alexandraki KI, Grossman AB. The ectopic ACTH syndrome. Rev Endocr Metab Disord 2010;11:117–26.

[41] Stewart PM, Walker BR, Holder G, et al. 11-Beta-hydroxysteroid dehydrogenase activity in Cushing's syndrome: explaining the mineralocorticoid excess state of the ectopic adrenocorticotropin syndrome. J Clin Endocrinol Metab 1995;80:3617–20.

[42] Lacroix A. Heredity and cortisol regulation in bilateral macronodular adrenal hyperplasia. N Engl J Med 2013;369:2147–9.

[43] Assie G, Libe R, Espiard S, et al. ARMC5 mutations macronodular adrenal hyperplasia with Cushing's syndrome. N Engl J Med 2013;369:2105–14.

[44] Yanovski JA, Cutler GB Jr. Perils in the use of inferior petrosal sinus sampling for the diagnosis of Cushing's syndrome. Endocrinologist 1994;4:245–51.

[45] Orth DN, DeBold CR, DeCherney GS, et al. Pituitary microadenomas causing Cushing's disease respond to corticotropin-releasing factor. J Clin Endocrinol Metab 1982;55:1017–9.

[46] Nieman LK, Cutler GB Jr, Oldfield EH, et al. The ovine corticotropin-releasing hormone (CRH) stimulation test is superior to the human CRH stimulation test for the diagnosis of Cushing's disease. J Clin Endocrinol Metab 1989;69:165–9.

[47] Nieman LK, Oldfield EH, Wesley R, et al. A simplified morning ovine corticotropin-releasing hormone stimulation test for the differential diagnosis of adrenocorticotropin-dependent Cushing's syndrome. J Clin Endocrinol Metab 1993;77:1308–12.

[48] Newell-Price J, Morris DG, Drake WM, et al. Optimal response criteria for the human CRH test in the differential diagnosis of ACTH-dependent Cushing's syndrome. J Clin Endocrinol Metab 2002;87:1640–5.

[49] Aron DC, Raff H, Findling JW. Effectiveness versus efficacy: the limited value in clinical practice of high dose dexamethasone suppression testing in the differential diagnosis of adrenocorticotropin-dependent Cushing's syndrome. J Clin Endocrinol Metab 1997;82:1780–5.

[50] Oldfield EH, Doppman JL, Nieman LK, et al. Petrosal sinus sampling with and without corticotropin-releasing hormone for the differential diagnosis of Cushing's syndrome. N Engl J Med 1991;325:897–905.

[51] Doppman JL, Chang R, Oldfield EH, et al. The hypoplastic inferior petrosal sinus: a potential source of false-negative results in petrosal sampling for Cushing's disease. J Clin Endocrinol Metab 1999;84:533–40.

[52] Wind JJ, Lonser RR, Nieman LK, et al. The lateralization accuracy of inferior petrosal sinus sampling in 501 patients with Cushing's disease. J Clin Endocrinol Metab 2013;98:2285–93.

[53] Findling JW, Kehoe ME, Raff H. Identification of patients with Cushing's disease with negative pituitary adrenocorticotropin gradients during inferior petrosal sinus sampling: prolactin as an index of pituitary venous effluent. J Clin Endocrinol Metab 2004;89:6005–9.

[54] Sharma ST, Raff H, Nieman LK. Prolactin as a marker of successful catheterization during IPSS in patients with ACTH-dependent Cushing's syndrome. J Clin Endocrinol Metab 2011;96:3687–94.

[55] Nieman LK, Chrousos GP, Oldfield EH, et al. The ovine corticotropin-releasing hormone stimulation test and the dexamethasone suppression test in the differential diagnosis of Cushing's syndrome. Ann Intern Med 1986;105:862–7.

[56] Ciric I, Zhao JC, Du H, et al. Transsphenoidal surgery for Cushing disease: experience with 136 patients. Neurosurgery 2012;70:70–81.

[57] Chowdhury IN, Sinaii N, Oldfield EH, et al. A change in pituitary magnetic resonance imaging protocol detects ACTH-secreting tumours in patients with previously negative results. Clin Endocrinol (Oxf) 2010;72:502–6.

[58] Patronas N, Bulakbasi N, Stratakis CA, et al. Spoiled gradient recalled acquisition in the steady state technique is superior to conventional postcontrast spin-echo technique for magnetic resonance imaging detection of adrenocorticotropin-secreting pituitary tumors. J Clin Endocrinol Metab 2003;88:1565–9.

[59] Ejaz S, Vassilopoulou-Sellin R, Busaidy NL, et al. Cushing syndrome secondary to ectopic adrenocorticotropic hormone secretion: the University of Texas MD Anderson Cancer Center Experience. Cancer 2011;117:4381–9.

[60] Ilias I, Torpy DJ, Pacak K, et al. Cushing's syndrome due to ectopic corticotropin secretion: twenty years' experience at the National Institutes of Health. J Clin Endocrinol Metab 2005;90:4955–62.

[61] de Herder WW, Krenning EP, Malchoff CD, et al. Somatostatin receptor scintigraphy: its value in tumor localization in patients with Cushing's syndrome caused by ectopic corticotropin or corticotropin-releasing hormone secretion. Am J Med 1994;96:305–12.

[62] Zemskova MS, Gundabolu B, Sinaii N, et al. Utility of various functional and anatomic imaging modalities for detection of ectopic adrenocorticotropin-secreting tumors. J Clin Endocrinol Metab 2010;95:1207–19.

[63] Kayani I, Conry BG, Groves AM, et al. A comparison of 68Ga-DOTATATE and 18F-FDG PET/CT in pulmonary neuroendocrine tumors. J Nucl Med 2009;50:1927–32.

[64] Jindal T, Kumar A, Venkitaraman B, et al. Role of (68)Ga-DOTATOC PET/CT in the evaluation of primary pulmonary carcinoids. Korean J Intern Med 2010;25:386–91.

[65] Conti PS, Lilien DL, Hawley K, et al. PET and [18F]-FDG in oncology: a clinical update. Nucl Med Biol 1996;23:717–35.

[66] Pacak K, Ilias I, Chen CC, et al. The role of [(18)F]fluorodeoxyglucose positron emission tomography and [(111)In]-diethylenetriaminepentaacetate-D-Phe-pentetreotide scintigraphy in the localization of ectopic adrenocorticotropin-secreting tumors causing Cushing's syndrome. J Clin Endocrinol Metab 2004;89:2214–21.

[67] Isidori AM, Sbardella E, Zatelli MC, et al. Conventional and nuclear medicine imaging in ectopic Cushing's syndrome: a systematic review. J Clin Endocrinol Metab 2015;100:3231–44.

6

Surgical Treatment of Cushing's Disease

E.R. Laws, Jr., MD, FACS*,**, J.A. Jane, Jr., MD†

*Harvard Medical School, Boston, MA, United States; **Neuro-Endocrine/Pituitary Program, Department of Neurosurgery, Brigham and Women's Hospital, Boston, MA, United States; †Department of Neurological Surgery, University of Virginia Health System, Charlottesville, VA, United States

1 INDICATIONS FOR SURGERY

1.1 Signs and Symptoms

Patients with unequivocal progressive signs and symptoms of Cushing's disease often merit consideration for surgical management. At present, surgery offers the only opportunity for a prompt "cure" (remission) and is usually considered first-line therapy, especially in patients with severe debilitating disease or failure of medical therapy (see Chapter 7

TABLE 6.1   Characteristics of 93 Adult Patients with Surgically Proven Cushing's Disease

Characteristics	Number of patients
Female/male	75/18
Obesity/weight gain	77
Hypertension	72
Moon facies	72
Hirsutism	72
Dorsal fat pad	68
Weakness/proximal myopathy	63
Ruddy complexion (plethora)	62
Bruising/ecchymoses	61
Depression/moodiness	59
Striae	52
Headache	45
Edema	37
Diabetes mellitus	29
Visual disturbances	25
Osteopenia/pathological fractures	25
Acne	24
Hyperpigmentation	19
Menstrual disorder (premenopausal women)	86%
Impotence/sexual dysfunction (men)	65%
Balding/hair loss (women)	28%

Adapted from Laws ER, Reitmeyer M, Thapar K, et al. Cushing's disease resulting from pituitary corticotrophic microadenoma. Neurochirurgie 2002; 48: 294–299.

for details of medical management) [1,2]. Because the evolution of this disease is often indolent and because the symptoms can be relatively nonspecific, many patients are evaluated by a series of different health care professionals before the actual diagnosis is even considered or made. The classic signs and symptoms include weight gain; depression; emotional and cognitive changes; excess body hair; generalized weakness and fatigue; diabetes mellitus, which is frequently difficult to control; elevated blood pressure, which also may be difficult to manage; characteristic round face, often with rosy cheeks; thin skin that easily bruises and heals poorly; acne and other infections; pigmented stretch marks on the abdomen and elsewhere (striae); excess collection of fat over the back of the neck (buffalo hump) and anteriorly with enlargement of the supraclavicular fat pads; pathologic fractures (osteoporosis); and occasional cardiovascular difficulties (Table 6.1). Once the diagnosis is made, the various symptoms and signs define a clinical picture that is typical of Cushing's disease [3].

TABLE 6.2   Standard Tests for the Diagnosis of Cushing's Disease

LABORATORY TESTS AND IMAGING
Serum cortisol determination (fasting)
Salivary cortisol (11 pm) measurement (performed twice)
Serum ACTH level
24-hour urinary free cortisol measurement (performed twice)
Low-and high-dose dexamethasone suppression testing
MRI of the pituitary
FURTHER TESTING[a]
Dexamethasone/corticotropin-hormone testing
Inferior petrosal sinus sampling
CT/MRI of chest, abdomen, and pelvis
Octreotide/PET imaging of chest, abdomen and pelvis

CT, Computed tomography; MRI, magnetic resonance imaging; and PET, positron emission tomography.
a See Chapter 5

1.2 Diagnostic Laboratory Studies and Imaging

Clinical suspicion of the diagnosis of Cushing's disease leads to a spectrum of laboratory tests that are used to confirm the diagnosis (Chapter 5). The definition of Cushing's disease depends on the demonstration of central adrenocorticotropic hormone (ACTH) related elevation in circulating cortisol. Accordingly, measurements of cortisol in the blood, saliva, and urine can confirm the diagnosis (Table 6.2). Additional testing can evaluate the levels of ACTH, which should not be excessively high. Markedly elevated ACTH levels are often associated with so-called ectopic sources of ACTH, such as bronchogenic cancer and carcinoid tumors.

The most common cause of Cushing's disease is a small benign tumor in the pituitary gland. The pituitary tumor secretes ACTH, which, in turn, stimulates the adrenal glands to secrete excess levels of cortisol. In most cases, the tumor cells have lost their responsiveness to external signals, which is the basis of dexamethasone suppression testing (Chapter 5). Further testing may be done in cases where the results of the standard evaluation (Table 6.2) are either confusing or inconsistent (Chapter 5).

Once there is significant suspicion of the presence of Cushing's disease from a pituitary source, current practice mandates the evaluation of the pituitary gland, using high-resolution focused magnetic resonance imaging (MRI). Computed tomography of the head is inadequate for the evaluation of most patients, as the resolution of the images is not fine enough to demonstrate the very small tumors present in Cushing's disease. Evidence of the tumor may be seen on high-quality pituitary protocol MRI studies in about half of the patients (Fig. 6.1); however, Cushing's disease can be caused by a very small tumor that is difficult or impossible to see even on routine MRI studies. A negative imaging study, however, does not preclude the recommendation for pituitary surgery, so long as the clinical picture and laboratory studies are consistent with a pituitary source of the disease.

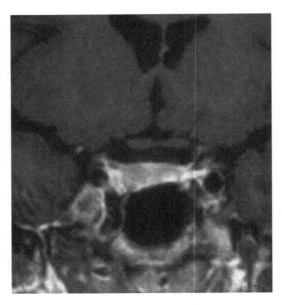

FIGURE 6.1   Coronal magnetic resonance imaging of a right-sided Cushing's microadenoma.

1.3 Ideal and Less Than Ideal Surgical Candidates

The differential diagnosis of Cushing's disease is complex and often confusing (Table 6.3). Because of the wide range of different entities, in different parts of the body, the presumptive diagnosis of Cushing's disease can be difficult and time-consuming. Some patients have classical signs and symptoms, with confirming laboratory tests, and are relatively straightforward. Others may have some components of the disease but might not benefit from surgical therapy focused on the pituitary. The ideal candidate for surgical management has clear and progressive symptoms and signs of Cushing's disease, classic alterations in the laboratory studies (Table 6.2), and a definitive, or at least suspicious, MRI study suggesting a pituitary tumor. Because of the nature of many of the symptoms and signs of Cushing's disease, making the diagnosis and considering a patient for surgery can be challenging.

The less than ideal candidate is the patient who may have some but not all of the classic symptoms, who may have some symptoms periodically, in a so-called "cyclical" fashion, or who may have been convinced for one reason or another that he or she is suffering from Cushing's disease. This latter group of patients can be very persistent, even fixated, and it is important for the surgeon to remain objective and to insist that at least minimum diagnostic criteria can be consistently met.

The majority of patients for whom pituitary surgery is recommended (>80%) fall into the pattern of the "ideal patient" if this definition includes a positive MRI scan. Patients who are significantly "less than ideal" or "cyclical" comprise less than 10% of most reported surgical series [4–6].

There are small number of patients who do have periodic manifestations of their disease, and there are some patients who are in excellent physical condition, performing regular

TABLE 6.3   Differential Diagnosis of Cushing's Disease

CUSHING'S DISEASE: ACTH-DEPENDENT (PITUITARY SOURCE)
Pituitary adenoma—ACTH secreting
Pituitary carcinoma—ACTH secreting
Primary pituitary—ACTH hyperplasia
CUSHING'S SYNDROME: EXTRA-PITUITARY SOURCES OF ACTH, CRH, OR CORTISOL
Small cell carcinoma of the lung
Carcinoid tumors (pulmonary, abdominal)
Pancreatic islet cell tumors
Medullary carcinoma of the thyroid
Pheochromocytoma
Adrenal adenoma
Adrenal carcinoma
Nodular adrenal hyperplasia
Exogenous steroids (medications, injections, factitious)
PSEUDO-CUSHINGOID STATES
Depression
Alcoholism
Obesity
Polycystic ovarian syndrome
Diabetes mellitus

ACTH, Adrenocorticotropic hormone; and CRH, corticotropin-releasing hormone.

exercise, and eating well who do not exhibit the typical body changes characteristic of Cushing's disease. Before recommending surgery in these equivocal patients, it is our usual practice to be certain that the patient has had at least two abnormal cortisol determinations, preferably with late-night (11 p.m.) salivary cortisol or 24-h urinary free cortisol determinations, a positive inferior petrosal sinus sampling study, and at least some suggestion of an abnormality on imaging in the pituitary region.

2 PREOPERATIVE CONSIDERATIONS

For the patient who is scheduled for pituitary surgery, there are a series of steps that should be taken preoperatively to ensure an optimal outcome from surgery. The first of these is to manage, correct, and optimize the frequent comorbidities of Cushing's disease. Hypertension should be diagnosed and controlled. The patient's cardiac status should be evaluated thoroughly and treated if necessary. Because diabetes mellitus is so common, glucose metabolism must be thoroughly evaluated, and appropriate diabetes management should be instituted and maintained throughout surgery and the recovery period. Many patients with Cushing's disease have sleep apnea or other respiratory problems. These must be evaluated and treated when necessary. Pulmonary function is an important part of successful anesthesia and surgery. Some patients with Cushing's disease have disorders of electrolyte status, particularly hypokalemia (low potassium), which must be corrected before surgery. Although blood transfusions are rarely needed in surgery for Cushing's disease, the coagulation status of the patient should be measured before the operation. Patients with Cushing's disease often have peripheral edema and may have superficial infections, such as acne or fungal infections. Management of all these conditions is important for the well-being of the patient and for successful surgery. On rare occasions the psychological side effects of Cushing's disease may impact the patient's state of mind regarding surgery. Appropriate reassurance and occasional psychoactive drug therapy may be indicated.

Technical aspects of the anesthetic phase of surgery include the use of monitoring when it is necessary for the patient under anesthesia. In those individuals who have hypertension or cardiac disease that is difficult to control, an arterial line and the measurement of central venous pressure may be necessary. In every case, very cautious and compulsive measuring of intravenous fluid input and urinary output during the operation and in the postoperative period is necessary. Our standard practice is to cautiously anticipate intraoperative and postoperative problems. We routinely use measures to prevent deep venous thrombosis (prevention of blood clots). Although significant blood loss is not anticipated, it is prudent as a precaution in the rare instance where a transfusion might be necessary to have the patient's blood type and crossmatch performed. Most patients who have surgery for Cushing's disease do not require care in the intensive care unit (ICU), but it is available for patients with complex problems if they occur.

Because of the possibility of an intraoperative cerebrospinal fluid (CSF) leak after removal of the pituitary tumor, steps are taken to have the abdomen available for harvesting of an abdominal fat graft to fill the space left by removal of the tumor and to prevent a postoperative CSF leak when necessary.

3 OPERATIVE CONSIDERATIONS

3.1 Transsphenoidal Surgery

Our patients are given general anesthesia with medications that have very little in the way of side effects or risks. Additionally, patients are closely monitored throughout the procedure for any of the uncommon adverse events or reactions that may be related to anesthesia [7,8]. Anesthesia is administered through an endotracheal tube, and the patient is asleep throughout the entire procedure, which usually lasts 2–3 h (or longer in patients who have had prior surgery). Blood transfusions are rarely needed, and most patients have minimal surgery-related pain on awakening.

Careful attention is paid to the positioning of the patient for the surgical procedure. The patient is well padded where there is any opportunity for pressure points to cause pain or skin complications after the procedure. The head is fixed in position so that it does not move during surgery and so that the computer guidance system can be used during surgery to ensure optimal safety. Computerized image guidance has all but replaced the former use of intraoperative fluoroscopy.

Our patients are in a "beach chair" position with the chest elevated to lower venous pressure. If a fat graft becomes necessary to fill the empty space left by removing the tumor or to treat an intraoperative CSF leak, the area of the abdomen just below the belly button (umbilicus) is prepared for a small incision used to obtain the graft. We almost never employ an intraoperative or postoperative lumbar drain, as we do not find that lowering intracranial pressure is necessary or desirable; we use it rarely to inject air to increase intracranial pressure to force soft suprasellar tumor (macroadenomas) downward into the surgical field.

With the patient asleep, a nasogastric tube is placed to prevent secretions associated with surgery from entering the stomach. It is used to remove such secretions at the end of the procedure and is removed before the patient is awakened. The typical operating time is 2–3 h, for routine first-time cases, and most patients who have uncomplicated surgery can be monitored without admittance to the ICU. The nurses on the neurosurgical floor are regularly instructed on the care and precautions related to our pituitary tumor patients, with particular attention paid to the patients with Cushing's disease [9].

3.2 Bilateral Adrenalectomy

Another method of dealing with ineffectively treated Cushing's disease or Cushing's syndrome is bilateral adrenalectomy. Currently, this is considered a radical step that is generally employed as a method of last resort. The indications for this operation are usually restricted to patients who are seriously ill, and progressively suffering, from the effects of elevated serum cortisol. Because cortisol is secreted from the adrenal glands, their removal, when complete, effectively eliminates the problem. In Cushing's disease, especially when its effects are poorly controlled, a source of excess ACTH (a pituitary adenoma) remains, and thus, the negative feedback of cortisol produced by the adrenal glands is no longer present. In Cushing's disease, this can result in a proliferation of the tumor in the pituitary, which often becomes more aggressive and is associated with Nelson's syndrome (Chapter 9). Currently, surgery for adrenalectomy is performed using laparoscopic techniques, which have made the operation less dangerous and more effective than previously. Despite this advance in surgical technique, the postoperative management of the patient with no functioning adrenal glands is complex and requires continuous monitoring. There are few large contemporary series of adrenal surgery for Cushing's syndrome of any cause. Most show almost complete elimination of circulating cortisol; however, long-term results and the effects on quality of life are not available.

4 POTENTIAL COMPLICATIONS OF SURGERY

As with any surgical procedure, complications can occur. Serious complications of the operation are uncommon [10,11]. The overall complications are listed in Table 6.4, which summarizes our experience in a series of 68 patients who had surgery for presumed Cushing's disease. Vascular injuries and postoperative death are no longer likely in the hands of experienced pituitary surgeons. Minor complications include temporary sinus and nasal discomfort and minor bleeding and discharge from the nose. A postoperative CSF leak may predispose patients to meningitis; however, this is unlikely but can be managed effectively in most cases.

TABLE 6.4   Complications of Pituitary Surgery for Cushing's Disease in 68 Consecutive Patients, 2008–14

Complications	Number of patients diagnosed
MINOR COMPLICATIONS	
Epistaxis (nosebleed)	1
Sinus problems	3
Aseptic meningitis	1
Transient hyponatremia (SIADH)	3
Transient diabetes insipidus	16
MAJOR COMPLICATIONS	
Carotid artery injury (repaired)	1
Epistaxis requiring exploration	1
Cerebrospinal fluid leak	0
Meningitis	0
Mortality	0

SIADH, Syndrome of inappropriate antidiuretic hormone.

5 SURGICAL TECHNIQUES

Essentially all of our operations for Cushing's disease are done using the transnasal transsphenoidal endoscopic technique, currently with a 3-D endoscope [12–14]. Former methods, using the operating microscope and sublabial or transnasal approaches, remain in use and are also effective surgical techniques.

With our preferred endoscopic method, there are no external incisions. The nasal turbinates are gently displaced laterally, and topical anesthetic and epinephrine are applied to prevent mucosal bleeding. The ostia of the sphenoid sinus are the connections between the nasal passages and the sphenoid sinus, which is the gateway to the pituitary region. These ostia are surgically enlarged and form the posterior limit of what is termed a posterior septectomy, where a portion of the nasal septum running back to the sphenoid sinuses is removed. Once the sphenoid sinus is entered, the anterior sphenoid wall is partially resected to give access to the sella turcica.

Landmarks are confirmed with the computerized image guidance system, to be sure that the operation respects the midline and does not endanger the carotid arteries on either side. The optic nerves and optic chiasm are rarely at risk in operations for Cushing's disease, except in cases of macroadenomas. The visualization obtained through the endoscope is correlated with the MRI imaging studies. The sella turcica is opened in the midline so that the dural envelope that contains the pituitary is fully visualized from one cavernous sinus to the other. Once the dura is exposed, the ultrasonic Doppler microprobe is used to investigate the dura and to be sure that the carotid arteries are not in danger. In Cushing's disease, the sella turcica is usually fairly small and has not been enlarged by the presence of a sizeable tumor. The uncommon ACTH-secreting macroadenomas are handled in the same fashion as other large pituitary adenomas [15]. Once the face of the pituitary dura is fully exposed and hemostasis is perfect, the dura is opened in the fashion of an X, or in a cruciate fashion. Even with small tumors within the sella turcica, some evidence of dural invasion may be present, and any involved dura should be removed if possible. A subdural dissection of the face of the pituitary gland often shows a bulge from the tumor, or the typical tumor tissue is readily apparent in the subdural plane. If it is not and if inferior petrosal sinus sampling has lateralized to one side or the other, a paramedian vertical incision is made; with deeper dissection, the capsule of the tumor may be discovered, or the tumor itself may extrude. Ideally, an extracapsular dissection of the tumor, using small pledgets of a gelatin sponge material (Gelfoam), and careful microdissection technique can result in elegant removal of the lesion [16]. Even if this occurs, it is our practice to remove a rim of the normal gland against the tumor capsule to be certain that no tumor cells have infiltrated the surrounding normal tissue. If, despite these maneuvers, the surgeon detects no obvious signs of tumor, the following steps are recommended: Since the majority of corticotrophs are in the central mucoid wedge of the pituitary gland, the first step is to remove the central anterior portion, taking the removal back to the pars intermedia and the thin membrane that sometimes separates the posterior pituitary; if this tissue does not appear abnormal, then our practice is to mobilize the lateral lobes of the pituitary gland by subdural dissection, one after the other, to dissect them away from the cavernous sinus and to inspect them and excise any suspicious areas; if these steps do not reveal tumor and if the imaging studies show no suggestion of either so-called ectopic cavernous sinus or suprasellar extension of a pituitary tumor, we prefer not to do a total hypophysectomy but to leave a thin rim of the superior aspect of the pituitary gland attached to the pituitary stalk. Vigorous dissection in the small confined space of the normal sella turcica can often increase the risks of an intraoperative CSF leak through the diaphragm or damage to the posterior pituitary or the pituitary stalk. It is our practice to repair a CSF leak by using abdominal fat placed to occlude the aperture in the roof of the sella turcica and held in place with a reconstruction of the sellar floor, using bone, cartilage, or an artificial plate. In the absence of a CSF leak, it is our practice to place Gelfoam within the tumor cavity. With the current technique, we usually can avoid packing the nostrils, as was routinely done with the microscopic approach.

6 POSTOPERATIVE ROUTINES

The patient should emerge from anesthesia fairly promptly and with good responses and normal vision unless previously impaired. Temperature, pulse, and blood pressure should be normal, although blood pressure control can sometimes be a problem in patients with Cushing's disease. Because of the possibility of damage to the posterior pituitary or the pituitary stalk, the entire patient care team must be alert for the possibility of diabetes insipidus, which presents as excessive thirst and frequent and excessive urination. Therefore, intake and output are strictly measured and kept in balance. The serum sodium level is monitored every 6 h for the first 2 days in order to avoid either hyper- or hyponatremia. Disturbances in sodium levels occur in about 9% of postoperative pituitary surgery patients. Both high- and low-sodium levels can be dangerous and must be corrected carefully [17–19]. Many patients with Cushing's disease have diabetes mellitus that is difficult to control; they should be carefully monitored for blood sugar concentrations and treated accordingly, with insulin if necessary. In cases of successful removal of an ACTH-secreting adenoma in Cushing's disease, the ideal response for a patient in remission is the development of signs and symptoms of adrenal insufficiency. Our patients are warned about this preoperatively. The early signs of low cortisol include headache, nausea, vomiting, profound fatigue, and hypothermia. As soon as these signs appear and adrenal insufficiency is suspected, an urgent serum cortisol level is obtained in addition to the routine cortisol checks every 6 h for the first 3 days after surgery. Stress-dose steroids may be necessary, but rapid conversion to routine replacement is desirable as soon as this is safe. We encourage early ambulation and the use of prophylaxis against deep vein thrombosis; we routinely give low-dose aspirin therapy to our patients with Cushing's disease, starting within the first 2 days postsurgery.

7 DISCHARGE AND POSTDISCHARGE CARE

Most of our patients with Cushing's disease can be discharged from the hospital 3 or 4 days after surgery, depending on whether they are in remission or not. We would like them to be on a steady pituitary hormone-replacement schedule, with care taken to adjust the management of diabetes mellitus, diabetes insipidus, or hypertension as necessary. Nasal care in the form of saline spray to help remove any crusting and to improve the healing of the nasal mucosa is begun a day after surgery and continues 2- or 3 times a day in each nostril for the first several weeks. If patients develop nasal congestion following surgery, they can treat this conservatively with Afrin or Sudafed or other relatively mild decongestants. Heavy lifting, bending over, and excessive physical activity that produces fatigue are discouraged, as full healing of the operative intervention may take approximately 6 weeks. We evaluate the patients in our clinic 1 week after surgery and at that time, check the serum sodium level and attend to any other symptoms or complaints. At 6 weeks postsurgery, patients are seen in conjunction with our endocrinologists, and a full pituitary laboratory evaluation is performed. In most patients, we defer the postoperative MRI scan, which is used as a baseline for the future, to the 3-month visit, as previous studies have shown that the postoperative imaging changes take about 3 months to resolve [20]. Endocrine follow-up to evaluate and treat remission is arranged as necessary. We emphasize the fact that many patients in remission will take a long time to feel normal again, and they often need a great deal of encouragement (Chapter 10). Once stable, annual reevaluation is recommended, as the recurrence rate for patients with Cushing's disease in remission after surgery increases steadily over time postoperatively.

8 OUTCOMES OF SURGERY FOR CUSHING'S DISEASE

The desired outcomes after surgery for Cushing's disease are the removal of the ACTH-secreting tumor and the restoration or preservation of otherwise normal pituitary function. The best results over the long-term occur in patients whose postoperative cortisol levels become quite low. This is a result of the tumor suppressing the output of the normal corticotroph cells in the normal pituitary; they often take many months to recover. To some degree, the longer the patient requires cortisol support after surgery, the better the long-term outcome.

Obtaining the ideal outcome depends on many factors: the size of the tumor, whether or not it is atypical or invasive, how long the patient has had symptoms and signs of Cushing's disease, how severe the symptoms and comorbidities are, the completeness of removal of the lesion, and the skill and experience of the surgeon and the multidisciplinary team caring for the patient. The removal of the tumor and lowering the excess circulating cortisol usually result in improved control of diabetes mellitus and improved management of hypertension. Other symptoms and signs slowly return to normal in most patients, although eliminating the excess weight present in most patients with Cushing's disease can be a major struggle. Cushing's disease is uncommon in children; however, the developing child has additional issues relative to growth, to diagnosis, and to management postoperatively. These are discussed in Chapter 11.

There are many excellent reviews of the outcomes of patients who have had transsphenoidal surgery for Cushing's disease, and they deal with several subcategories of pathologic presentation. The outcomes tend to be fairly similar [21–25], with better outcomes in patients with microadenomas rather than macroadenomas, with a definitive ACTH-staining tumor found at surgery, and with noninvasive tumors. In addition, outcomes are significantly more reliable in patients who have a dramatic fall in serum cortisol immediately after surgery [26]. In those reported series where the follow-up has been relatively long, it is clear that recurrences of the ACTH-secreting tumors are quite common and that the possibility of recurrence increases over time following what appears to be successful surgery.

In general, the initial postoperative results following removal of an ACTH-secreting microadenoma are 80–90% successful. A satisfactory result is found in approximately 50% of patients with ACTH macroadenomas. Recurrence rates for microadenomas are about 12% at 10 years and over 20% at 20 years [27]. Recurrence rates for macroadenomas are significantly higher. Those patients who do develop recurrent tumors after initial surgery can be treated with repeat surgery, radiation therapy, or radiosurgery [28], and occasionally with medical therapy, which is discussed in Chapter 7.

The goal for all of our patients is to achieve a satisfactory and nearly normal quality of life and life expectancy [29]. To a large degree this depends on reversal of the comorbidities associated with Cushing's disease. Follow-up care and management by a skilled multidisciplinary team are essential in achieving these goals (Chapter 9 [30]).

References

[1] Biller BMK, Grossman AB, Stewart PM, et al. Treatment of adrenocortin-dependent Cushing's syndrome: a consensus statement. J Clin Endocrinol Metabol 2008;93:2454–62.

[2] Nieman LK, Biller BMK, Findling JW, et al. Treatment of Cushing's syndrome: an Endocrine Society Guideline. J Clin Endocrinol Metabol 2015;100:2807–31.

[3] Iuliano SL, Laws ER. Early recognition of Cushing's disease: a case study. J Am Assoc Nurse Pract 2013;325:402–6.

[4] Alexandraki KI, Kaltsas GA, Isidori AM, et al. The prevalence and characteristic features of cyclicity and variability in Cushing's disease. Eur J Endocrinol 2009;160(6):1011–8.

[5] Yamada S, Fukuhara N, Nishioka H, et al. Surgical management and outcomes in patients with Cushing's disease with negative pituitary magnetic resonance imaging. World Neurosurg 2012;77(3–4):525–32.

[6] Semple PL, Vance ML, Findling J, et al. Transsphenoidal surgery for Cushing's disease: outcome in patients with a normal magnetic resonance imaging scan. Neurosurgery 2000;46:553–9.

[7] Dunn LK, Nemergut EC. Anesthesia for transsphenoidal pituitary surgery. Curr Opin Anaesthesiol 2013;26(5):549–54.

[8] Burton CM, Nemergut EC. Anesthetic and critical care management of patients undergoing pituitary surgery. Front Horm Res 2006;34:236–55.

[9] Jane JA Jr, Thapar K, Kaptain GJ, et al. Pituitary surgery: transsphenoidal approach. Neurosurgery 2002;51(2): 435–42.

[10] Semple PL, Laws ER Jr. Complications in a contemporary series of patients who underwent transsphenoidal surgery for Cushing's disease. J Neurosurg 1999;91(2):175–9.

[11] Smith TR, Hulou MM, Huang KT, et al. Complications after transsphenoidal surgery for patients with Cushing's disease and silent corticotroph adenomas. Neurosurg Focus 2015;38(2):E12.

[12] Dallapiazza RF, Oldfield EH, Jane JA Jr. Surgical management of Cushing's disease. Pituitary 2015;18:211–6.

[13] Laws ER, Starke RM, Reames DL, et al. Endoscopic transsphenoidal surgery for Cushing's disease. Neurosurgery 2013;72:420–7.

[14] Sratke RM, Reames DL, Chen C-J, et al. Neurosurgery 2013;72:240–7.

[15] De Tommasi C, Vance ML, Okonkwo DO, et al. Surgical management of adrenocorticotrophic hormone–secreting macroadenomas: outcome and challenges in patients with Cushing's disease or Nelson's syndrome. J Neurosurg 2005;103(5):825–30.

[16] Oldfield EH, Vortmeyer AO. Development of a histological pseudocapsule and its use as a surgical capsule in the excision of pituitary tumors. J Neurosurg 2006;104:7–19.

[17] Burton CM, Nemergut EC. Anesthetic and critical care management of patients undergoing pituitary surgery. Front Horm Res 2006;34:236–55.

[18] Nemergut EC, Zuo Z, Jane JA Jr, et al. Predictors of diabetes insipidus after transsphenoidal surgery: a review of 881 patients. J Neurosurg 2005;103(3):448–54.

[19] Kristof RA, Rother M, Neuloh G, et al. Incidence, manifestations, and course of water and electrolyte metabolism disturbances following transsphenoidal pituitary adenoma surgery: a prospective observational study. J Neurosurg 2009;111(3):555–62.

[20] Kremer P, Forsting M, Ranaei G, et al. Magnetic resonance imaging after transsphenoidal surgery of clinically non-functioning macroadenomas. Acta Neurochir 2002;144(5):433–43.

[21] Chandler WF, Barkan A, Hollon T, et al. Outcome of transsphenoidal surgery for Cushing disease: a single center experience over 32 years. Neurosurgery 2016;78:216–23.

[22] Kelly DF. Transsphenoidal surgery for Cushing's disease: a review of success rates, remission predictors, management of failed surgery, and Nelson's syndrome. Neurosurg Focus 2007;23:E5.

[23] Pouratian N, Prevedello DM, Jagannathan J, et al. Outcomes and management of patients with Cushing's disease without pathological confirmation of tumor resection after transsphenoidal surgery. J Clin Endocrinol Metab 2007;92(9):3383–8.

[24] Prevedello DM, Pouratian N, Sherman J, et al. Management of Cushing's disease: outcome in patients with microadenoma detected on pituitary magnetic resonance imaging. J Neurosurg 2008;109(4):751–9.

[25] Reitmeyer M, Vance ML, Laws ER Jr. The neurosurgical management of Cushing's disease. Mol Cell Endocrinol 2002;197(1–2):73–99.

[26] Simmons NE, Alden TD, Thorner MO, et al. Serum cortisol response to transsphenoidal surgery for Cushing disease. J Neurosurg 2001;95(1):1–8.

[27] Patil CG, Prevedello DM, Lad SP, et al. Late recurrences of Cushing's disease after initial successful transsphenoidal surgery. J Clin Endocrinol Metab 2008;93(2):358–62.

[28] Jagannathan J, Sheehan JP, Pouratian N, et al. Gamma knife surgery for Cushing's disease. J Neurosurg 2007;106(6):980–7.

[29] Patil CG, Lad SP, Harsh GR, et al. National trends, complications, and outcomes following transsphenoidal surgery for Cushing's disease from 1993 to 2002. Neurosurg Focus 2007;23(3):E7.

[30] McLaughlin N, Laws ER, Oyesiku N, et al. Pituitary centers of excellence. Neurosurgery 2012;71:916–26.

Medical Treatment of Cushing's Disease

S. Hopkins, MD*, M. Fleseriu, MD**

*Department of Medicine (Endocrinology), and Northwest Pituitary Center, Oregon Health & Science University, Portland, OR, United States; **Department of Medicine (Endocrinology), Department of Neurological Surgery, and Northwest Pituitary Center, Oregon Health & Science University, Portland, OR, United States

OUTLINE

1 OVERVIEW OF MEDICAL THERAPY AND ITS ROLE IN THE MANAGEMENT OF CUSHING'S DISEASE

Although surgery remains the primary treatment of choice for Cushing's disease, medical therapy plays an important role in select patient groups, either as a primary or adjunctive therapy [1]. Medical therapy is used most commonly in patients with evidence of persistent or recurrent disease following surgery, either in addition to, or as an alternative to, radiation

Cushing's Disease. http://dx.doi.org/10.1016/B978-0-12-804340-0.00007-3

therapy. Alternatively, in patients at high risk of surgical complications, including patients with multiple comorbidities and life-threatening Cushing's syndrome, or in patients in whom the source of excess adrenocorticotropic hormone (ACTH) is unknown, medical treatments may be used as first-line therapy [1–3].

2 CLASSIFICATION OF MEDICAL THERAPIES USED IN THE TREATMENT OF CUSHING'S DISEASE

Medical therapies used in the treatment of Cushing's disease fall into three categories: (1) pituitary-directed neuromodulators of ACTH release, (2) adrenal steroidogenesis inhibitors, and (3) glucocorticoid receptor blockers. The physiology, efficacy, and side effects of the drugs most commonly employed within these three categories are reviewed in Table 7.1.

2.1 Pituitary-directed Neuromodulators of ACTH Release

Cushing's disease, by definition, results from an overproduction of ACTH by the pituitary gland, usually harboring an ACTH-secreting benign adenoma. It would follow that the most effective treatment should inhibit ACTH production at the level of the pituitary. Two medications that act at the level of the pituitary are most frequently employed in the treatment of Cushing's disease: pasireotide, a somatostatin analog, and cabergoline, a dopamine agonist.

2.1.1 Pasireotide

Pasireotide is a somatostatin receptor ligand approved by the European Medicines Agency (EMA) and the U.S. Food and Drug Administration (FDA) for treatment of Cushing's disease. Somatostatin is mainly a somatotropin release-inhibiting factor. At the level of the anterior pituitary, somatostatin inhibits secretion of ACTH in addition to growth hormone (GH), prolactin, and thyrotropin. Peripherally, it acts at the level of the gastrointestinal tract to slow gastric motility, and at the pancreas to inhibit release of insulin, glucagon, and pancreatic polypeptide [4–7].

There are five somatostatin receptor subtypes (SSTR1–SSTR5) [8,9]. Each subtype is expressed in varying amounts throughout the body, and they are variably expressed in different tumors. The SSTR5 is the predominant receptor type expressed by corticotrope adenomas, while the predominant receptor type expressed by GH-producing adenomas is SSTR2 [4,7,10,11].

Somatostatin has a very short half-life (approximately 3 min), thus precluding its use as a long-term suppressive therapy. Over the last several decades, somatostatin analogs with longer half-lives have been developed. Octreotide and lanreotide predominantly bind to SSTR2 and have been used successfully in the treatment of acromegaly and secretory neuroendocrine tumors of the gut and pancreas [12], but they rarely have been effective in Cushing's disease [11,13]. Pasireotide exhibits high affinity binding to SSTR5 as well as SSTR1, SSTR2, and SSTR3. Pasireotide has a 40-fold greater affinity for SSTR5 compared to other somatostatin receptor ligands, and correspondingly demonstrates greater efficacy in the treatment of Cushing's disease [8,14–18].

TABLE 7.1 Medical Therapies Used in Cushing's Disease

Drug class	Chemical name	Trade name	Molecular structure	Mechanism of action	Dose	Adverse effects
Pituitary-directed ACTH neuromodulators	Pasireotide	SOM 230		Somatostatin receptor agonist	600–1200 mcg; 2 times daily	Hyperglycemia; nausea/vomiting/diarrhea; Biliary sludge/gallstones; LFT elevations; QTc prolongation
	Cabergoline	Dostinex		Dopamine agonist	0.5–7 mg/week	Cardiac valve disease; asthenia; hypotension

(Continued)

TABLE 7.1 Medical Therapies Used in Cushing's Disease (cont.)

Drug class	Chemical name	Trade name	Molecular structure	Mechanism of action	Dose	Adverse effects
Adrenal steroidogenesis inhibitors	Ketoconazole	Ketoconazole		Inhibition of 11β-hydroxylase, cholesterol side chain, and 17,20 lyase	200–400 mg 2–3 times daily	Hepatotoxicity; adrenal insufficiency; gynecomastia; testosterone deficiency; vitamin D deficiency
	Levoketoconazole	COR-003		Inhibition of 11β-hydroxylase, cholesterol side chain, and 17,20 lyase	Titration dose	Hepatotoxicity; adrenal insufficiency; gynecomastia; testosterone deficiency; vitamin D deficiency
	Metyrapone	Metopirone		Inhibition of 11β- and 18β-hydroxylase	250–1500 mg; 4 times daily	adrenal insufficiency; hypertension; hypokalemia; hirsutism; acne; GI side effects
	Mitotane	Lysodren		1. Inhibition of 11β- and 18β-hydroxylase, and cholesterol side arm cleavage 2. Atrophy of adrenal cortex 3. Increase CYP3A4 → Decrease cortisol bioavailability	500–1000 mg; 3 times daily	Adrenal insufficiency anorexia, nausea, vomiting, and diarrhea Dysarthria, ataxia, confusion, dizziness, and paresthesias

Etomidate		Inhibition of 11β-hydroxylase cholesterol and side arm cleavage	0.03 mg/kg IV bolus followed by 0.1–0.3 mg/kg/h	Adrenal insufficiency; nephrotoxicity; sedation; nausea/vomiting; hiccups/coughing; anaphylaxis; myoclonus
LCI699 Osilodrostat		Inhibition of 18β and 11β-hydroxylase	10–20 mg/day; 2 times daily	Adrenal insufficiency; nausea/diarrhea; asthenia; nasopharyngitis; hirsutism; acne
Glucocorticoid receptor blockers	Mifepristone Korlym		Glucocorticoid and progesterone receptor antagonist	300–1200 mg; daily	Adrenal insufficiency; hypokalemia; endometrial thickening/vaginal bleeding; ACTH elevation → possible tumor growth

LFTs, Liver function tests; IV, intravenous; and GI, gastrointestinal.

Information in the table was taken from the following references: Cuevas-Ramos D, Fleseriu M. Treatment of Cushing's disease: a mechanistic update. J Endocrinol 2014; 223(2): R19–R39; Colao A, Petersenn S, Newell-Price J, et al. A 12-month phase 3 study of pasireotide in Cushing's disease. N Engl J Med 2012; 366 (10): 914–924; Godbout A, Manavela M, Danilowicz K, et al. Cabergoline monotherapy in the long-term treatment of Cushing's disease. Eur J Endocrinol 2010; 163 (5): 709–716; Biller BMK, Grossman AB, Stewart PM, et al. Treatment of adrenocorticotropin-dependent Cushing's syndrome: a consensus statement. J Clin Endocrinol Metab 2008; 93 (7): 2454–2462; Bertagna X, Pivonello R, Fleseriu M, et al. LCI699, a potent 11β-hydroxylase inhibitor, normalizes urinary cortisol in patients with Cushing's disease: results from a multicenter, proof-of-concept study. J Clin Endocrinol Metab 2014; 99 (4): 1375–1383; Fleseriu M, Molitch ME, Gross C, et al. A new therapeutic approach in the medical treatment of Cushing's syndrome: glucocorticoid receptor blockade with mifepristone. Endocr Pract 2013; 19 (2): 313–326.

An initial phase 2 trial with pasireotide [5] showed good short-term efficacy: 22 patients (76%) showed a reduction in urinary free cortisol (UFC) levels, of whom 5 (17%) had normal UFC levels (responders), after 15 days of treatment. Serum cortisol levels and plasma ACTH levels were also reduced. Responders had greater pasireotide exposure than patients who did not respond.

In a phase 3, double-blind study of 162 patients with Cushing's disease, treatment with pasireotide at doses of 600 µg (82 patients) and 900 µg (80 patients) twice daily resulted in improvements in biochemical and clinical parameters, as well as a decrease in tumor volume [14]. The primary end-point of the study was a UFC level at/or below the upper limit of the normal (ULN) range at month 6 without an increase in dose.

More than half of the patients had either normalization of, or a more than 50% reduction in UFC levels at 6 months. A total of 12 of the 82 patients in the 600-µg group and 21 of the 80 patients in the 900-µg group met the primary end point. In particular, UFC normalization was noted in 50% of patients who had mild pretreatment elevations in UFC. Significant improvements were also observed in the classic signs and symptoms of Cushing's syndrome, including decreases in systolic and diastolic blood pressure, low-density lipoprotein, and weight, as well as improvements in quality of life scores. These benefits were not limited to patients with normalization of UFC, suggesting that even modest declines in UFC levels may result in clinical benefit [14].

Patients with higher baseline UFC levels were less likely to respond to pasireotide. In those patients who did respond, a clinically significant response to pasireotide was evident and stable within 1–2 months of starting the medication. Therefore, the selection of those patients most likely to benefit from continued therapy may be predicted early in the treatment course [14].

Additionally, pasireotide has been demonstrated to have significant effects on tumor growth [19]. Of those patients with a measurable pituitary tumor at baseline, tumor volume was reduced 9.1% in the 600-µg group and 43.8% in the 900-µg group at 12 months in the phase 3 study [14]. In a single center study of 16 patients, a more than 25% reduction in tumor size was shown in all patients, and a more than 50% reduction in tumor volume was found in 57% of patients [20].

Of note, distinct from other somatostatin analogs, pasireotide may be associated with significant hyperglycemia. In the phase 3 study discussed earlier, 78% of patients experienced at least one hyperglycemia-related adverse event. Mean hemoglobin A1c (HbA1c) values increased by about 1.5%, and 48% of patients without a prior diagnosis of diabetes had an elevated HbA1c of 6.5% or greater after 12 months of therapy. Patients with baseline-impaired fasting glucose were most at risk [14]. Studies with pasireotide in healthy volunteers suggest that hyperglycemia is the result of a decreased release of insulin and glucagon-like peptide-1 (GLP-1) by beta cells of the pancreas and intestine, respectively, while hepatic and peripheral insulin sensitivities appear to remain intact [21]. Based on the previous observations, close monitoring for the development or worsening of hyperglycemia following initiation and dose adjustments of pasireotide is recommended [22]. Furthermore, first-line therapy for hyperglycemia should include metformin followed by the addition of an incretin-based therapy, such as a dipeptidyl peptidase-4 (DPP-4) inhibitor or GLP-1 agonist [21,22].

Reductions in mean UFC and improvements in clinical signs of Cushing's disease have been maintained over 24 months of pasireotide use in a recent clinical trial [20]. Patients who derived benefit from pasireotide in the phase 3 trial continued the same dose of pasireotide at the end of the core study as in the extension study (300–1,200 µg twice daily). Dose titration was allowed, however, was according to efficacy or drug-related adverse events. Of the patients who entered the extension, 50.0% (29/58) and 34.5% (20/58) had controlled UFC (i.e., UFC is less than or equal to the ULN) at months 12 and 24, respectively. The mean percentage decrease in UFC was 57.3% ($n = 52$) and 62.1% ($n = 33$) after treatment for 12 and 24 months, respectively. Improvements in clinical signs of Cushing's disease were sustained up to 24 months. Hyperglycemia was seen in almost 40% of patients, but no new safety issues were identified during the extension study [23]. Cases with even longer-term treatment have also been reported up to 5 years [24].

Additional adverse effects of pasireotide are similar to other somatostatin analogs, and predominantly include gastrointestinal side effects, such as nausea, vomiting, diarrhea, biliary sludge, gallstones, transient elevations of liver function tests (LFTs), and the risk of QT prolongation on electrocardiogram (ECG) [14]. With these adverse effects in mind, baseline assessment includes: LFTs, thyroid function tests, insulin-like growth factor 1 (IGF-1) levels, fasting plasma glucose levels, HbA1c, right upper quadrant ultrasound, and an ECG. Fingerstick blood glucose should be measured frequently during the first week of therapy in all patients and then tailored based on the degree of hyperglycemia and the need for treatment. Additional parameters listed should then be reassessed at 3–4-month intervals based on the patients' symptoms or dose adjustments [25].

Although the large phase 3 trial showed that patients with mild UFC elevation responded better, there have been other attempts to predict the response to pasireotide. The acute pasireotide suppression test (PST) has been suggested as a useful option [26] in predicting response to medium- or long-term treatment in Cushing's disease. A total of 19 patients with active Cushing's disease were prospectively investigated at two referral centers, and follow-up data (median 6 months; range 1–9 months) were available for 16 patients. All patients received a single subcutaneous (SC) injection of 600 µg of pasireotide in the morning. Serum cortisol and plasma ACTH were measured before and after pasireotide administration. Late-night salivary cortisol was also measured before and after pasireotide administration. After an acute PST, all patients were continued on pasireotide, 600 µg SC twice a day. Pasireotide treatment was associated with a normalization of 24-h UFC at last follow-up in 68% of patients. A decrease of over 27% of late-night salivary cortisol during the PST was the best parameter in predicting a positive response to treatment with pasireotide (i.e., positive predictive value 100%; negative predictive value 75%) [26]. Further studies are needed to elucidate clearly, which patients will benefit the most from using a somatostatin analog as first-line medical treatment.

2.1.2 Cabergoline

Cabergoline is a dopamine agonist commonly used in the medical treatment of prolactinomas. It has been suggested that cabergoline may play a role in the treatment of Cushing's disease [25]. Pathology specimen analysis suggests that the expression of the D2 dopamine receptor may be present in up to 80% of Cushing's disease pituitary adenomas [27]. Furthermore, in vitro and in vivo studies demonstrate that D2 receptor expression can help predict treatment response to cabergoline as measured by both declines in cortisol and ACTH levels [27,28].

In a study of 20 patients with persistent disease following pituitary surgery, cabergoline used at doses of 1–7 mg/week resulted in short-term response (defined as a >25% reduction in UFC) in 75% of patients at 3 months and in 40% of patients at 2 years. Mild hyperprolactinemia was present in 45% of the patients and was highly predictive of their response to cabergoline treatment at 3 months, but not at 2 years. Clinical improvements were also observed at 2 years, including a 25% decrease in the prevalence rates of being overweight or obese, a 50% decrease in the prevalence of hypertension, and a 17.5% decline in the prevalence of impaired fasting glucose or diabetes. Tumor shrinkage of over 25% was seen in four (50%) of the responsive patients [29].

In another study of 30 patients with Cushing's disease (27 postsurgery and 3 treatment naive), a short-term response with cabergoline doses of 1–6 mg/week was observed in only 50% of patients at 3 months, with 36.6% demonstrating normalization of UFC. However, 30% demonstrated sustained responses at a mean of 36 months. In this study, there was no correlation between hyperprolactinemia and treatment response. In fact, the three patients with baseline hyperprolactinemia had no response to cabergoline treatment [30].

Cabergoline was generally well tolerated in the studies noted previously. Hypotension and severe asthenia, leading to study withdrawal, were observed in 2 of 20 patients in the first study and not observed in the second study. Notably, neither study demonstrated significant cardiac valve effects, with only one patient demonstrating slight worsening of mild mitral regurgitation.

Although Cushing's disease patients do require considerably higher cabergoline doses than prolactinoma patients, the doses remain quite modest in comparison to the doses and long-term exposure of dopamine agonists used in the treatment of Parkinson's disease. This difference in total exposure may explain the absence of cardiac valve effects seen in association with cabergoline use in Cushing's disease as compared to the rates observed in Parkinson's disease patients [29,30].

The efficacy of cabergoline in Cushing's disease was recently found to be lower than initially thought in a 6-month prospective study [29–31]. Cabergoline was administered in increasing doses of 0.5–5 mg/week over 6 weeks in 20 patients (19 surgery naive and 1 recurrent). The median cabergoline dose at the end of the study was 5 mg (range 2.5–5 mg/week). During treatment, hypercortisolism varied, but gradual and dose-dependent reductions in UFC were not seen. A total of five patients had a 50% or more decrease of UFC, but three had a 50% or more rise of UFC. The prolactin levels were suppressed in all patients, which confirmed compliance with the study drug.

Currently, cabergoline is not FDA approved for use in the treatment of Cushing's disease; studies, including monotherapy and combination therapy with cabergoline, are ongoing. Monitoring should include periodic cardiac examinations and echocardiograms, especially if high doses are required [32].

2.2 Adrenal Steroidogenesis Inhibitors

Adrenal steroidogenesis inhibitors have played a role in the treatment of Cushing's disease for many years. Several different steroidogenesis inhibitors are available, but there are no large phase 3 studies, yet that have assessed short- and long-term response rates [15,25,33]. Additionally, variability in study designs prohibits direct comparison among steroidogenesis inhibitors. That being said, data currently available on the most commonly used steroidogenesis inhibitors as relevant to the treatment of Cushing's disease are discussed later in the chapter. Please refer to Fig. 7.1 for the site of action of each agent.

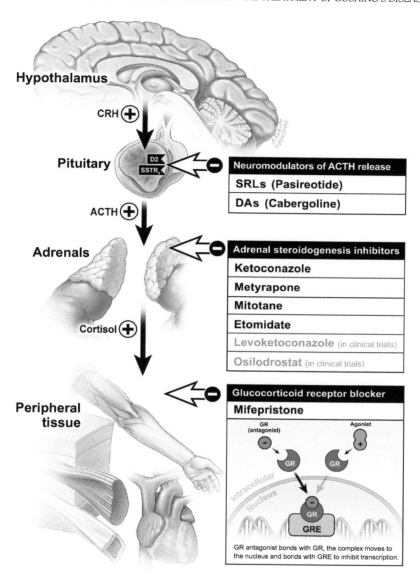

FIGURE 7.1 **Mechanism of action and targets for therapy in Cushing's disease.** *ACTH,* Adrenocorticotropic hormone; *CRH,* corticotropin-releasing hormone; *DA,* dopamine agonist; *GR,* glucocorticoid receptor; *GRE,* glucocorticoid response element; and *SRL,* somatostatin receptor ligand. *Source: Adapted with permission from Fleseriu M. Medical management of persistent and recurrent Cushing's disease. Neurosurg Clin N Am 2012; 23(4): 657. Published by Elsevier.*

2.2.1 Ketoconazole

Although principally employed as an antifungal agent, the inhibitor effects of ketoconazole on cortisol production have been recognized for several decades. Concerns regarding ketoconazole hepatotoxicity led to an FDA and an EMA warning in 2013 [34]. However, the EMA approved ketoconazole for the treatment of Cushing's syndrome in 2014 [35].

Ketoconazole most potently inhibits 11β-hydroxylase and cholesterol side chain cleavage but also has effects on other p450 enzymes, including inhibition of 17,20 lyase, which leads to low testosterone levels [36]. Additionally, for reasons that are poorly understood, despite ketoconazole causing adrenal enzyme inhibition, its use rarely results in ACTH elevation [15,37,38].

A retrospective study by Castinetti et al. sought to describe the efficacy and safety of ketoconazole for use in the Cushing's disease population [39]. They undertook a retrospective study of 200 Cushing's disease patients treated with ketoconazole as presurgical treatment, primary treatment, or secondary treatment following surgery or radiation therapy. Typically, ketoconazole was started at a dose of 200 mg daily with treatment-effective doses ranging from 600 to 1200 mg daily. Overall, at the time of last follow up, 49.3% of patients had normal UFC levels, 25.6% had at least a 50% decline in UFC, and 25.4% had no change in UFC levels. Normalization of UFC levels was approximately 50% in all three treatment groups, while partial response rates were greatest in the presurgical group (38.4%) and least in the postsurgery or radiation group (22.2%). All groups demonstrated significant clinical improvements in rates of hypertension, hypokalemia, and diabetes. Fifty-one patients were treated for over 24 months with ketoconazole, with 64.7 and 23.5% demonstrating normalization of UFC and an over 50% decline in UFC at last follow up, respectively. Notably, sex was the only baseline characteristic predictive of improved response rates, with women demonstrating a greater response than men. There was no significant relationship between age at diagnosis, initial UFC, baseline tumor characteristics, nor prior treatment or responses to treatment [39].

Hepatotoxicity, defined as less than 5 times or more than 5 times elevation in liver enzyme levels was observed in 30 (15.1%) and 5 (2.6%) patients, respectively. One patient demonstrated a 40-fold increase in aspartate transaminase (AST) and alanine transaminase (ALT), but this patient was also consuming alcohol and using acetaminophen. All increases in liver enzyme levels were apparent within 1 month of treatment initiation or dose increase. In all patients but one, liver enzymes returned to normal within 2–4 weeks of a dose reduction of 200 mg/day or drug withdrawal. Liver enzymes returned to normal after 3 months in the patient with a 40-fold increase. There was no relationship between ketoconazole dose and liver toxicity [39].

An additional noteworthy adverse effect is adrenal insufficiency, which was observed in approximately 5% of patients treated with ketoconazole. Less common side effects include gynecomastia, testosterone and vitamin D deficiencies, pruritus, fatigue, hair loss, edema, muscle pain, dizziness, dyspnea, hypertriglyceridemia, neutropenia, and elevated creatinine levels [4–7,39]. Of note, ketoconazole absorption requires an acidic environment and, therefore, commonly employed treatments for gastroesophageal reflux disease, such as H2 blockers and proton pump inhibitors, must be stopped before the initiation of use [6,15,25].

With these adverse effects in mind, clinic visits should include assessment for signs and symptoms of adrenal insufficiency or liver toxicity. Furthermore, LFTs should be checked at baseline and monitored closely for 1 month after initiation of therapy or dose increase and every 3 months thereafter. In the event of a less than 5 times ULN rise in liver enzymes, the ketoconazole dose should be reduced by at least 200 mg/day and should be stopped altogether in response to more than 5 times ULN elevation of liver enzymes. In the event of adrenal insufficiency, the medication can be stopped; or as part of a block and replace strategy, ketoconazole can be continued, and patients can be started on hydrocortisone replacement [15].

2.2.2 Levoketoconazole

Levoketoconazole is a 2S,4R-enantiomer of ketoconazole, an inhibitor of the cytochrome P450 family 11 subfamily B polypeptide 1 (CYP11B1), CYP17A1, and CYP21A2. After having been previously studied in patients with diabetes mellitus type 2, a large phase 3 international study is ongoing to evaluate the efficacy and safety of levoketoconazole in patients with Cushing's disease [40].

2.2.3 Metyrapone

Metyrapone inhibits cortisol synthesis through inhibition of 11β- and 18β-hydroxylase activity [41]. Metyrapone is rapidly effective and can lead to cortisol reductions within a few hours of the first dose. The dose required to shut down cortisol production can vary greatly among patients, with effective doses ranging from 500 mg to 6 g daily. To ensure blockade of cortisol synthesis, the dose must be titrated up quickly, typically starting at 250 mg every 6 h [42].

In studies seeking to exploit the rapid cortisol-lowering effects of metyrapone, short-term use of the drug has been shown to be an effective bridging tool, while patients await surgery [43]. Additionally, in a small group of patients with severe Cushing's disease, combination therapy with ketoconazole and mitotane was an effective alternative to bilateral adrenalectomy (discussed below in Section 3.1) [44].

Although metyrapone can clearly be effective in the short-term, and a few studies have demonstrated long-term control of hypercortisolemia [43], its role as a long-term therapeutic agent remains to be defined. With prolonged use (>1 month), lack of cortisol feedback can lead to marked ACTH elevations. The ACTH elevations can then result in breakthrough hypercortisolemia as well as a buildup of androgenic and mineralocorticoid precursors, leading to hirsutism, acne, hypertension, and hypokalemia [45]. Additionally, metyrapone can cause adrenal insufficiency for which cortisol replacement may need to be administered as part of a block and replace strategy [43,45]. Other adverse effects include gastrointestinal side effects, which are common but can be mediated by taking the medication with food; rare side effects include ataxia, lethargy, and dizziness [43,46].

Lastly, several drugs alter the metabolism of metyrapone. Phenytoin and phenobarbital increase and estrogen decreases metyrapone metabolism; therefore, close monitoring is required any time these medications are introduced or adjusted [47].

2.2.4 Mitotane

Mitotane at high doses has long been used in the treatment of adrenocortical carcinoma, but can also be effective as combination therapy in the treatment of Cushing's disease. Mitotane works in three ways to curb steroid production [48]: (1) Mitotane administration leads to lipid accumulation within and resultant atrophy of the adrenal cortex. (2) Mitotane modifies steroid metabolism by stimulating CYP3A4 expression, thereby reducing cortisol bioavailability.

(3) Mitotane directly inhibits steroid synthesis by inhibiting 11β- and 18β-hydroxylation as well as side arm cleavage.

Although mitotane does exhibit similar enzymatic inhibition to ketoconazole and metyrapone, the onset of action is much slower, with full inhibitory effects typically seen after 2–3 months of therapy. Adrenolytic properties, however, prevent breakthrough ACTH and hypercortisolemia seen with metyrapone and allow for long-term control of hypercortisolemia. Therefore, in contrast to other cortisol synthesis inhibitors, mitotane has a slow onset but a long duration of activity [6,49].

In a retrospective study looking at the use of mitotane as first-line or second-line therapy after surgery in 67 patients with Cushing's disease, normalization of UFC was achieved in 72% of patients after a median treatment time of 6.7 months. In an additional 9 patients, mitotane effectively normalized UFC before transsphenoidal surgical resection. The serum mitotane concentration required to normalize UFC was 8.5 mg/L. This is markedly decreased from target mitotane concentrations in adrenocortical carcinoma treatment (14–20 mg/L) and may allow for lower total mitotane exposure and decreased rates of adverse effects. In 24 patients in whom mitotane was discontinued and an alternative treatment not pursued, 17 (71%) developed a recurrence of hypercortisolism with a median-time-to-recurrence of 13.2 months. Also of note, in 12 patients with initial tumor-negative magnetic resonance imaging (MRI), a pituitary lesion became apparent following treatment, allowing for surgical resection [50].

The most notable adverse effect is the risk of adrenal insufficiency despite typical hydrocortisone replacement doses. Mitotane accelerates steroid metabolism and, therefore, increased hydrocortisone (HC) replacement doses are required to treat the induced adrenal insufficiency [49,51].

Gastrointestinal and neurological side effects are most frequent, reportedly occurring in 47 and 30% of patients, respectively. Typical gastrointestinal side effects include anorexia, nausea, vomiting, and diarrhea, while neurological signs included dysarthria, ataxia, confusion, dizziness, and paresthesias. Twenty-eight percent of patients demonstrated serious side effects, leading to treatment withdrawal [50]. Other rare side effects, such as gynecomastia, rash, increases in liver transaminases, and hypercholesterolemia, have also been reported [52].

This medication should not be used in women considering pregnancy within the next 5 years, as mitotane has been shown to be stored in adipose tissue for up to 2 years. In women of childbearing age who are treated with mitotane, control of hypercortisolemia may result in restoration of fertility, and therefore, contraception may be necessary [52].

The use of mitotane requires close monitoring of mitotane blood levels. Although specific target mitotane levels have not been established for the treatment of Cushing's disease, levels of 10 mg/dL have been demonstrated to control hypercortisolism in most patients. A typical starting dose is 500 mg, 3 times a day [53]. Mitotane levels should be checked every 4–8 weeks initially until target levels are reached, and then every 3 months once a therapeutic level is reached. Serum cortisol levels are not reliable, as mitotane can increase corticosteroid-binding globulin (CBG) levels, and 24-h UFC levels should be monitored instead. Thyroid-stimulating hormone (TSH) and free T_4 levels should also be monitored regularly [54].

2.2.5 Etomidate

Etomidate is an imidazole-containing agent that is most commonly used as an anesthetic agent secondary to its rapid onset of action and minimal cardiac side effects. In the 1980s, prolonged etomidate exposure was found to be associated with increased mortality rates secondary to adrenal suppression and impaired ACTH response. Ultimately, etomidate was discovered to inhibit 11β-hydroxylase as well as cholesterol side arm cleavage at high doses [37,55].

Etomidate is the only parenteral steroidogenesis inhibitor that provides rapid control of hypercortisolemia [25]. A 3–5 mg (or 0.03 mg/kg) bolus followed by continuous infusion at a rate of 0.3 mg/kg/h has been shown to cause a significant reduction in serum cortisol levels within 5 h of initiation, with peak effects seen at 11 h [56]. The doses needed to control cortisol levels have not been associated with altered mental status or sedation. That said, etomidate use requires close monitoring in an intensive care unit (ICU). Cortisol levels must be monitored every 4–6 h. Doses can be increased 0.01–0.02 mg/kg/h to a maximum dose of 0.3 mg/kg/h. Due to its rapid effects, steroid replacement should be initiated after 24 h of treatment or when serum cortisol levels drop below 18–30 mg/dL in the ICU, to prevent adrenal insufficiency; often intravenous cortisol replacement is necessary [57].

Although rapidly effective because of the need for intravenous administration and close monitoring, the use of etomidate is reserved for life-threatening hypercortisolism, such as sepsis, respiratory failure, or severe psychosis [25]. In such severe cases, etomidate may serve to stabilize a patient's condition sufficiently in order to proceed with surgery.

2.2.6 Osilodrostat

Osilodrostat (LC1699) is an oral inhibitor of aldosterone synthase (18β-hydroxylase) as well as 11β-hydroxylase at higher concentrations. Initial investigations focused on its use in the treatment of hypertension as an alternative to spironolactone or eplerenone. During these studies, higher doses were associated with an abnormal response to ACTH stimulation [58]. For this reason, Bertagna et al. designed a proof of concept study (LINC 1) to investigate the role of LCI699 in the treatment of Cushing's disease. Twelve patients with Cushing's disease and a UFC of ≥1.5 times the ULN, were treated with LCI699 at doses starting at 4 mg, titrating up to a maximum dose of 100 mg/day every 14 days, (a much higher dose range than that was used in the hypertension trials, up to 3 mg higher). Seventy days into treatment, all 12 patients achieved at least a 50% reduction in baseline UFC and 11 (92%) achieved normalization of UFC [59].

In a follow-up study (LINC 2), 4 patients controlled during the LINC 1 study and 15 new patients were treated with the same protocol. At 10 and 22 weeks, normalization of UFC was achieved in 89.5 and 78.9%, respectively. In regards to the effects on other hormones, at week 22 ACTH levels increased 4-fold, 11-deoxycorticosterone levels rose 11-fold, and testosterone levels rose to over the ULN in 75% of women, while aldosterone levels predictably declined to below the lower limit of normal (LLN) [16,52].

Clinical outcomes differed between the two studies. In LINC 1, reductions in systolic and diastolic blood pressure were observed, but there was a 3.5-kg increase in mean weight. In LINC 2, however, no significant changes were noted in weight, body mass index, and systolic or diastolic blood pressure. Mild decreases were seen in fasting plasma glucose and HbA1c. Reasons for these discrepancies are unclear, but may relate to differences in treatment modalities for hypertension and diabetes [16,52,59].

The most common adverse effects included nausea, diarrhea, asthenia, nasopharyngitis, and adrenal insufficiency. Additionally, those women with elevated testosterone levels did report new or worsening hirsutism or acne. Overall, only 1 patient discontinued the LINC 2 study secondary to an adverse effect, and 16/17 patients elected to continue on LCI699 as part of an optional extension study [16,52,59].

Overall, LC1699 demonstrated very good efficacy with a satisfactory safety profile, showing promise for the future treatment of patients with Cushing's disease. A phase 3 study is ongoing and will determine the place of osilodrostat in the medical treatment of Cushing's disease.

2.2.7 Levoketoconazole

A phase 3 study is in progress, however, no data is available, to date, in patients with Cushing's syndrome [40].

2.3 Glucocorticoid Receptor Blockers

2.3.1 Mifepristone

Mifepristone (RU486) is a synthetic steroid analog with antagonistic activity at progesterone and glucocorticoid receptors [60]. Mifepristone was first used to induce menses or to terminate pregnancies. Women who received this medication were found to have elevated cortisol levels. In a study designed to describe further the effects of mifepristone on the hypothalamic-pituitary-adrenal axis (HPAA), medical students were administered mifepristone at doses ranging from 100 to 400 mg at 2 a.m. It was discovered that mifepristone administration resulted in elevations of both cortisol and ACTH that were not suppressed by a dexamethasone challenge. In other words, mifepristone, through its direct effect on glucocorticoid receptors, blocks the negative feedback of cortisol, leading to elevations in both cortisol and ACTH [60,61]. There are now many case reports of patients with Cushing's disease treated with mifepristone [62,63].

In a phase 3, multicenter, open-label Study of the Efficacy and Safety of Mifepristone in the Treatment of Endogenous Cushing's Syndrome (SEISMIC) of 50 patients with endogenous Cushing's syndrome (43 Cushing's disease) with diabetes who had failed prior therapy, 24 weeks of mifepristone at 300–1200 mg daily resulted in significant clinical improvements and diabetes outcomes. A total of 60% demonstrated an over 25% decline in the area under the curve during a 2-h oral glucose tolerance test. Mean reductions in HbA1c and fasting plasma glucose were 1.14 and 44.3%, respectively [64]. Improvements in diastolic blood pressure, waist circumference, weight, and quality of life were also significant, with an overall clinical response rate of 87% [64,65].

Determinants of a positive global clinical response included change in weight, blood pressure, glucose levels, and appearance [65]. Based on these results, mifepristone was approved by the FDA in 2012 for treatment of hyperglycemia associated with Cushing's syndrome.

Adverse effects were present in up to 88% of patients during the SEISMIC trial. The most severe adverse effects included two patients who developed adrenal insufficiency, one severe case of hypokalemia, and one case of persistent vaginal bleeding, which led to protocol interruptions in four patients. Adrenal insufficiency during mifepristone use must be treated with high levels of glucocorticoid to overcome the glucocorticoid receptor blockade. Dexamethasone is preferred, and typically doses from 2 to 8 mg daily might be required. Hypokalemia, an expected complication based on the resultant rise in aldosterone levels secondary to a lack of negative feedback, as well as hypertension and edema, can be treated with potassium supplementation or spironolactone [63]. Through its action at the progesterone receptor, mifepristone can cause endometrial thickening and vaginal bleeding, and overall 38% of women enrolled in the SEISMIC study had one or both complications [64]. Other common side effects include nausea, fatigue, headache, vomiting, and peripheral edema [64].

Due to theoretical concerns that the rise in ACTH levels seen with mifepristone use may, in turn, promote tumor growth and Nelson's syndrome (a rare disorder that occurs in some Cushing's disease patients as a result of removing both adrenal glands), secondary analysis of the SEISMIC trial focused on ACTH levels and MRI findings in 27 patients with Cushing's disease treated with mifepristone for a median of 11.3 (range 0.5–42) months. Seventy-two percent of patients demonstrated an over twofold increase in ACTH levels. Levels of ACTH rose within 2 weeks of starting treatment, plateaued between weeks 10 and 24, and declined to baseline levels within 6 weeks of stopping mifepristone. Furthermore, log regression analysis demonstrated that ACTH change from baseline correlated with the mifepristone dose. In regard to tumor growth, four patients demonstrated gradual tumor enlargement over 20–36 months. Three of these patients had macroadenomas at baseline and one had no prior visible tumor. No relationship was found between the degree of ACTH elevation and tumor progression. Two patients demonstrated tumor regression and 30 patients had no significant change in tumor size [66].

Mifepristone has many drug–drug interactions, and caution is recommended when statins and other medications are started [63]. An ECG is recommended at the beginning of the treatment and after starting the drug. Potassium should also be normalized if possible before starting therapy; spironolactone has been helpful in addition to potassium supplementation to normalize potassium after starting mifepristone. Due to significant improvements in diabetes control, medications for diabetes have to be adjusted, sometimes immediately. During treatment with mifepristone, cortisol measurements in plasma, saliva, and urine are not reliable due to the mechanism of action of the drug.

Many patients treated with mifepristone in the phase 3 trial have noted significant clinical improvement [65]. However, its antiprogesterone effects might limit its use in some women, and the lack of reliable biochemical markers of response complicates evaluation for response and titration of therapy [25].

2.4 Combination Therapies

No single treatment option, as yet, has demonstrated overwhelming efficacy, and at higher doses the risk of serious adverse effects increases. For these reasons, some studies have sought to determine the benefit of combining treatments with differing mechanisms of action (e.g., somatostatin analogs, dopamine agonists, and steroidogenesis inhibitors) in patients who have failed surgery or are not candidates for surgery.

2.4.1 Cabergoline and Ketoconazole

In a study of cabergoline use in 12 patients with persistent Cushing's disease following unsuccessful surgery, the addition of ketoconazole (200–400 mg daily) led to normalization of UFC in 6 of 9 (66.6%) patients who were not controlled with the use of cabergoline alone after 6 months. Additionally, in two of these patients, the addition of ketoconazole allowed for a cabergoline dose reduction from 3 to 2 mg at 6 months. The three patients who were not controlled on dual therapy did demonstrate a 44.4–51.7% reduction from baseline UFC. Adverse effects included moderate dizziness or nausea in 25% of patients on cabergoline, and 11.1% demonstrated mild transaminase elevations with the addition of ketoconazole. Notably, no hypoglycemia or cardiac events were observed. Overall, all patients reported significant improvement in clinical symptoms, and overall the combination treatment was well tolerated, without interruptions of treatment. None of the patients demonstrated treatment escape, although larger long-term studies are needed [67]. In a follow-up study comparing the addition of ketoconazole to cabergoline versus the addition of cabergoline to ketoconazole therapy in patients with Cushing's disease, 79% demonstrated normalization of UFC in both groups. However, late-night salivary cortisol remained above normal in most patients, which may indicate a failure of the HPA to return to normal [68].

2.4.2 *Pasireotide, Cabergoline, and Ketoconazole*

Feelders and coworkers described the effects of step-up therapy over an 80-day trial in 17 patients with Cushing's disease [69]. Patients were initially treated with pasireotide (100 µg up to 250 µg, 3 times daily), followed by the addition of cabergoline (0.5 mg up to 1.5 mg every other day) at day 15 if UFC remained elevated, followed by the addition of 200 mg of ketoconazole at day 60 if UFC remained elevated. A total of 5 of 17 (29%) patients demonstrated normalization of UFC with pasireotide alone. A total of 4 of 17 (24%) demonstrated normalization of UFC following the addition of cabergoline. Of the remaining 8 patients with persistent UFC elevations at 60 days of treatment, the addition of ketoconazole led to normalization of UFC in 6 (75%). The overall response rate at day 80 was 88%. Improvements in UFC were accompanied by weight loss, decreased waist circumference, as well as decreased systolic and diastolic blood pressures. Adverse effects noted were an increase in HbA1c by 0.9% and a decrease in IGF-1 levels to below the LLN in 9 of 17 patients [69]. A prospective study of combination pasireotide and cabergoline is ongoing.

3 SPECIAL POPULATIONS

3.1 Life-threatening Hypercortisolism

In critically ill patients with uncontrolled hypercortisolism thought unfit to undergo pituitary surgery, bilateral adrenalectomy has traditionally been employed to control cortisol levels quickly. However, both open and laparoscopic adrenalectomy procedures are not without risk in this patient population and ultimately lead to the need for lifelong glucocorticoid and mineralocorticoid replacement, as well as the risk of Nelson's syndrome. As discussed briefly earlier, medical therapy may serve as a bridge to curative surgery and negate the need for adrenalectomy, but the medications used must have immediate and sustained effects.

In a study of 11 patients with ACTH-dependent Cushing's syndrome (four with Cushing's disease) and severe hypercortisolism, combination therapy of metyrapone, ketoconazole, and mitotane, led to significant declines in cortisol levels by 24–28 h of treatment in all 11 patients, from a median baseline value of 2737 µg/24 h to a median UFC with treatment of 50 µg/24 h. Patients also demonstrated improvements in clinical parameters, including successful control of infection, weight loss, decreased blood pressure, reduced antihypertensive medication, improved fasting plasma glucose, improved HbA1c, and reduced diabetes medication. Combination therapy was continued for 1–9 months. Metyrapone and ketoconazole were discontinued in 7 of 11 patients after an average of 3.5 months (range 3–6). Mitotane was continued for a median period of 3 months (range 2–27) with sustained normalization of UFC during monotherapy. Ultimately, all four patients with Cushing's disease underwent pituitary surgery, three with sustained remission and one requiring the addition of mitotane for a postoperative recurrence [44].

Nausea and vomiting were the most frequently reported adverse effects, present in 11 of 17 (63%) patients. These gastrointestinal side effects were mild, improved with splitting up the drugs throughout the day, and did not lead to treatment interruption. Other more serious complications included liver toxicity, hypokalemia, and acute adrenal insufficiency. Transaminase levels were also elevated with gamma-glutamyl transferase (GGT) elevations being most common (9/17 patients). Liver dysfunction led to ketoconazole dose reductions in two patients and withdrawal in one patient. Hypokalemia, likely resulting from deoxycorticosterone elevations secondary to metyrapone, was present in all patients and easily treated with a combination of potassium replacement and spironolactone. Acute adrenal insufficiency developed in four patients. The study protocol required the initiation of hydrocortisone replacement at a median dose of 32.5 mg/day to prevent iatrogenic adrenal insufficiency. However, acute adrenal insufficiency resulted from the failure to transition to intravenous HC administration during episodes of vomiting and intentional HC withdrawal in a fourth patient [44].

3.2 Medical Treatment of Patients with Cushing's Disease in Pregnancy

Pregnancy is rare in Cushing's syndrome, as cortisol excess results in androgen excess, leading to hypogonadotropic hypogonadism and infertility [25,53]. Additionally, the diagnosis of Cushing's disease can be difficult, as pregnancy is naturally accompanied by elevations in corticotropin-releasing hormone, ACTH, total cortisol, and to a lesser degree free cortisol, as the amount of free cortisol is mediated by a concurrent rise in CBG [70]. Interestingly, the causes of Cushing's syndrome in pregnancy differ from nonpregnant women in that adrenal Cushing's (Cushing's syndrome) is more prevalent than pituitary Cushing's (Cushing's disease). Regardless, when present, hypercortisolism can cause significant risks to both the fetus and mother [71].

For treatment of Cushing's disease in pregnancy, data are limited. However, in a review of the literature, if treatment is necessary, pituitary surgery typically remains first line and is performed, when possible, near the end of the first trimester and the beginning of second trimester. In regard to medical therapy, metyrapone has been used in 69% of cases in which medical therapy was employed and successfully controlled cortisol levels. Metyrapone does cross the placenta, but it has not been associated with neonatal abnormalities [72]. The greatest concern surrounding its use is the risk of adrenal insufficiency, as well as a rise in 11-deoxycorticosterone, which can lead to worsening hypertension and the risk of preeclampsia. Ketoconazole has not been used frequently, secondary to the risk of antiandrogenic activity and teratogenic effects seen in animal models. Pituitary-directed medical therapies have not been studied in pregnancy, with the exception of patients treated with cabergoline [71].

4 CONCLUSIONS

Medical therapy remains an important treatment component in Cushing's disease when pituitary surgery is neither an option, nor curative. For some patients, it can also play a role as preoperative treatment. Currently available treatments target one of three sites: (1) pituitary-directed ACTH secretion, (2) adrenal corticosteroid synthesis, and (3) glucocorticoid receptors. The somatostatin receptor ligand; pasireotide is often a first-line agent for its direct action at the pituitary, its efficacy, and its tolerability profile. That said, complete biochemical response rates are not very high, and hyperglycemia is often encountered. However, many patients benefit (both clinically and biochemically), and assessment of response can be done in 2–3 months. Studies with dopamine agonists, such as cabergoline, had contradictory results. Adrenal steroidogenesis inhibitors have been the first medications available, but are all used "off label" in the United States. Knowing each drug in detail, starting from the mechanism of action and potential adverse effects, ensures maximizing their efficacy and safety. For example, metyrapone is preferred in men, while ketoconazole would be the preferred drug for women because of changes in testosterone. Similarly, for patients who have had gastric bypass, ketoconazole, which needs gastric acidity for absorption, is not a good option. In patients with diabetes and absence of severe hypokalemia or vaginal bleeding, treatment with a glucocorticoid receptor blocker can be an initial option, with immediate improvement in hyperglycemia and clinical features. However, cortisol cannot be measured as a marker and patients require close monitoring.

Thus, combination therapies are often required both for long-term and immediate control of hypercortisolism in life-threatening Cushing's disease. As such, continued efforts in large clinical trials to investigate the efficacy and safety of specific therapies, such as osilodrostat and levoketoconazole, as well as early studies of other molecules being developed with different mechanisms of action, will be of great importance in increasing our ability to treat this difficult disease.

References

[1] Lacroix A, Feelders RA, Stratakis CA, et al. Cushing's syndrome. Lancet 2015;386(9996):913–27.
[2] Aghi MK. Management of recurrent and refractory Cushing disease. Nat Clin Pract Endocrinol Metab 2008;4(10):560–8.
[3] Sundaram NK, Carluccio A, Geer EB. Characterization of persistent and recurrent Cushing's disease. Pituitary 2013;17(4):381–91.
[4] Batista DL, Zhang X, Gejman R, et al. The effects of SOM230 on cell proliferation and adrenocorticotropin secretion in human corticotroph pituitary adenomas. J Clin Endocrinol Metab 2006;91(11):4482–8.
[5] Boscaro M, Arnaldi G. Approach to the patient with possible Cushing's syndrome. J Clin Endocrinol Metab 2009;94(9):3121–31.
[6] Cuevas-Ramos D, Fleseriu M. Treatment of Cushing's disease: a mechanistic update. J Endocrinol 2014;223(2):R19–39.
[7] Hofland LJ, van der Hoek J, Feelders R, et al. The multi-ligand somatostatin analogue SOM230 inhibits ACTH secretion by cultured human corticotroph adenomas via somatostatin receptor type 5. Eur J Endocrinol 2005;152(4):645–54.
[8] Cuevas-Ramos D, Fleseriu M. Somatostatin receptor ligands and resistance to treatment in pituitary adenomas. J Mol Endocrinol 2014;52(3):R223–40.
[9] Miller GM, Alexander JM, Bikkal HA, et al. Somatostatin receptor subtype gene expression in pituitary adenomas. J Clin Endocrinol Metab 1995;80(4):1386–92.

[10] de Bruin C, Pereira AM, Feelders RA, et al. Coexpression of dopamine and somatostatin receptor subtypes in corticotroph adenomas. J Clin Endocrinol Metab 2009;94(4):1118–24.

[11] Nielsen S, Mellemkjær S, Rasmussen LM, et al. Expression of somatostatin receptors on human pituitary adenomas in vivo and ex vivo. J Endocrinol Invest 2001;24(6):430–7.

[12] Lamberts SW. Somatostatin analogs in the management of gastrointestinal tumors. Horm Res 1988;29(2–3):118–20.

[13] van der Hoek J. Distinct functional properties of native somatostatin receptor subtype 5 compared with subtype 2 in the regulation of ACTH release by corticotroph tumor cells. Am J Physiol Endocrinol Metab 2005;289(2):E278–87.

[14] Colao A, Petersenn S, Newell-Price J, et al. A 12-month phase 3 study of pasireotide in Cushing's disease. N Engl J Med 2012;366(10):914–24.

[15] Fleseriu M, Petersenn S. Medical management of Cushing's disease: what is the future? Pituitary 2012;15(3): 330–41.

[16] Pivonello R, De Leo M, Cozzolino A, et al. The treatment of Cushing's disease. Endocr Rev 2015;36(4):385–486.

[17] Tritos NA, Biller BM. Advances in medical therapies for Cushing's syndrome. Discov Med 2012;13(69):171–9.

[18] Murray RD, Kim K, Ren SG, et al. The novel somatostatin ligand (SOM230) regulates human and rat anterior pituitary hormone secretion. J Clin Endocrinol Metab 2004;89(6):3027–32.

[19] Shimon I, Rot L, Inbar E. Pituitary-directed medical therapy with pasireotide for a corticotroph macroadenoma: pituitary volume reduction and literature review. Pituitary 2012;15(4):608–13.

[20] Simeoli C, Auriemma RS, Tortora F, et al. The treatment with pasireotide in Cushing's disease: effects of long-term treatment on tumor mass in the experience of a single center. Endocrine 2015;50(3):725–40.

[21] Henry RR, Ciaraldi TP, Armstrong D, et al. Hyperglycemia associated with pasireotide: results from a mechanistic study in healthy volunteers. J Clin Endocrinol Metab 2013;98(8):3446–53.

[22] Colao A, De Block C, Gaztambide MS, et al. Managing hyperglycemia in patients with Cushing's disease treated with pasireotide: medical expert recommendations. Pituitary 2014;17(2):180–6.

[23] Schopohl J, Gu F, Rubens R, et al. Pasireotide can induce sustained decreases in urinary cortisol and provide clinical benefit in patients with Cushing's disease: results from an open-ended, open-label extension trial. Pituitary 2015;18(5):604–12.

[24] Trementino L, Cardinaletti M, Concettoni C, et al. Up to 5-year efficacy of pasireotide in a patient with Cushing's disease and pre-existing diabetes: literature review and clinical practice considerations. Pituitary 2015;18(3):359–65.

[25] Nieman LK, Biller BM, Findling JW, et al. Treatment of Cushing's syndrome: an Endocrine Society Clinical Practice Guideline. J Clin Endocrinol Metab 2015;100(8):2807–31.

[26] Trementino L, Cardinaletti M, Concettoni C, et al. Salivary cortisol is a useful tool to assess the early response to pasireotide in patients with Cushing's disease. Pituitary 2015;18(1):60–7.

[27] Stefaneanu L, Kovacs K, Horvath E, et al. Dopamine D2 receptor gene expression in human adenohypophysial adenomas. Endocrine 2001;14(3):329–36.

[28] Pivonello R, Ferone D, de Herder WW, et al. Dopamine receptor expression and function in human normal adrenal gland and adrenal tumors. J Clin Endocrinol Metab 2004;89(9):4493–502.

[29] Pivonello R, De Martino MC, Cappabianca P, et al. The medical treatment of Cushing's disease: effectiveness of chronic treatment with the dopamine agonist cabergoline in patients unsuccessfully treated by surgery. J Clin Endocrinol Metab 2009;94(1):223–30.

[30] Godbout A, Manavela M, Danilowicz K, et al. Cabergoline monotherapy in the long-term treatment of Cushing's disease. Eur J Endocrinol 2010;163(5):709–16.

[31] Burman P, Eden-Engstrom B, Ekman B, et al. Limited value of cabergoline in Cushing's disease: a prospective study of a 6-week treatment in 20 patients. Eur J Endocrinol 2016;174(1):17–24.

[32] Auriemma RS, Pivonello R, Ferreri L, et al. Cabergoline use for pituitary tumors and valvular disorders. Endocrinol Metab Clin North Am 2015;44(1):89–97.

[33] Gadelha MR, Vieira Neto L. Efficacy of medical treatment in Cushing's disease: a systematic review. Clin Endocrinol (Oxf) 2014;80(1):1–12.

[34] Greenblatt HK, Greenblatt DJ. Liver injury associated with ketoconazole: review of the published evidence. J Clin Pharmacol 2014;54(12):1321–9.

[35] European Medicines Agency. Ketoconazole HRA recommended for approval in Cushing's syndrome. http://www.ema.europa.eu/ema/index.jsp?curl=pages/news_and_events/news/2014/09/news_detail_002174.jsp&mid=WC0b01ac058004d5c1; 2014.

[36] Pont A, Williams PL, Azhar S, et al. Ketoconazole blocks testosterone synthesis. Arch Intern Med 1982;142(12):2137–40.

[37] Feldman D. Ketoconazole and other imidazole derivatives as inhibitors of steroidogenesis. Endocr Rev 1986;7(4):409–20.

[38] Sonino N. The use of ketoconazole as an inhibitor of steroid production. N Engl J Med 1987;317(13):812–8.

[39] Castinetti F, Guignat L, Giraud P, et al. Ketoconazole in Cushing's disease: is it worth a try? J Clin Endocrinol Metab 2014;99(5):1623–30.

[40] Salvatori R, DelConte A, Geer E, et al. An open-label study to assess the safety and efficacy of levoketoconazole (COR-003) in the treatment of endogenous Cushing's syndrome. The Endocrine Society's 97th Annual Meeting. San Diego, California; 2015.

[41] Gower DB. Modifiers of steroid-hormone metabolism: a review of their chemistry, biochemistry and clinical applications. J Steroid Biochem 1974;5(5):501–23.

[42] Verhelst JA, Trainer PJ, Howlett TA, et al. Short and long-term responses to metyrapone in the medical management of 91 patients with Cushing's syndrome. Clin Endocrinol (Oxf) 1991;35(2):169–78.

[43] Daniel E, Aylwin S, Mustafa O, et al. Effectiveness of metyrapone in treating Cushing's syndrome: a retrospective multicenter study in 195 patients. J Clin Endocrinol Metab 2015;100(11):4146–54.

[44] Kamenicky P, Droumaguet C, Salenave S, et al. Mitotane, metyrapone, and ketoconazole combination therapy as an alternative to rescue adrenalectomy for severe ACTH-dependent Cushing's syndrome. J Clin Endocrinol Metab 2011;96(9):2796–804.

[45] Vilar L, Naves LA, Machado MC, et al. Medical combination therapies in Cushing's disease. Pituitary 2015;18(2):253–62.

[46] Valassi E, Crespo I, Gich I, et al. A reappraisal of the medical therapy with steroidogenesis inhibitors in Cushing's syndrome. Clin Endocrinol (Oxf) 2012;77(5):735–42.

[47] Jubiz W, Levinson RA, Meikle AW, et al. Absorption and conjugation of metyrapone during diphenylhydantoin therapy: mechanism of the abnormal response to oral metyrapone. Endocrinology 1970;86(2):328–31.

[48] Nieman LK. Medical therapy of Cushing's disease. Pituitary 2002;5(2):77–82.

[49] van Erp NP, Guchelaar HJ, Ploeger BA, et al. Mitotane has a strong and a durable inducing effect on CYP3A4 activity. Eur J Endocrinol 2011;164(4):621–6.

[50] Baudry C, Coste J, Bou Khalil R, et al. Efficiency and tolerance of mitotane in Cushing's disease in 76 patients from a single center. Eur J Endocrinol 2012;167(4):473–81.

[51] Robinson BG, Hales IB, Henniker AJ, et al. The effect of o,p'-DDD on adrenal steroid replacement therapy requirements. Clin Endocrinol (Oxf) 1987;27(4):437–44.

[52] Fleseriu M. Medical treatment of Cushing disease: new targets, new hope. Endocrinol Metab Clin North Am 2015;44(1):51–70.

[53] Biller BMK, Grossman AB, Stewart PM, et al. Treatment of adrenocorticotropin-dependent Cushing's syndrome: a consensus statement. J Clin Endocrinol Metab 2008;93(7):2454–62.

[54] Veytsman I, Nieman L, Fojo T. Management of endocrine manifestations and the use of mitotane as a chemotherapeutic agent for adrenocortical carcinoma. J Clin Oncol 2009;27(27):4619–29.

[55] Lambert A, Mitchell R, Frost J, et al. Direct in vitro inhibition of adrenal steroidogenesis by etomidate. Lancet 1983;322(8358):1085–6.

[56] Schulte HM, Benker G, Reinwein D, et al. Infusion of low-dose etomidate: correction of hypercortisolemia in patients with Cushing's syndrome and dose-response relationship in normal subjects. J Clin Endocrinol Metab 1990;70(5):1426–30.

[57] Preda VA, Sen J, Karavitaki N, et al. Etomidate in the management of hypercortisolaemia in Cushing's syndrome: a review. Eur J Endocrinol 2012;167(2):137–43.

[58] Calhoun DA, White WB, Krum H, et al. Effects of a novel aldosterone synthase inhibitor for treatment of primary hypertension: results of a randomized, double-blind, placebo- and active-controlled phase 2 trial. Circulation 2011;124(18):1945–55.

[59] Bertagna X, Pivonello R, Fleseriu M, et al. LCI699, a potent 11β-hydroxylase inhibitor, normalizes urinary cortisol in patients with Cushing's disease: results from a multicenter, proof-of-concept study. J Clin Endocrinol Metab 2014;99(4):1375–83.

[60] Bertagna X, Bertagna C, Luton J-P, et al. The new steroid analog RU 486 inhibits glucocorticoid action in man. J Clin Endocrinol Metab 1984;59(1):25–8.

[61] Bertagna X, Bertagna C, Laudat MH, et al. Pituitary-adrenal response to the antiglucocorticoid action of RU 486 in Cushing's syndrome. J Clin Endocrinol Metab 1986;63(3):639–43.

[62] Castinetti F, Conte-Devolx B, Brue T. Medical treatment of Cushing's syndrome: glucocorticoid receptor antagonists and mifepristone. Neuroendocrinology 2010;92(1):125–30.

[63] Fleseriu M, Molitch ME, Gross C, et al. A new therapeutic approach in the medical treatment of Cushing's syndrome: glucocorticoid receptor blockade with mifepristone. Endocr Pract 2013;19(2):313–26.

[64] Fleseriu M, Biller BM, Findling JW, et al. Mifepristone, a glucocorticoid receptor antagonist, produces clinical and metabolic benefits in patients with Cushing's syndrome. J Clin Endocrinol Metab 2012;97(6):2039–49.

[65] Katznelson L, Loriaux DL, Feldman D, et al. Global clinical response in Cushing's syndrome patients treated with mifepristone. Clin Endocrinol (Oxf) 2014;80(4):562–9.

[66] Fleseriu M, Findling JW, Koch CA, et al. Changes in plasma ACTH levels and corticotroph tumor size in patients with Cushing's disease during long-term treatment with the glucocorticoid receptor antagonist mifepristone. J Clin Endocrinol Metab 2014;99(10):3718–27.

[67] Vilar L, Naves LA, Azevedo MF, et al. Effectiveness of cabergoline in monotherapy and combined with ketoconazole in the management of Cushing's disease. Pituitary 2010;13(2):123–9.

[68] Barbot M, Albiger N, Ceccato F, et al. Combination therapy for Cushing's disease: effectiveness of two schedules of treatment: should we start with cabergoline or ketoconazole? Pituitary 2014;17(2):109–17.

[69] Feelders RA, de Bruin C, Pereira AM, et al. Pasireotide alone or with cabergoline and ketoconazole in Cushing's disease. N Engl J Med 2010;362:1846–8.

[70] Nieman LK, Biller BM, Findling JW, et al. The diagnosis of Cushing's syndrome: an Endocrine Society Clinical Practice Guideline. J Clin Endocrinol Metab 2008;93(5):1526–40.

[71] Bronstein MD, Machado MC, Fragoso MC. Management of endocrine disease: management of pregnant patients with Cushing's syndrome. Eur J Endocrinol 2015;173(2):R85–91.

[72] Blanco C, Maqueda E, Rubio JA, et al. Cushing's syndrome during pregnancy secondary to adrenal adenoma: metyrapone treatment and laparoscopic adrenalectomy. J Endocrinol Invest 2006;29(2):164–7.

Multidisciplinary Management of Cushing's Disease: Centers of Excellence Approach

D.F. Kelly, MD*, W. Sivakumar, MD**,
G. Barkhoudarian, MD*

*Pacific Brain Tumor Center and Pituitary Disorders Center, Providence Saint John's
Health Center and John Wayne Cancer Institute, Santa Monica, CA, United States;
**Department of Neurosurgery University of Utah, Salt Lake City, UT, United States

O U T L I N E

Cushing's Disease. http://dx.doi.org/10.1016/B978-0-12-804340-0.00008-5

1 INTRODUCTION

Cushing's disease is a complex endocrinopathy that poses significant challenges for clinicians in both diagnosis and treatment. As has been shown with other disorders, it is clear that optimal care of the Cushing's patient is best provided in a multidisciplinary collaborative environment led by experienced pituitary practitioners in endocrinology and neurosurgery, as well as other specialties that typically include radiation oncology, diagnostic and interventional neuroradiology, endocrine surgery, neuropathology, and neuropsychology. This chapter highlights the rationale for a center of excellence (COE) approach to Cushing's disease with the overall goal of using state-of-the-art techniques to confirm the presence or absence of the disease and to provide safe and effective treatment for each patient. Such COEs should also offer medical education in the management of Cushing's disease through conferences, residency or fellowship training, and patient education events; they should also contribute to research in advancing the diagnosis and treatment of Cushing's disease.

2 BRIEF HISTORY OF COEs IN MEDICINE

The term COE has been given numerous definitions often without clear consensus on its meaning. For the purposes of this chapter, we define a COE as a "cohesive team of specialists that promote collaboration and apply best practices around a specific focus area to improve results and overall outcomes" [1]. The term COE was first used in health care in 1991 by the Centers for Medicare and Medicaid Services when it started its Medicare Participating Heart Bypass Center Demonstration project aimed at lowering health care costs [2]. Since then the COE model has been successfully applied to several other major areas of medicine, including bariatric surgery [3–7], trauma [8–12], and stroke [13–16]. It is now well documented that establishing criteria and a formalized verification process for Trauma Center and Stroke Center designation has proven to be highly beneficial in improving the delivery of care to trauma and stroke victims.

3 RATIONALE FOR COE MODELS IN PITUITARY TUMOR MANAGEMENT

Given the success of COE models in other areas of medicine, numerous neurosurgeons and endocrinologists have advocated over the years for a similar approach to treating patients with pituitary tumors. In 2012, we published our article "Pituitary Centers of Excellence," which provided a detailed rationale and framework for formally establishing such centers [1]. We stressed that the complexities of diagnosing and treating patients with pituitary tumors and the need to involve multiple subspecialties in optimally treating them, mandates a comprehensive team approach of experienced clinicians. We also provided data from several studies documenting better clinical outcomes and lower complication rates for specialized high-volume surgeons in general and for transsphenoidal pituitary surgeons in particular [1,17–29]. As shown in the treatment of acromegaly, the importance of the experience of the neurosurgeon may be particularly applicable in patients with Cushing's disease who in many

TABLE 8.1 Cushing's Disease Centers of Excellence Team Roster

Team captains	Diagnostic specialties	Diagnostic and interventional specialties
Endocrinology	Diagnostic neuroradiology	Primary care
Neurosurgery	Interventional neuroradiology	Neuropsychology
	Neuroophthalmology	Otolaryngology
	Neuropathology	Radiation oncology
		Medical oncology
		Endocrine surgery

instances have small, difficult to find, and potentially invasive adenomas [17–22]. We also emphasized that further advances in the field of pituitary medicine through research and clinical trials, as well as in clinician education and patient support can best be facilitated by established pituitary COEs that routinely treat a high volume of pituitary patients.

4 ESSENTIAL COMPONENTS OF A TEAM APPROACH TO CUSHING'S DISEASE

Since most patients with Cushing's disease are diagnosed by an endocrinologist and treated surgically by a neurosurgeon, these two clinicians should be the team leaders of any COE with a focus on Cushing's disease. However, given the broad clinical manifestations of Cushing's disease and the multiple diagnostic and treatment options available for Cushing's patients, other key practitioners are needed to provide a comprehensive team approach. As shown in Table 8.1, in addition to the "team captains" from endocrinology and neurosurgery, other key specialties should include radiation oncology, diagnostic and interventional neuroradiology, medical oncology, neuroophthalmology, otolaryngology, endocrine surgery, and neuropathology. Given the psychosocial stresses and neurocognitive issues that face many Cushing's disease patients both before and after treatment, a neuropsychologist should also be part of the Cushing's team of experts. Finally, since Cushing's disease impacts so many areas of an individual's health, close involvement by a patient's primary care physician is also strongly encouraged.

The optimal level of experience and expertise that each team member of a pituitary COE should have remains unclear and controversial [1]. Considering the five major subspecialties involved in diagnosing and treating Cushing's disease (i.e., neurosurgery, endocrinology, interventional neuroradiology, radiation oncology, and endocrine surgery), as noted earlier, there are data that support the simple concept of "more is better" when it comes to experience and patient outcomes [21,23,29]. Regarding neurosurgical expertise, each center should ideally have at least one neurosurgeon with extensive transsphenoidal surgical experience after completing residency training, a substantial center case volume of pituitary adenoma surgery, and a demonstrated interest in Cushing's disease [1,17–21]. As to what this surgical volume should be is unclear, but a reasonable threshold would be a minimum of 50 pituitary adenoma surgeries a year [24–30]. Ideally, the endocrinologist team captain should have a majority, or significant minority, of their clinical practice in treating patients with pituitary tumors, specifically Cushing's disease [31]. The interventional neuroradiologist and their interventional team who may perform inferior petrosal sinus sampling (IPSS), should also have a significant track record in this procedure, which calls for precision catheter placement, injection of provocative hormones, as well as precise timing and collection of central and peripheral blood specimens for assessment of adrenocorticotropic hormone (ACTH) levels [32]. The radiation oncologists and their team should also be highly experienced, particularly in the treatment of sellar and parasellar tumors, using both stereotactic radiosurgery (SRS) and stereotactic radiotherapy (SRT) [33]. Tumor targeting and treatment planning of SRS and SRT should ideally be done in collaboration with the neurosurgeon who performed the patient's pituitary surgery. Finally, the endocrine surgeon who may perform bilateral adrenalectomy (BLA) should ideally be fellowship trained in endocrine surgery and have a substantial track record and expertise in performing minimally invasive laparoscopic adrenalectomy [34].

5 TEAM MANAGEMENT OF THE CUSHING'S DISEASE PATIENT OVER TIME

To understand why a team approach to Cushing's disease is essential, it is helpful to consider Cushing's disease as a chronic condition that may require ongoing diagnostic and interventional management over many years. As such, Cushing's disease patients need care from when the disease is first considered based on signs and symptoms, through diagnostic evaluations, definitive treatment, and short- and long-term follow-up. Given the potential for disease recurrence many years after initial remission, long-term surveillance of all Cushing's disease patients is essential [31]. If recurrence does occur, then several treatment options are available, which may involve multiple other specialists. Finally, psychosocial support should also be available for Cushing's disease patients even after achieving disease remission as the lingering neurobehavioral effects of the disease may persist for years or be lifelong.

As shown in Fig. 8.1, the management of Cushing's disease patients involves multiple practitioners at various times, providing different but essential aspects of care. Initially, when the diagnosis is first being considered, the key practitioners will be the primary care physician and the endocrinologist. Once the suspicion of Cushing's syndrome is confirmed and Cushing's disease is strongly considered, then input from diagnostic neuroradiology and neurosurgery is typically warranted. If a patient is confirmed to have ACTH-dependent Cushing's disease and the endocrinologist is trying to distinguish between Cushing's disease and ectopic Cushing's, interventional neuroradiology may be needed to perform IPSS. If the patient is shown to have a macroadenoma causing optic apparatus compression or has visual complaints unexplained by neuroimaging, then a neuroophthalmological evaluation would be warranted. Finally, if there are significant neuropsychiatric issues and the patient is amenable to an evaluation and possible counseling, then input from a neuropsychologist or other mental health specialist would be reasonable.

Once the diagnosis of Cushing's disease is established and it has been jointly decided by an endocrinologist and a neurosurgeon that transsphenoidal adenoma removal is indicated, the patient should have the appropriate preoperative medical evaluations and clearances, which may include a cardiologist or other specialists, depending on the patient's comorbidities. For

Time-line of the team approach for Cushing's disease

Diagnosis	Transsph surgery	Post op follow-up	Disease recurrence	Medical therapy	Radio surgery	BLA	Long-term follow-up
Primary care Endocrinology Neurosurgery Dxic NeuroRad Inter NeuroRad Neuropsych Neuroophthalmology[a]	Neurosurgery Otolaryngology Endocrinology Neuropathology	Endocrinology Neurosurgery Otolaryngology Primary care Neuropsych	Endocrinology Neurosurgery Dxic NeuroRad Inter NeuroRad Neuropsych Medical oncology[b]	Endocrinology Medical oncology[b]	Radiation oncology Neurosurgery Dxic NeuroRad Endocrinology	Endocrinology Endocrine surg Pathology	Endocrinology Primary care Neurosurgery Dxic NeuroRad Neuropsych

FIGURE 8.1 **Timeline of the team approach for Cushing's disease.** *BLA*, Bilateral adrenalectomy; *Dxic neurorad*, diagnostic neuroradiology; *inter neurorad*, interventional neuroradiology; *neuropsych*, neuropsychology; *surg*, surgery; *transsph*, transsphenoidal. [a]For patients with macroadenomas causing optic apparatus compression. [b]For patients with refractory or atypical adenomas who may be candidates for tumor profiling, chemotherapy, and or clinical trials.

most patients undergoing transsphenoidal adenomectomy, a neurosurgeon and an endocrinologist handle the in-hospital perioperative management. The key immediate postoperative issues that endocrinology and neurosurgery jointly manage are monitoring early remission status (i.e., documenting subnormal serum cortisol levels) and the need for replacement glucocorticoids, as well as monitoring and treating diabetes insipidus and other fluid/electrolyte abnormalities [35–36]. Currently, at many centers performing endonasal endoscopic pituitary surgery, an otolaryngologist will also be involved in both the surgery and perioperative care [37]. Neuropathology also has a key role at this time, confirming the diagnosis of Cushing's disease based upon histopathology and immunostaining tests.

During the first several postoperative weeks after hospital discharge, a neurosurgeon, endocrinologist, otolaryngologist, and primary care physician will lead patient management. A neuropsychologist may also be involved, depending on the patient's postoperative emotional state. A neurosurgeon sees the patient at least once during this period and monitors for any postoperative complications (e.g., cerebrospinal fluid leak or meningitis). An otolaryngologist, if involved, typically sees the patient at least twice during this period to monitor sinonasal healing, perform nasal debridements, and address any related complications, such as sinusitis or epistaxis. An endocrinologist and a neurosurgeon jointly monitor glucocorticoid replacement in patients achieving early remission; delayed hyponatremia, which occurs in up to 10% of patients within a week after surgery; and possible diabetes insipidus [38]. An endocrinologist also monitors the patient for the development of new postoperative anterior hormone deficiencies and the need for new hormone replacement therapies. For Cushing's disease patients with preoperative hypertension and diabetes mellitus, the endocrinologist and primary care physician monitor and adjust the need for antihypertensive therapy and diabetes medications, both of which typically decrease significantly after successful surgery.

Over the first 6–12 months after transsphenoidal surgery for Cushing's disease, the endocrinologist has the primary role of managing the patient's glucocorticoid taper and establishing whether remission has been achieved. The primary care physician and the neurosurgeon typically see the patient on an as-needed basis during this period. Once remission is established, the endocrinologist continues to monitor remission status (as described in Chapter 9) typically by measuring 24-h urinary free cortisol levels and serum ACTH and cortisol levels at least every 6 months as well. The neurosurgeon typically continues to see the patient at least annually. Both the endocrinologist and the neurosurgeon should carefully assess the patient at each visit for possible symptoms and signs of Cushing's disease recurrence (as described in Chapter 3). If there is a clinical suspicion of recurrence, then the appropriate testing (as described in Chapter 5) is performed.

For patients with Cushing's disease recurrence or for those patients who never achieved remission after initial transsphenoidal surgery, a "team" consensus is necessary as to the next course of treatment. Whether to have repeat transsphenoidal surgery, medical therapy, radiosurgery, bilateral adrenalectomies, or to continue to observe, is a complex decision and typically requires the input of not only endocrinology and neurosurgery but also of neuroradiology, radiation oncology, and in some cases, medical oncology and endocrine surgery. Once a treatment approach is chosen and performed, the endocrinologist and other involved treating physicians closely monitor the patient for evidence of remission and treatment-related complications or side effects. For patients undergoing medical therapy, this monitoring is done almost exclusively by an endocrinologist and a primary care physician. For patients undergoing radiosurgery, the radiation oncologist, neurosurgeon, and endocrinologist are primarily involved. For patients undergoing bilateral adrenalectomy, the endocrine surgeon and endocrinologist are primarily involved. The psychological toll of Cushing's disease recurrence should also be anticipated; distress screening and appropriate interventions by a neuropsychologist or other mental health professional should be available to these patients.

In summary, the long-term management of Cushing's disease needs to be overseen by the endocrinologist and neurosurgeon. However, input from multiple specialists is essential to the successful treatment of these patients, particularly for those who may have persistent or recurrent Cushing's disease after initial surgery. Close surveillance of all Cushing's disease patients should continue for well over a decade even after initially successful transsphenoidal surgery, given that recurrence of disease can occur in up to 25% of patients [39].

6 THE ROLE OF PITUITARY COEs IN ADVANCING EDUCATION AND RESEARCH IN CUSHING'S DISEASE

As the title of this book indicates, Cushing's disease may be uncommon, but it is certainly not rare. Epidemiological data in fact suggest that a major challenge in the overall treatment of Cushing's disease is shortening the delays in diagnosis and definitive treatment that are so common (Chapter 5). Once diagnosed, finding an experienced team to treat Cushing's disease effectively is the next challenge. Given these deficiencies in the broader population health picture of treating Cushing's disease, pituitary COEs should take the lead in (1) raising awareness within the medical community of the symptom complex of Cushing's disease, and (2) expanding expertise in the comprehensive treatment of Cushing's disease. To raise Cushing's disease awareness, pituitary COEs should be involved in regular continuing medical education events for physicians, nurses, and mental health providers and should provide easily accessible clinical information on their web sites about the diagnostic workup and treatments available for Cushing's disease patients. To expand the expertise of treating patients with Cushing's disease, pituitary COEs should also be involved in training and education in pituitary medicine with a focus on Cushing's disease. Such activities can be part of a residency training program in neurosurgery or fellowship training in neurosurgery, endocrinology, radiation oncology, interventional neuroradiology, or endocrine surgery. It is critical that the trainees understand the importance of this multidisciplinary approach to managing pituitary disorders in general and Cushing's disease in particular. Finally, to raise public awareness, pituitary COEs should provide community outreach related to pituitary hormonal disorders in general and Cushing's disease in particular, including patient education events and support groups.

Given the complexities and insufficiencies in diagnosing and treating patients with Cushing's disease, pituitary COEs should also lead the way in helping advance the field of pituitary hormonal medicine as it relates specifically to this disorder. Pituitary COEs can do so by participating in Cushing's disease–related research, which may include basic or translational research efforts, involving adenoma specimen collection, epidemiological studies, clinical outcome studies, and clinical trials. To achieve this goal, all pituitary COEs should be encouraged to establish consistent clinical treatment protocols, maintain a detailed clinical outcomes database, and have an adenoma tissue repository if sufficient tissue is available at surgery. Replicated around the country, this effort could result in a highly valuable national clinical registry to assess efficacy and safety of new surgical, radiation, or endocrine interventions and in helping to conduct clinical trials. Having a nationwide tissue repository could be used to understand the genomics of typical and atypical subtypes of ACTH-secreting pituitary adenomas and the rare pituitary carcinomas and to help create targeted therapies for these refractory adenoma subtypes. Notably, many of these efforts are currently ongoing at established pituitary centers, but coordination and collaboration of these efforts are needed. An excellent example of an active multicenter clinical research effort in endoscopic pituitary surgery is that lead by Dr. Little and his coworkers [40].

7 THE FUTURE OF PITUITARY CENTERS OF EXCELLENCE AND WORKING WITH AVAILABLE EXPERTISE

While the criteria for establishment of pituitary COEs was proposed several years ago, and there appears to be strong interest and support for this effort, particularly among those practitioners who regularly treat pituitary patients, the actual implementation of COE criteria and a verification process within the organized societies of endocrinology and neurosurgery has lagged. This lack of progress is related in part to frank opposition to establishing rigid criteria for pituitary COEs, which critics claim have the potential for being too exclusive, restricting the scope of practice for some clinicians and lacking the "data" that clearly show the superiority of such a pituitary COE model [1]. If a verification process for pituitary COEs is to occur, it is also unclear which organizations should lead this effort: the Pituitary Society, the Endocrine Society, the American Association of Neurological Surgeons, the International Society of Pituitary Surgeons, or a combination of these societies.

In the meantime, to provide optimal care for Cushing's disease patients specifically and for pituitary patients in general, clinicians involved in their care should strive to create an experienced multidisciplinary team as we have described in this chapter. For a pituitary practitioner who has limited experience in treating patients with Cushing's disease, partnering with an established COE should be encouraged. If the team leaders of endocrinology and neurosurgery are working well together but a given area of expertise is lacking (e.g., interventional neuroradiology to perform IPSS or an experienced endocrine surgeon to perform BLA), then such collaborators at other centers should be sought. Ultimately, by using this team approach to treat and monitor Cushing's disease, whether all practitioners are within the same center or are regionally connected, patients can receive the best possible care.

References

[1] McLaughlin N, Laws ER, Oyesiku NM, et al. Pituitary centers of excellence. Neurosurgery 2012;71(5):916–24.

[2] Hamilton JF. Centers of excellence: an evolving concept and controversy. Bull AAOS 2006;54(1.). Available from: http://www2.aaos.org/bulletin/feb06/fline8.asp.

[3] Champion JK, Pories WJ. Centers of excellence for bariatric surgery. Surg Obes Relat Dis 2005;1(2):148–51.

[4] Hollenbeak CS, Rogers AM, Barrus B, et al. Surgical volume impacts bariatric surgery mortality: a case for centers of excellence. Surgery 2008;144(5):736–43.

[5] Kohn GP, Galanko JA, Overby DW, et al. High case volumes and surgical fellowships are associated with improved outcomes for bariatric surgery patients: a justification of current credentialing initiatives for practice and training. J Am Coll Surg 2010;210(6):909–18.

[6] Pratt GM, McLees B, Pories WJ. The ASBS Bariatric Surgery Centers of Excellence program: a blueprint for quality improvement. Surg Obes Relat Dis 2006;2(5):497–503.

[7] DeMaria EJ, Pate V, Warthen M, et al. Baseline data from American Society for Metabolic and Bariatric Surgery–designated Bariatric Surgery Centers of Excellence using the Bariatric Outcomes Longitudinal Database. Surg Obes Relat Dis 2010;6(4):347–55.

[8] Jurkovich GJ. Systematic review of trauma system effectiveness based on registry comparisons. J Trauma 1999;47(Suppl. 3):S46–55.

[9] Mann NC, MacKenzie EJ, Jurkovich GJ, et al. Systematic review of published evidence regarding trauma system effectiveness. J Trauma 1999;47(Suppl. 3):S25–33.

[10] Kelly DF. Advances in management of neurosurgical trauma: USA and Canada. World J Surg 2001;25(9):1979–85.

[11] Sampalis JS, Lavoie A, Fréchette P, et al. Trauma care regionalization: a process-outcome evaluation. J Trauma 1999;46(4):579–81.

[12] Chiara O. Organized trauma care: does volume matter and do trauma centers save lives. Curr Opin Crit Care 2003;9(6):510–4.

[13] Alberts MJ, Latchaw RE, Jagoda A, et al. Recommendations for the establishment of primary stroke centers. Brain Attack Coalition. JAMA 2000;282(23):3102–9.

[14] Alberts MJ, Selman WR, Shephard T, et al. Recommendations for comprehensive stroke centers: a consensus statement from the Brain Attack Coalition. Stroke 2005;36(7):1597–616.

[15] Lichtman JH, Wang Y, Watanabe E, et al. Stroke patient outcomes in US hospitals before the start of the Joint Commission Primary Stroke Center certification program. Stroke 2009;40(11):3574–9.

[16] Lichtman JH, Wang Y, Watanabe E, et al. Outcomes after ischemic stroke for hospitals with and without Joint Commission–certified primary stroke centers. Neurology 2011;76(23):1976–82.

[17] Yamada S, Aiba T, Takada K, et al. Retrospective analysis of long-term surgical results in acromegaly: preoperative and postoperative factors predicting outcome. Clin Endocrinol (Oxf) 1996;45(3):291–8.

[18] Gittoes NJ, Sheppard MC, Johnson AP, et al. Outcome of surgery for acromegaly—the experience of a dedicated pituitary surgeon. QJM 1999;92(12):741–5.

[19] Erturk E, Tuncel E, Kiyici S, et al. Outcome of surgery for acromegaly performed by different surgeons: importance of surgical experience. Pituitary 2005;8(2):93–7.

[20] Bates PR, Carson MN, Trainer PJ, et al. Wide variation in surgical outcomes for acromegaly in the UK. Clin Endocrinol (Oxf) 2008;68(1):136–42.

[21] Shahlaie K, McLaughlin N, Kassam AB, et al. The role of outcomes data for assessing the expertise of a pituitary surgeon. Curr Opin Endocrinol Diabetes Obes 2010;17(4):369–76.

[22] Swearingen B. Update on pituitary surgery. J Clin Endocrinol Metab 2012;97(4):1073–81.

[23] Ciric I, Ragin A, Baumgartner C, et al. Complications of transsphenoidal surgery: results of a national survey, review of the literature, and personal experience. Neurosurgery 1997;40(2):225–36.

[24] Barker FG 2nd, Klibanski A, Swearingen B. Transsphenoidal surgery for pituitary tumors in the United States, 1996–2000: mortality, morbidity, and the effects of hospital and surgeon volume. J Clin Endocrinol Metab 2003;88(10):4709–19.

[25] Ahmed S, Elsheikh M, Stratton IM, et al. Outcome of transsphenoidal surgery for acromegaly and its relationship to surgical experience. Clin Endocrinol (Oxf) 1999;50(5):561–7.

[26] Fatemi N, Dusick JR, Mattozo C, et al. Pituitary hormonal loss and recovery after transsphenoidal adenoma removal. Neurosurgery 2008;63(4):709–18.

[27] Jane JA Jr, Laws ER Jr. The surgical management of pituitary adenomas in a series of 3,093 patients. J Am Coll Surg 2001;193(6):651–9.

[28] Laws ER, Jane JA Jr. Pituitary tumors—long-term outcomes and expectations. Clin Neurosurg 2001;48:306–19.

[29] Wilson CB. Surgical management of pituitary tumors. J Clin Endocrinol Metab 1997;82(8):2381–5.

[30] Hammer GD, Tyrrell JB, Lamborn KR, et al. Transsphenoidal microsurgery for Cushing's disease: initial outcome and long-term results. J Clin Endocrinol Metab 2004;89(12):6348–57.

[31] Psaras T, Milian M, Hattermann V, et al. Aftercare in patients with Cushing's disease and acromegaly: is there room for improvement? Acta Neurochir (Wien) 2010;152(2):271–8.

[32] Pecori Giraldi F, Cavallo LM, Tortora F, et al. The role of inferior petrosal sinus sampling in ACTH-dependent Cushing's syndrome: review and joint opinion statement by members of the Italian Society for Endocrinology, Italian Society for Neurosurgery, and Italian Society for Neuroradiology. Neurosurg Focus 2015;38(2):E5.

[33] Tritos NA, Biller BM. Update on radiation therapy in patients with Cushing's disease. Pituitary 2015;18(2):263–8.

[34] Reincke M, Ritzel K, Osswald A, et al. A critical reappraisal of bilateral adrenalectomy for ACTH-dependent Cushing's syndrome. Eur J Endocrinol 2015;173(4):M23–32.

[35] McLaughlin N, Cohan P, Barnett P, et al. Early morning cortisol levels as predictors of short-term and long-term adrenal function after endonasal transsphenoidal surgery for pituitary adenomas and Rathke's cleft cysts. World Neurosurg 2013;80(5):569–75.

[36] Esposito F, Dusick JR, Cohan P, et al. Clinical review: early morning cortisol levels as a predictor of remission after transsphenoidal surgery for Cushing's disease. J Clin Endocrinol Metab 2006;91(1):7–13.

[37] Lobo B, Heng A, Barkhoudarian G, et al. The expanding role of the endonasal endoscopic approach in pituitary and skull base surgery: a 2014 perspective. Surg Neurol Int 2015;6:82.

[38] Cote DJ, Alzarea A, Acosta MA, et al. Predictors and rates of delayed symptomatic hyponatremia after transsphenoidal surgery: a systematic review. World Neurosurg 2016;88:1–6.

[39] Patil CG, Prevedello DM, Lad SP, et al. Late recurrences of Cushing's disease after initial successful transsphenoidal surgery. J Clin Endocrinol Metab 2008;93(2):358–62.

[40] Little AS, Kelly DF, Milligan J, et al. Comparison of sinonasal quality of life and health status in patients undergoing microscopic and endoscopic transsphenoidal surgery for pituitary lesions: a prospective cohort study. J Neurosurg 2015;123(3):799–807.

Posttreatment Management of Cushing's Disease

A. Prete, MD*, R. Salvatori, MD**

*Unit of Endocrinology, Faculty of Medicine, Catholic University of the Sacred Heart, Rome, Italy; **Pituitary Center, Department of Medicine, Division of Endocrinology, Diabetes, and Metabolism, Johns Hopkins University School of Medicine, Baltimore, MD, United States

O U T L I N E

1 INTRODUCTION

Transsphenoidal surgery, aiming to completely remove the adrenocorticotropic hormone–(ACTH-) secreting pituitary tumor, is the first-line treatment for Cushing's disease. The initial overall remission rates for primary pituitary surgery range between 25% and 100%, according to case series, with a recurrence rate of 0–51.2% for all patients [1]. Time to recurrence is highly variable, ranging between months to several years after primary surgery, explaining the need for lifelong follow-up. Numerous factors have been associated with the outcome of pituitary surgery for Cushing's disease (Table 9.1) [2,3].

Unsuccessful pituitary surgery is a major problem in the management of patients with Cushing's disease. The approach to recurrent and persistent disease encompasses a wide range of clinical challenges, including laboratory confirmation of recurrent or persistent disease, the choice of which second-line (and sometimes third-line) therapy is best for the patient, as well as the management of adverse events and complications associated with different therapeutic approaches.

Follow-up of patients who achieve persistent remission poses several management issues as well, such as dosing of ongoing glucocorticoid replacement therapy, assessment of the recovery of normal adrenal function, and timing for clinical, biochemical, and radiological studies throughout long- and short-term follow-up.

TABLE 9.1 Factors Related to Cure After Pituitary Surgery for Cushing's Disease

Development of adrenal insufficiency	The development of adrenal insufficiency and the degree of hypocortisolism are the most useful tools for predicting remission and recurrence.
Nonprovocative and provocative laboratory tests	(Tables 9.2 and 9.3)
Patient and biochemical features	• Male gender is associated with local aggressiveness of tumors and negative preoperative pituitary imaging • Cyclic Cushing's disease is more likely to relapse
Tumor features	Factors associated with a higher risk of recurrence or persistent disease: • No tumor identification at preoperative MRI • Pituitary adenoma > 2 cm • Suprasellar extension • Cavernous sinus invasion • Involvement of the pituitary intermediate lobe • Ectopic pituitary adenoma (cavernous sinus, suprasellar, pituitary stalk)
Surgery	• Tumor identification at surgical intervention • Surgeon's experience
Pathological findings	Factors associated with a higher risk of recurrence or persistent disease: • No tumor confirmation at final histology • Pituitary hyperplasia at final histology • Absence of peritumoral Crooke's cells[a] • Presence of intratumoral Crooke's cells (Crooke's cell adenomas)[b]

ACTH, Adrenocorticotropic hormone; and MRI, magnetic resonance imaging.
[a]*Crooke's cells (also known as basophil cell hyaline degeneration) are large corticotroph cells with an intracytoplasmic hyaline ring (keratin filaments), paranuclear vacuoles (lysosomes), and secretory granules. These cells are typically observed in both endogenous and exogenous Cushing's syndrome [2]. Absence of Crooke's cells in the paraadenomatous tissue may be a sign of incomplete tumor removal.*
[b]*Crooke's cell adenoma is a very rare and locally aggressive subtype of ACTH-secreting pituitary adenomas [3].*

2 DEFINITIONS: CURED, PERSISTENT, AND RECURRENT CUSHING'S DISEASE

No clear criteria have been established to define "cured," "persistent," and "recurrent" Cushing's disease after surgical treatment. Two major problems account for the lack of consensus in the literature. On the one hand, biochemical and clinical parameters used for classifying a patient's response after treatment (especially primary pituitary surgery) vary among studies, making it hard to compare data adequately. On the other hand, duration of follow-up is highly variable in different studies: this may account for some of the differences among outcomes in case series, underlying the importance of long-term ongoing evaluation in patients treated for Cushing's disease.

"Cured" Cushing's disease means that the patient has gone into persistent remission, defined either as normalization of the hypothalamic-pituitary-adrenal axis (HPAA) after surgery or radiotherapy (RT), or as hypoadrenalism following pituitary surgery or bilateral adrenalectomy (BLA). Positive clinical and biochemical responses with cortisol-lowering medications cannot be considered "curative," as withholding the drug causes Cushing's disease to relapse and clinical and biochemical data to worsen. Lifelong follow-up is mandatory for patients who undergo "curative" neurosurgery, since they can present with a relapse of Cushing's disease many years after pituitary surgery. In fact Cushing's disease recurs in 3–22% of patients after more than 3 years of follow-up and in 20–25% of patients at 10 years [4]. Recurrence of Cushing's disease has been reported up to 29 years after "curative" surgery [5]. Longstanding surveillance is also required for patients subjected to "curative" RT and BLA in order to detect potential long-term consequences (e.g., delayed hypopituitarism after RT or tumor growth after adrenal surgery).

"Persistent" Cushing's disease is defined as sustained hypercortisolism requiring further treatment after pituitary surgery. Diagnosing the persistence of Cushing's disease after RT (conventional RT or radiosurgery [RS]) requires longer follow-up, as this approach can lead to progressive disease control over a period of several months or years. "Recurrent" Cushing's disease is defined as hypercortisolism requiring further treatment, occurring after transient resolution of the abnormal cortisol secretion. Residual corticotroph tumor cells within the pituitary gland or surrounding structures cause both persistent and recurrent Cushing's disease. In recurrent Cushing's disease, a near-total pituitary tumor removal leads to a sudden decrease of ACTH plasma levels with temporary eucortisolemia or even adrenal insufficiency; when remaining tumor cells start producing enough ACTH to over stimulate the adrenal glands, Cushing's disease relapses [6]. Very rarely, persistent and recurrent Cushing's disease can be seen after BLA: this might be caused by the presence of adrenal gland remnants, accessory adrenal glands, or ectopic adrenal tissue [7].

Establishing remission after pituitary surgery for Cushing's disease can be challenging. Although the development of adrenal insufficiency and the duration of exogenous glucocorticoid requirement after surgery are usually seen as a positive predictive factor, other biochemical data may be used [8]. Several nonprovocative and provocative laboratory tests have been proposed (both alone and in combination), but wide heterogeneity exists among studies. No clear consensus exists about which test is more accurate, when to perform laboratory evaluation, and how to interpret the results [1,8].

TABLE 9.2 Criteria for Establishing Remission After Pituitary Surgery: Nonprovocative Tests

Test	When to Perform	Proposed Cutoffs	Features
Postsurgical morning serum cortisol	1–7 days after pituitary surgery[a]	<1.8 µg/dL (50 nmol/L): remission very likely <5 µg/dL (138 nmol/L): remission likely >7.2 µg/dL (200 nmol/L): recurrence likely	• Easy to perform • No clear cutoff values • No consensus on ideal time for collection • It can be influenced by preoperative medical treatment[b] and postoperative exogenous glucocorticoid administration[a] • It can be influenced by CBG levels: patients having high CBG levels are likely to have high postsurgical serum cortisol values
Late-night salivary cortisol	Within 3 months after pituitary surgery	<1.9 nmol/L (0.7 ng/mL): remission likely >7.4 nmol/L (2.7 ng/mL): recurrence likely	• Easy to perform • Little data • Limited availability of salivary cortisol assays • No clear cutoff values
24-h UFC	1–7 days after pituitary surgery[a]	<28–56 nmol/day (10–20 µg/day)	• No clear cutoff values • No consensus on ideal time for collection • It requires patients' compliance and longstanding exogenous glucocorticoid withholding
Plasma ACTH	12–24 h or days after pituitary surgery	<20 pg/mL or decrease > 40% compared to baseline: remission likely	• Easy to perform • Little data • Conflicting results • No clear cutoff values

Note. This table reports the most frequent and recent findings. Differences among studies do occur.

ACTH, Adrenocorticotropic hormone; CBG, corticosteroid-binding globulin; and UFC, urinary free cortisol.

[a]*Some authors suggest that late measurement of morning serum cortisol (1–6 months after pituitary surgery) and 24-h UFC (>6 weeks after pituitary surgery) better predict remission. It has been hypothesized that, due to longstanding Cushing's disease and adrenal overstimulation, an autonomous adrenal cortisol production could be expected for weeks to months after surgery despite a drop in ACTH plasma levels, leading to potential false-positive results of laboratory tests soon after surgery. Conversely, exogenous glucocorticoid administration in the immediate postoperative period could inhibit ACTH secretion by a residual adenoma, masking endogenous hypercortisolism and leading to potential false-negative results of morning serum cortisol and 24-h UFC.*

[b]*Use of cortisol-lowering or blocking drugs before surgery may derepress normal ACTH-secreting cells, leading to adrenal stimulation with detectable morning serum cortisol after surgery.*

2.1 Nonprovocative Tests

Several nonprovocative laboratory tests have been proposed for the diagnosis of "cured," "persistent," and "recurrent" Cushing's disease after neurosurgery (Table 9.2).

Postsurgical morning serum cortisol is the most used and investigated test to establish remission, while late-night salivary cortisol is considered the easiest and most accurate tool to screen for Cushing's disease persistence or recurrence after pituitary surgery. "Inappropriately low" bedtime salivary cortisol, however, shows promising results in predicting remission [8–10]. Successive laboratory confirmation can be obtained with other strategies, such as overnight or classical 2-day low-dose dexamethasone suppression testing (DST) and 24-h urinary free cortisol (UFC). The 24-h UFC assessment by mass spectrometry is more analytically specific as compared to traditional immunoassays, is currently considered the "gold standard" for biochemical evaluation [11], and is used with increasing frequency in clinical settings [8].

It is worth noting that none of the nonprovocative tests shows reliable accuracy in predicting long-term remission. For example, very low or undetectable postsurgical morning serum cortisol is observed in approximately 10% of patients who will later relapse, and conversely, some patients with elevated or normal postsurgical morning serum cortisol will go into persistent remission [12]. Moreover, in mild forms of Cushing's disease, including de novo, persistent, or recurrent disease, levels of 24-h UFC may be within the reference range [13,14]. A possible explanation for this phenomenon is that adrenal steroid production has fluctuations during the day both in normal subjects and in patients with Cushing's disease, often causing an overlap between normal and pathological conditions [15]. In addition, patients with active Cushing's disease present an intrapatient variability of approximately 50% in 24-h UFC [16]. A minimum of two 24-h UFC samples should be obtained for validating the diagnosis of cortisol excess [8]. All of this emphasizes the importance of longstanding surveillance in all patients who undergo apparently curative surgery.

2.2 Provocative Tests

Several provocative laboratory tests have been proposed for the diagnosis of "cured," "persistent," and "recurrent" Cushing's disease after neurosurgery (Table 9.3) [17].

A clear role for provocative tests has not been established in patients surgically treated for Cushing's disease, and to date, they do not appear to offer advantages over nonprovocative tests, especially morning serum cortisol and late-night salivary cortisol.

3 MANAGEMENT OF PERSISTENT AND RECURRENT CUSHING'S DISEASE

The first step when evaluating a patient with persistent or recurrent ACTH-dependent hypercortisolism following pituitary surgery is to ask if the diagnosis of Cushing's disease is correct. Most of the time laboratory evaluation and neuroimaging obtained at baseline clearly indicate that ACTH is of pituitary origin. Ectopic sources of ACTH (and, rarely, corticotropin-releasing hormone [CRH]) can mimic the presentation of ACTH-secreting pituitary adenomas both on a clinical and biochemical basis [18]. Similarly, pseudo-Cushing's may mimic Cushing's disease, with inferior petrosal sinus sampling (IPSS) pointing to the pituitary as the source of ACTH. Therefore, when persistent or recurrent Cushing's disease is suspected, we suggest a careful reexamination of all existing clinical, laboratory, radiological, and histopathological data and retesting the patient, if there are any doubts.

When the diagnosis of persistent or recurrent Cushing's disease is established, magnetic resonance imaging (MRI) of the pituitary gland should be performed to detect residual or recurrent disease. Bilateral IPSS is not needed if abnormal pituitary ACTH secretion has already been confirmed previously (by previous IPSS or positive pathology), given that accuracy of

TABLE 9.3   Establishing Remission after Pituitary Surgery: Provocative Tests

Test	When to Perform	Proposed Cutoffs	Features
Low-dose DST	Days or months after pituitary surgery	*After 1-mg overnight low-dose DST:* Remission has been considered likely for cortisol levels < 5 µg/dL (138 nmol/L). The most stringent proposed cutoff is cortisol < 1.8 µg/dL (50 nmol/L). *After 2-mg overnight low-dose DST:* Remission is likely for cortisol levels < 2 µg/dL (55 nmol/L). *After 2-mg 2 days low-dose DST:* Remission has been considered likely for cortisol levels < 5 µg/dL (138 nmol/L). The most stringent proposed cutoff is cortisol < 2.2 µg/dL (60 nmol/L).	• No consensus on dexamethasone dose and on the time to perform the test • No consensus on cutoff values • Dexamethasone metabolism can be influenced by several drugs affecting its hepatic clearance • Serum cortisol is influenced by drugs affecting CBG levels
CRH testing	Days or months after pituitary surgery	Blunted responses of plasma ACTH and serum cortisol after CRH administration predict remission (significant differences in terms of cutoffs have been reported).[a]	• Expensive test • Different protocols using either human or animal CRH • No consensus on timing to perform the test • No consensus on cutoff values
DDAVP testing	Days or months after pituitary surgery	No response of plasma ACTH and serum cortisol levels after DDAVP administration predicts remission.[a]	• Little data • The specificity and positive predictive value are low
Metyrapone testing	Two weeks after surgery	Serum 11-deoxycortisol < 150 nmol/L: remission is likely.	• Little data • Low specificity

ACTH, Adrenocorticotropic hormone; CBG, corticosteroid-binding globulin; CRH, corticotropin-releasing hormone; DDAVP, desmopressin acetate; HPAA, hypothalamic-pituitary-adrenal axis; and DST, dexamethasone suppression testing.
[a]*In control subjects a normal response of plasma ACTH and serum cortisol to CRH is observed (integrity of HPAA), whereas the response to DDAVP is little or absent (upregulation of the V3 receptor on tumor corticotroph cells only). Therefore, in the case of long-term remission, response to DDAVP tends to remain blunted during follow-up, whereas a gradual recovery of response to CRH is typically observed. According to Barbot et al. [17], the presence of ACTH hyperresponsiveness to both DDAVP (ACTH plasma levels > 9 pg/mL) and CRH (ACTH plasma levels > 36.7 pg/mL) 6 months after surgery gives positive and negative predictive values for recurrence of approximately 100%. The authors suggest performing DDAVP testing as a first step, using CRH stimulation in case of borderline ACTH responses to DDAVP.*

lateralization is limited [19] and surgery can alter sellar anatomy and venous drainage of the pituitary gland, possibly leading to misinterpretation of the results [20].

The decision regarding the best treatment for patients who relapse after primary pituitary surgery is complex. Several options are available (e.g., an initial wait-and-see approach, neurosurgical reintervention, RT, medical treatment, or BLA), and the choice has to be tailored to each patient, taking into account the severity of symptoms, comorbidities, neuroimaging, surgical risks, desire for pregnancy, response and tolerance to medical treatment, and patients' preferences.

We believe that surgical reintervention (when feasible) should be the first step in cases of relapse after primary surgery. If surgery is not a viable option or is expected to be unsuccessful,

TABLE 9.4 Strategies for Managing Persistent and Recurrent Cushing's Disease: Repeat Pituitary Surgery

When to consider?	Disease control rate	Risk of recurrence	Features
Surgical reintervention should be the first step in case of noncurative primary surgery. If surgery is not feasible or is expected to be unsuccessful as judged by an experienced pituitary surgeon, second-line options should be considered. *Factors associated with favorable outcomes:* Evidence of recurrent or persistent resectable, noninvasive tumor at postoperative MRI. *Factors associated with unfavorable outcomes:* Lack of visible tumor, evidence of cavernous sinus invasion, extrasellar extension, or bone invasion are likely to reduce the efficacy of repeat surgery	30–87.5% (mean 58%)	0–60% (mean 16%)	• The success rate of surgical reintervention is lower than for primary surgery • Repeat surgery harbors a higher risk of hypopituitarism (9–78.5%, mean 38%) • Repeat surgery has been associated with a higher risk of surgical complications (e.g., CSF leakage and diabetes insipidus). The risk seems to be higher for delayed intervention, possibly related to the formation of scar tissue

Note. This table reports the most frequent and recent findings. Differences among studies do occur.
CSF, Cerebrospinal fluid; and MRI, magnetic resonance imaging.

second-line options should to be considered. Favorable outcomes often result from a combination of different second- and third-line approaches.

3.1 Wait-and-see

A wait-and-see approach with repeated clinical and laboratory evaluation over time can be considered when the postoperative clinical picture improves but biochemical tests are unclear. In fact, a delayed remission may be achieved months after primary surgery in approximately 5% of patients, and immediate postoperative laboratory data may be misleading [21].

3.2 Surgical Reintervention

A detailed description of the surgical approach to the pituitary gland is reviewed elsewhere (Chapter 6). This chapter focuses on features of surgical reintervention with relapse after primary pituitary surgery (Table 9.4).

A major indication for repeat surgery is the postoperative evidence on MRI of a clear, resectable, and noninvasive tumor, particularly if the initial surgery was not performed by an experienced pituitary surgeon [8]. Repeat pituitary surgery includes selective adenomectomy, partial hypophysectomy, and total hypophysectomy [22]: the decision concerning the most appropriate surgical approach depends on several aspects, including primary tumor location, postoperative MRI, intraoperative findings, and the surgeon's expertise [4]. A very important consideration is that tumor recurrence is expected to occur at the same site of the primary tumor, making selective adenomectomy a potentially successful option. Nonetheless, in some patients, there is no radiological evidence of recurrence after primary surgery, and a more aggressive surgical approach, including partial or total hypophysectomy may be considered a possibility [20].

The success rate of surgical reintervention is lower than that for primary pituitary surgery [1], and repeat neurosurgery is associated with a higher risk of complications and hypopituitarism (especially if hypophysectomy, instead of selective adenomectomy, is performed) [23]. Pituitary reintervention, if feasible and expected to be successful, should be planned as soon as the recurrence or persistence of Cushing's disease is confirmed. When the clinical picture improves and laboratory tests are unclear after primary surgery, a wait-and-see approach of weeks to months before reconsidering reintervention can be followed.

3.3 Radiotherapy and Radiosurgery

A detailed description of the RT approach to the pituitary gland is reviewed elsewhere (Chapter 7). This section focuses on features of conventional RT and RS with relapse of Cushing's disease after primary pituitary surgery (Table 9.5) [24–27].

Conventional fractionated RT was widely used to treat Cushing's disease up until the 1970s [28]. In recent years, conventional fractionated RT has been progressively replaced by more accurate stereotactic techniques, including fractionated stereotactic RT (SRT) and RS (SRS) [e.g., gamma-knife, cyberknife linear accelerator-based therapies, and proton beam therapy]. Today RT is generally considered as a second- or third-line treatment for Cushing's disease after unsuccessful pituitary surgery or medical therapy, as adjuvant therapy to control residual tumor growth (after pituitary surgery), or to prevent Nelson's syndrome (NS) after BLA.

It is difficult to compare results among clinical studies and case series, regarding the outcomes of different RT approaches, because of differences in terms of patient selection; timing of RT; total radiation dose; margin radiation dose; concomitant medical treatment; duration of follow-up; and criteria to define disease control, recurrence, and side-effects. It can be said, however, that SRT techniques offer comparable results in terms of disease control rates as compared to conventional fractionated RT, achieving remission earlier and with a smaller risk of optic chiasm involvement. Moreover, stereotactic techniques may seem to have a slightly reduced risk of late-onset hypopituitarism, which yet remains a major clinical problem in the management and follow-up of patients undergoing RT [1].

Another consideration is that, regardless of the RT technique employed, an extended time to remission is expected (months to years). Therefore, after RT, long-term "bridge" therapy with cortisol-lowering medications is required before obtaining Cushing's disease remission. We advise ascertaining that medical therapy is well-tolerated, not contraindicated, and effective in controlling hypercortisolism before considering RT as a second- or third-line therapy to resolve Cushing's disease [8].

3.4 Medical Therapy

A detailed description of medical therapies for Cushing's disease is reviewed elsewhere (Chapter 7). Table 9.6 highlights some particular aspects of the use of medical therapy after unsuccessful primary pituitary surgery [1,8,29–31].

Medications currently prescribed for patients with Cushing's disease include adrenal steroidogenesis inhibitors, pituitary-addressed drugs, and a glucocorticoid-receptor antagonist (mifepristone). Medical therapy is considered as a second-line strategy in patients who have unsuccessful surgery, have contraindications to surgery, or refuse surgery. Medical therapy

TABLE 9.5   Strategies for Managing Persistent and Recurrent Cushing's Disease: RT and RS

When to consider?	Disease control rate	Risk of recurrence	Features

• *Second-line treatment:* Consider RT or RS when surgical reintervention is not indicated or has failed in controlling the disease
• *Third-line treatment:* Consider RT or RS after unsuccessful pituitary surgery and if following medical therapy is ineffective, contraindicated, or not tolerated
• Consider RT or RS especially when a clear target is visible on MRI[a]
• Consider RT or RS when a noninvasive approach is preferred (e.g., major contraindications to surgery)
• Consider RT or RS as a viable strategy to reduce the chance of residual tumor regrowth (after surgical reexploration) and of developing NS (after BLA)
Factors associated with favorable outcomes of RT and RS:
Small tumors far from the optic chiasm
Factors associated with unfavorable outcomes of RT and RS:
• Residual tumor after surgery > 10 mm
• Tumor distance from optic chiasm < 5 mm (can be less in case of fractionated stereotactic RT)
• No target at MRI
• Use of hormone suppressive medications when starting RT[b]
	39–84% (mean 64% for conventional fractionated RT)
	75% (for fractionated stereotactic conformal RT)
	17–100% (mean 59% for gamma-knife RS)
	22–100% (mean 62% for linear accelerator)
	52–86% (mean 71% for proton-beam RT)
		0 (for conventional fractionated RT)
		0–100% (mean 13% for gamma-knife RS)
		0–23.5% (mean 14.5% for linear accelerator)
		0–15% (mean 6% for proton beam RT)
			• RS appears to provide earlier remission than conventional fractionated RT
			• RS reduces margin radiation dose and the risk of hypopituitarism and optic chiasm involvement
			• A long time to remission is expected (months to years). Medical "bridge" therapy is needed before achieving remission
			• Higher radiation doses are associated with a higher remission rates, but they can negatively affect the safety of RT and RS
			• There is a high risk of late-onset hypopituitarism (21–78% for conventional RT; 0–69% for RS)
			• Factors associated with the risk of hypopituitarism after RT or RS include:
			  • Radiation dose
			  • Radiation margin
			  • Volume and location of the irradiated area
			  • Suprasellar extension of RT
			  • Surgery before RT or RS
			  • Cavernous sinus invasion of the tumor

Note. This table reports the most frequent and recent findings. Differences among studies do occur.

ACTH, Adrenocorticotropic hormone; BLA, bilateral adrenalectomy; CRH, corticotropin-releasing hormone; MRI, magnetic resonance imaging; NS, Nelson's syndrome; RS, radiosurgery; and RT, radiotherapy.

[a]*Some experts advise using RT (especially RS) even if a clear target is not visible. RT should be addressed to the whole sella and a few millimeters beyond, as an "equivalent" to total hypophysectomy [24].*

[b]*It has been observed that the use of ketoconazole when starting RT for Cushing's disease potentially impairs the efficacy of RT [25], as has been suggested in patients with acromegaly treated with octreotide before RT [26]. This might be due to a radioprotective effect of ketoconazole (e.g., a decreased proliferation of corticotroph adenomatous cells?), as suggested by one study in the rat where ketoconazole inhibits CRH-stimulated ACTH release [27]. Data regarding the potential effects on RT outcomes of neoadjuvant therapy with the pituitary-directed drug pasireotide are lacking.*

TABLE 9.6　Strategies for Managing Persistent and Recurrent Cushing's Disease: Medical Therapy

When to consider?	Which drug?	Features
• Consider medical therapy when surgical reintervention is not indicated or has been unsuccessful in controlling the disease • Consider medical therapy as a "bridge" treatment after RT or RS, while awaiting remission • Consider medical therapy when the patient refuses other second-line strategies or in case of a high surgical risk • Consider medical therapy in patients with pituitary carcinoma and metastases	*Pasireotide:* • This has been approved for patients with Cushing's disease after surgery has failed or is not an option • This pituitary-directed drug can lead to tumor shrinkage [29]. This can be useful in case of large tumors with compression/infiltration of surrounding structures *Cabergoline:* • Its use is off-label in patients with Cushing's disease • This pituitary-directed drug can cause tumor volume reduction, as with pasireotide (see above) [30] *Ketoconazole:* • It is approved by the EMA for patients over the age of 12 years with Cushing's syndrome • It is used off-label in the United States • Invisible pituitary tumors can appear during ketoconazole treatment, and patients can, therefore, be sent to surgery. This wait-and-see approach could be considered in patients with mild Cushing's disease *Metyrapone:* • It is approved by the EMA for patients with Cushing' syndrome. It is difficult to obtain in the United States *Mifepristone:* • It is approved by the FDA to treat hyperglycemia in patients with Cushing's syndrome and type 2 diabetes, glucose intolerance after unsuccessful surgery, or if surgery is not an option *Mitotane:* • It is approved to treat adrenal cancer. Its use is off-label in patients with Cushing's syndrome not caused by adrenal cancer	• Efficacy varies among different drugs, which can be used as single or combination therapies • Individual patient factors can influence drug choice (e.g., age, sex, desire for parenthood, concurrent diseases, and drug interactions) • Costs and drug availability should be considered in the management • Clinicians should be aware that some side effects of these drugs can resemble adrenal insufficiency. This is particularly important when waiting for disease control after RT or RS • Drugs should be withheld or doses reduced if adrenal insufficiency is suspected

EMA, European Medicines Agency; FDA, Food and Drug Administration; RS, radiosurgery; and RT, radiotherapy.

can be used as "bridge" therapy before pituitary surgery to ameliorate the clinical picture and reduce the surgical risk, or after RT while awaiting Cushing's disease control.

The efficacy of medications in the control of hypercortisolism and its metabolic effects is undisputed, but positive clinical and biochemical responses during medical therapy cannot be considered "curative," as drug discontinuation results in the recurrence of symptoms [32]. Moreover, the efficacy and safety of long-term medical therapy are yet to be fully clarified. For example, it has been observed that patients with refractory ACTH-dependent Cushing's syndrome (of ectopic or pituitary origin) who are treated with adrenal steroidogenesis inhibitors only are more likely to die from hypercortisolism-related sequelae when compared to patients who are treated first with medical therapy and later with BLA [33].

3.5 Adrenal Surgery

Table 9.7 highlights some characteristics of the use of BLA after unsuccessful pituitary surgery or other second-line strategies (Chapter 6) [1,8,34]. The major advantage of BLA is that it provides an immediate and definitive resolution of hypercortisolism, with rapid improvement of the clinical picture, despite a lifelong need of glucocorticoid and mineralocorticoid replacement therapy and risk of NS. It is worth noting that patients with refractory Cushing's

TABLE 9.7 Strategies for Managing Persistent and Recurrent Cushing's Disease: BLA

When to consider?	Disease control rate	Risk of recurrence	Features
• Consider BLA in case of refractory Cushing's disease after first- and other second-line treatments • Consider BLA in case of persistent disease if other second-line strategies are contraindicated or not tolerated • Consider BLA in patients wishing to avoid radiation-induced hypopituitarism (e.g., in young female patients who wish to have children) • Consider BLA in patients with very severe disease who are likely to benefit from a rapid resolution of hypercortisolism (given they have no contraindications to adrenal surgery)	88–100%	0–12% (Only 1–2% of patients develop clinically evident hypercortisolism)	• Morbidity: 18% • Mortality: 3% (Most of deaths occur during the first year after surgery) • The shift from open to laparoscopic BLA has significantly improved surgical management • Laparoscopic BLA is associated with longer operative times as compared to the open technique, but it improves patients' recovery • There is a longstanding risk of developing NS • There is a lifelong need for glucocorticoid and mineralocorticoid therapy • The risk of recurrence is due to the continuous ACTH stimulation of adrenal remnants after surgery, accessory adrenal glands, or ectopic adrenal tissue

Note. This table reports the most frequent and recent findings. Differences among studies do occur.
ACTH, Adrenocorticotropic hormone; BLA, bilateral adrenalectomy; and NS, Nelson's syndrome.

disease have a higher surgical risk per se, such as comorbidities, decreased wound healing, and an increased likelihood of postsurgical infections and thromboembolic events [34].

4 POSTTREATMENT MANAGEMENT OF CUSHING'S DISEASE

Posttreatment management of patients with Cushing's disease is complex and depends intimately on the type of approach (or combination of approaches) used. The following sections analyze the medical problems with which clinicians are faced during the lifelong follow-up of patients treated for Cushing's disease with surgery, RT, or BLA. Management and follow-up of patients treated with medical therapy is reviewed elsewhere (Chapter 7).

4.1 After Pituitary Surgery

4.1.1 Central Adrenal Insufficiency

Development of adrenal insufficiency derives from endogenous hypercortisolism-induced HPAA suppression (e.g., hypothalamic CRH-producing neurons and normal pituitary corticotroph cell suppression) [35,36].

Adrenal insufficiency following successful pituitary surgery for Cushing's disease can be permanent or transient. A recent paper by Berr et al. [37] shows that only 58% of patients in a large case series recover from adrenal insufficiency within 5 years. The likelihood of adrenal function recovery was 100% in patients who had late Cushing's disease recurrence (2.4–14.4 years after surgery), 71% in patients with normal postoperative pituitary function and no recurrence during long-term follow-up, and very poor in patients showing postoperative insufficiency of two or more pituitary axes. Conversely, Alexandraki et al. [5] reported that all patients who experienced a recurrence of Cushing's disease showed HPAA recovery within 3 years of surgery: recovery within 6 months, 1 year, and 2 years had a positive predictive value of recurrence of 64%, 61%, and 59%, respectively. Our experience is that most patients who do not have postoperative panhypopituitarism do recover their HPAA. As a general rule, we can say that patients not showing HPAA recovery before 3 years are very likely to be permanently in remission; every patient in which adrenal function recovers before 3 years postoperatively is potentially at risk for late recurrence; the quicker the HPAA recovers, the higher the risk of recurrence.

When HPAA function recovers after successful pituitary surgery, the actual duration of adrenal insufficiency varies widely, with a median range between 13 and 25 months, depending on case series [5,37–41]. Several factors have been proposed as predictive of the probability and timing of HPAA recovery (Table 9.8) [37].

Medical treatment of central adrenal insufficiency involves the use of short-acting glucocorticoids (e.g., immediate-release hydrocortisone or cortisone acetate) or modified-release hydrocortisone (Table 9.9) [42]. Long-acting glucocorticoids should be avoided in this setting, as they can extend the duration of HPAA suppression [8].

In patients with central adrenal insufficiency, the possible presence of residual adrenal activity can lead to lower drug requirements in comparison to primary adrenal insufficiency (Table 9.16). Moreover, in the presence of mild central adrenal insufficiency (e.g., borderline results of the ACTH stimulation test for cortisol or other dynamic testing), a feasible option

TABLE 9.8 Factors Predicting the Probability and Timing of HPAA Recovery after Surgery

Patient features	Younger age is a positive predictive factor for HPAA recovery.
Surgery	• Repeated surgery is a negative predictive factor for HPAA recovery • The extent of pituitary exploration (selective adenomectomy vs. hypophysectomy) can be a predictive factor • Median localization of the tumor within the pituitary has been associated with a higher risk of permanent adrenal insufficiency
Biochemical features	• Postoperative insufficiency of ≥2 pituitary axes is a negative predictive factor for HPAA recovery • The severity and duration of Cushing's disease before surgery (?) can be a predictive factor
Pathological features	A larger proportion of Crooke's cells in the paraadenomatous tissue has been observed in long-term cortisol-insufficient patients. This might be linked to the duration of hypercortisolism before surgery, explaining widespread corticotroph cell degeneration.

HPAA, Hypothalamic-pituitary-adrenal axis.

is to prescribe a low dose of glucocorticoids (e.g., hydrocortisone, 10 mg/day) or to suggest glucocorticoid administration only in the case of stressful events.

An important clinical problem in the management of patients with adrenal insufficiency is the risk of adrenal crisis. It is a medical emergency and a potentially life-threatening event deriving from the inadequate response of HPAA to major stressful events (e.g., systemic infections, diarrhea, dehydration, trauma, burns, or acute myocardial infarction). It is characterized by acute impairment of the general state of health and requires a timely diagnosis and immediate treatment [42]. Table 9.10 illustrates the medical approach to an adrenal crisis and other stressful events.

Patients, their relatives, and caregivers should be instructed on how to recognize and treat an adrenal crisis, and they should be aware of the circumstances that potentially trigger acute hypoadrenalism. The patient should carry a kit of injectable emergency steroids when traveling far from medical facilities. Moreover, patients should have a medical alert tag (bracelet or necklace) with the diagnosis of adrenal insufficiency and the need for hydrocortisone to receive prompt assistance, especially in case of loss of consciousness [8].

A major issue in the postsurgical management of "cured" patients with Cushing's disease is how to evaluate the recovery of normal basal and stress-induced endogenous cortisol production, and, therefore, to possibly stop glucocorticoid replacement therapy. Establishing HPAA recovery after pituitary surgery can include measurement of both morning serum cortisol and plasma ACTH as well as dynamic laboratory evaluation to assess ACTH reserve (Table 9.11) [8,43–50]. The recovery pattern is highly variable in terms of duration, but the pattern always follows the same profile. The ACTH level needs to rise (sometimes above normal) before cortisol secretion by the adrenal glands normalizes. Therefore, our practice is to check morning pre-hydrocortisone serum cortisol and plasma ACTH every 8 weeks.

Another common clinical problem after successful pituitary surgery for Cushing's disease is the "glucocorticoid withdrawal syndrome." It is a self-limiting condition defined as the presence of symptoms resembling adrenal insufficiency despite adequate glucocorticoid replacement therapy: patients may experience asthenia, anorexia, weight loss, nausea, vomiting,

TABLE 9.9   Medical Treatment of Central Adrenal Insufficiency in Adults

Glucocorticoids	*Short-acting glucocorticoids hydrocortisone, 10–12 mg/m²/day (usually 15–20 mg orally/day):* • In two divided doses: 2/3 of the daily dose at awakening and 1/3 of the daily dose 6–8 h after the first administration • In three divided doses: 3/6 of the daily dose at awakening; 2/6 around midday; 1/6 late afternoon. The three-time administration mimics the endogenous cortisol production more physiologically • In the immediate postoperative period, some patients may benefit from higher doses of hydrocortisone to prevent the "glucocorticoid withdrawal syndrome" (see below); however, there is currently no consensus on this point, and the therapeutic decisions should be tailored to the patient's clinical picture • Evening and night administrations should be avoided because normal cortisol secretion rate is notably reduced between 6:00 p.m. and 3:00 a.m. *Cortisone acetate, usually 25–37.5 mg orally/day in two divided doses:* • It has a higher pharmacokinetic variability compared to hydrocortisone, since it has to be activated by hepatic 11β-hydroxysteroid dehydrogenase type I *Modified-release hydrocortisone:* It has an outer coat of immediate-release hydrocortisone and an inner core of slow-release hydrocortisone. Two different dosages are available: 20 mg and 5 mg. • It is given in one dose at awakening (usually 20–30 mg orally/day) • It is able to mimic accurately the endogenous cortisol production • Data show that this formulation can be superior to short- and long-acting glucocorticoids, concerning several outcomes (e.g., body composition, blood pressure, glycated hemoglobin, and bone resorption) • It is not available in the United States *Adrenal insufficiency and hypothyroidism* Starting LT₄ before correcting adrenal insufficiency may lead to an adrenal crisis. (Thyroid hormones enhance the clearance of corticosteroids) *Adrenal insufficiency and GH replacement therapy* Starting GH replacement in patients on glucocorticoid replacement therapy (especially cortisone acetate or prednisone) may lead to an adrenal crisis (GH inhibits the action of 11β-hydroxysteroid dehydrogenase type I, which converts cortisone to cortisol). Moreover, GH replacement therapy may unmask undiagnosed adrenal insufficiency *Adrenal insufficiency and diabetes insipidus* Starting glucocorticoids in central adrenal insufficiency can unmask central diabetes insipidus. Glucocorticoids reduce DDVAP secretion and action (in partial diabetes insipidus) and cause a rise in blood pressure and renal blood flow; these actions can all cause polyuria
Mineralocorticoids	Mineralocorticoid replacement is not necessary in central adrenal insufficiency. Deficiency of ACTH causes only cortisol deficiency, whereas adrenal mineralocorticoid secretion is preserved

ACTH, Adrenocorticotropic hormone; DDVAP, vasopressin acetate; GH, growth hormone; and LT4, levothyroxine.

dizziness, arthralgia, flu-like symptoms, and hypotension [51]. Some patients may also develop psychiatric symptoms, such as depression, anxiety, and panic attacks, all of which can last for 6–9 months after resolution of hypercortisolism [8]. The mechanism behind this syndrome is not fully understood. It has been hypothesized that a "relative adrenal insufficiency" can manifest when giving physiological doses of glucocorticoids because of the peripheral tolerance to glucocorticoids induced by the longstanding hypercortisolism [52]. A postoperative

TABLE 9.10   Management of Adrenal Crisis and Other Stressful Events

Adrenal crisis	• Clinical picture: The patient may experience profound asthenia, lethargy, confusion, loss of consciousness, sweating, abdominal pain, nausea, vomiting, or severe hypotension
	• Laboratory evaluation in central adrenal insufficiency may show hyponatremia, hypercalcemia, and hypoglycemia
	• Therapeutic management:
	  • Give parenteral fluids immediately: 0.9% saline solution
	  • Give hydrocortisone immediately: 100 mg of hydrocortisone intravenously and then every 6–8 h thereafter, then taper the dosage, according to the clinical picture
	  • If present, correct hypoglycemia, hyponatremia, and hypercalcemia
	  • Treat the triggering cause, if possible (e.g., infection)

Other stressful events	• For a surgical procedure, give hydrocortisone parenterally before and immediately after surgery. (The dose is determined on the basis of the clinical picture and the kind of surgery.) Taper parenteral hydrocortisone during the postoperative days, returning to the usual oral regimen as soon as the clinical picture improves. Excessive and extended administration of hydrocortisone perioperatively can mask signs and symptoms of complications (e.g., infection) and impair wound healing • For moderately stressful events (e.g., endoscopy procedures; medical procedures, requiring local anesthesia), give parenteral hydrocortisone immediately before the procedure. Repeat after 6–8 h, if needed • For minor stressful events (e.g., fever, diarrhea), the patient should be instructed to double or triple the usual oral dose of glucocorticoids for a maximum of 3 days.[a] If the disease worsen or persists for more than 3 days, the patient should see a physician • In the case of intense psychophysical stress (e.g., bereavement, strenuous exercise, or anticipated profuse sweating), take an extra dose of oral hydrocortisone immediately before • If vomiting is present, give hydrocortisone parenterally. • During the third trimester of pregnancy, a 30–50% increase of the usual dosage of hydrocortisone may be required. Patients with primary adrenal insufficiency may also need more fludrocortisone because of the anti-mineralocorticoid action of progesterone • During delivery, give hydrocortisone parenterally every 6 h in case of cesarean section or prolonged labor. Taper the dose returning to the usual oral regimen within 3 days

[a]*Patients taking modified-release hydrocortisone should be instructed to increase the usual oral regimen by increasing the frequency of daily administrations (every 8 ± 2 h) and not by increasing the morning dose. Alternatively, immediate-release hydrocortisone can replace modified-release hydrocortisone or can be given in addition to it during the intercurrent illness. Finally, it is important to note that diarrhea can alter the absorption of modified-release hydrocortisone. Administration of immediate-release hydrocortisone is advised in this setting.*

rise in the level of interleukin-6 has also been advocated as a potential triggering event [53]. Patients experiencing the glucocorticoid withdrawal syndrome may benefit from higher glucocorticoid dosing and slower tapering of glucocorticoids after pituitary surgery or from a temporary increase in the dose of replacement therapy [51].

Finally, it is not uncommon after resolution of Cushing's disease and the onset of adrenal insufficiency that patients develop or have a recurrence of autoimmune diseases (e.g. psoriasis, connective tissue diseases, or inflammatory bowel syndrome). This is probably the result of the derepression of disorders previously masked by hypercortisolism [54].

TABLE 9.11 Laboratory Assessment of HPAA Recovery

Basal evaluation	Morning serum cortisol on two or more occasions (before hydrocortisone administration):
	• Cortisol < 7.4 µg/dL (200 nmol/L): Adrenal insufficiency is likely. The patient should be kept on glucocorticoid replacement therapy and retested after several weeks
	• Cortisol 7.4–15 µg/dL (200–414 nmol/L): A dynamic test may be performed to assess ACTH reserve. It should be noted that morning serum cortisol > 10 µg/dL (275 nmol/L) usually predicts that HPAA has recovered or that the underlying partial adrenal insufficiency is not clinically relevant in basal conditions or for minor stressful events
	• Cortisol > 15 µg/dL (414 nmol/L): HPAA recovery is very likely, and further dynamic testing is unnecessary. A normal response of cortisol to the insulin-induced hypoglycemia test is expected in virtually all patients

Dynamic evaluation	**ACTH Stimulation test for cortisol**	**Pros of the test**	**Cons of the Test**
	• Give synthetic ACTH 1–24 (cosyntropin) parenterally, and measure serum cortisol 30 and 60 minutes after the injection	• Easy to perform	• The test may cause an overstimulation of the adrenal glands, leading to a "normal" response in patients with partial ACTH deficiency or recent (less than 1 month) pituitary damage (e.g., the adrenal glands are not completely atrophic)
	• If stimulated cortisol is ≥18 µg/dL (500 nmol/L), the patient's ACTH reserve and response to stress are considered normal	• Cost-effective	
		• It can be used in an outpatient setting	
	• Two versions of this test have been proposed: *standard-dose test* (250 µg of cosyntropin is given intravenously or intramuscularly) and *low-dose test* (1 µg of cosyntropin is given intramuscularly). If 1 mcg is used, a 30-minute time point *must* be checked	• Very low risks (only allergic reactions very rarely reported)	• Conflicting results regarding the higher sensibility of the low-dose test in comparison to the standard-dose test. A recent metaanalysis shows that both high- and low-dose tests have comparable diagnostic accuracy in patients with central adrenal insufficiency due to low sensitivity [50]
		• The low-dose test might provide advantages (higher sensibility) over the standard-dose test in patients with partial ACTH deficiency or recent pituitary damage because the stimulus is not supramaximal	
	Insulin-induced hypoglycemia test	**Pros of the test**	**Cons of the test**
	• Give insulin intravenously (usually 0.1 units kg of body weight), and measure serum cortisol and glucose before and 15, 30, 60, 90, and 120 min after the injection	• It is considered the gold standard to study HPAA response to stress	• It may be dangerous in the elderly and in patients with a history of cardiovascular, cerebrovascular, or seizure disorders
	• If glycemia falls to < 50 mg/dL (2.8 mmol/L) and the concomitant cortisol level is ≥18 µg/dL (498 nmol/L), the patient's ACTH reserve and response to stress are normal	• It performs very well in patients with partial ACTH deficiency or recent pituitary damage	• It requires close monitoring of the patient
			• It causes discomfort for the patient
	• Stop the test, and give glucose intravenously if severe neuroglycopenic symptoms develop or glycemia falls to < 35 mg/dL (1.9 mmol/L)		

Metyrapone test

- Give 750 mg of metyrapone orally every 4 hours for 24 h. If serum 11-deoxycortisol after 24 h is < 10 μg/dL (497 nmol/L), the patient's ACTH reserve is decreased, and response to stress can be impaired. Give 100 mg of hydrocortisone parenterally at the end of the test to avoid acute adrenal insufficiency. Stop the test, and give hydrocortisone if hypotension or other clinical signs of hypoadrenalism occur
- A short version of this test is the *overnight single-dose metyrapone test*: 30 mg of metyrapone per kg of body weight are given at midnight; the response to the test is considered normal if morning serum 11-deoxycortisol is 7–22 μg/dL (200–660 nmol/L)
- A morning serum cortisol < 5 μg/dL (138 nmol/L) confirms adequate drug-induced HPAA blockade

Pros of the test

- It is very reliable in predicting ACTH reserve and HPAA response to stressful events
- Metyrapone can be used in adults of any age
- It is a potential alternative when the insulin-induced hypoglycemia test is contraindicated

Cons of the Test

- Metyrapone not easily available in the United States
- Routine laboratory assessment of 11-deoxycortisol is not universally available
- Some think that it should be performed in an inpatient setting as it can cause hypotension and acute adrenal insufficiency
- Some drugs can enhance metyrapone metabolism (e.g., phenytoin and fosphenytoin), making the test unreliable unless the dosage is increased (e.g., 750 mg of metyrapone every 2 h)
- If given concurrently, metyrapone may increase the serum concentrations of paracetamol and its hepatotoxic metabolite

ACTH, Adrenocorticotropic hormone; and HPAA, hypothalamic-pituitary-adrenal axis.

4.1.2 *Central Diabetes Insipidus*

Central diabetes insipidus after pituitary surgery is caused by decreased or absent secretion of antidiuretic hormone (ADH) by the posterior pituitary, following damage to neurohypophyseal axons that derive from the magnocellular neurons of the supraoptic and paraventricular nuclei of the hypothalamus. Hypotonic polyuria (<300 mOsm/kg H_2O) with compensatory polydipsia (given that the thirst mechanism is preserved) is the presenting clinical picture of diabetes insipidus [55]. An unpredictable daily urine output (3–20 L/day) can be observed. The concomitant presence of serum hyperosmolality and hypernatremia strongly suggests the diagnosis of diabetes insipidus, but these laboratory alterations can be borderline or absent if the patient has an intact thirst mechanism and access to water [56]. Central diabetes insipidus can be acute or chronic (onset and duration of the disease), transient or permanent (duration of the disease), and partial or complete (decreased or absent ADH release), depending on the kind and extent of the damage to magnocellular neurons.

Central diabetes insipidus is a common clinical problem after pituitary surgery for Cushing's disease: the incidence of transient diabetes insipidus is reported to be similar between primary and repeated surgery (approximately 29% and 23%, respectively), whereas permanent diabetes insipidus is more common after repeated surgery (approximately 6% vs. 25%) [1]. The endoscopic transsphenoidal approach has been recently reported to be associated with a slightly higher frequency of permanent diabetes insipidus in patients with Cushing's disease and silent corticotroph adenomas, possibly because of greater manipulation of the pituitary gland in comparison to the microscopic approach [57].

Acute diabetes insipidus usually occurs 12–24 h after pituitary surgery and can be transient or evolve into chronic diabetes insipidus. Water metabolism derangement can manifest in a triphasic pattern (approximately 3% of patients): a polyuric phase, which develops within 24–48 h after surgery and is caused by the shock of neurohypophyseal axons, resulting in ADH secretion; an antidiuretic phase, which develops 4–8 days after surgery and lasts approximately 2–5 days, is caused by uncontrolled ADH release by deposits within degenerated neurohypophyseal axons (e.g., the patient is temporarily able to concentrate urine); and a later polyuric phase, which is caused by the depletion of ADH deposits [56]. Table 9.12 outlines the medical treatment and monitoring of central diabetes insipidus [58–60].

The antidiuretic phase described above (uncontrolled ADH release) is sometimes isolated and configures a picture of the syndrome of inappropriate ADH (SIADH) secretion with transient hyponatremia. This temporary, late-onset fall of blood sodium levels may be enhanced by concomitant hypocortisolism and is observed in 5–20% of all patients undergoing transsphenoidal surgery for Cushing's disease, with a peak incidence 7–8 days after surgery [57,61]. Other postsurgical causes of hyponatremia include parenteral administration of large amounts of fluids perioperatively, overtreatment with desmopressin (DDAVP) or 8l-8-L-arginine vasopressin (AVP), and cerebral salt wasting syndrome [56,57].

4.1.3 *Follow-Up*

Long-term follow-up of patients going into remission after pituitary surgery for Cushing's disease includes three main clinical issues: establishing the likelihood of HPAA recovery, monitoring for the risk of hypopituitarism (both anterior and posterior pituitary insufficiency), and early diagnosis and management of potential disease relapse (Table 9.13).

According to the 2015 Endocrine Society guidelines [8], clinicians are advised to measure morning serum cortisol (before the morning hydrocortisone dose) every 3–6 months after

TABLE 9.12 Management of Central Diabetes Insipidus

Acute diabetes insipidus	Treatment	<ul><li>*Liquid infusion (IV fluid that is hypoosmolar with respect to the patient's serum):* It may not be necessary if plasma sodium levels and plasma osmolality are normal, the patient is conscious, and the thirst mechanism is preserved</li><li>*DDAVP or AVP:* Drug doses have to be titrated cautiously, according to the clinical and biochemical response. In general, short-acting AVP is preferred in the immediate postoperative period because of the lower risk of overdosing (water intoxication)<ul><li>AVP: short-acting ADH analog. It can be administered IM or SC 5–10 U 2–3 times a day</li><li>DDAVP: long-acting ADH analog. It can be administered: 1. IV, IM, or SC: 0.5–2 μg 1–3 times a day; 2. Orally: 0.2–1.2 mg 1–3 times a day; 3. Sublingually: 120–720 μg 1–3 times a day; or 4. Intranasally: 10–60 μg 1–3 times a day</li></ul></li><li>Aim: to keep plasma sodium levels and plasma osmolality within reference ranges, avoiding "water intoxication"</li></ul>
	Monitoring	<ul><li>Water balance (liquid intake/urine output)</li><li>Body weight</li><li>Plasma and urine osmolality</li><li>Plasma sodium: If SIADH and hyponatremia develop, the first-line treatment is fluid restriction. If necessary, give hypertonic (3%) NaCl solution either via bolus or continuous IV infusion and adapt administration, according to sodium plasma levels. In cases of SIADH where hyponatremia persists and fluid restriction is ineffective, pharmacological therapy should be considered (e.g., demeclocycline, urea, or vasopressin receptor antagonists). Hyponatremia should not be corrected too rapidly because of the risk of osmotic demyelination syndrome</li></ul>
Chronic diabetes insipidus	Treatment	<ul><li>Mild, partial forms of diabetes insipidus with preserved thirst mechanism and a total urine output not causing discomfort for the patient may not require medical therapy</li><li>DDAVP: Drug doses have to be titrated cautiously, according to the clinical and biochemical response. They can be administered: 1. Orally: 0.2–1.2 mg 1–3 times a day; 2. Sublingually: 120–720 μg 1–3 times a day; or 3. Intranasally: 10–60 μg 1–3 times a day</li></ul>
	Monitoring	<ul><li>Water balance</li><li>Body weight</li><li>Plasma and urine osmolality</li><li>Plasma sodium</li></ul>During the first 6 months after pituitary surgery, DDAVP treatment should be stopped every so often (e.g., twice a month) to identify transient forms of diabetes insipidus. Monitoring is required monthly when starting DDAVP, changing the dose and route of administration, according to the clinical picture, the biochemical response, and the patient's preferences. When a fixed dose is identified, controls can be performed every 6–12 months. As a rule of thumb, patients should be instructed to:<ul><li>Drink only when thirsty.</li><li>Await the antidiuretic effect of DDAVP to end and polyuria to present before taking a new dose.</li><li>Keep urine output between 1–2 L/day.</li><li>Regularly check body weight as a sign of over- or under-treatment</li></ul>

ADH, antidiurectic hormone; AVP, 8l-8-L-arginine vasopressin; DDAVP, desmopressin; IM, intramuscular injection; IV, intravenous injection; NaCl, sodium chloride; SIADH, syndrome of inappropriate ADH secretion; and SC, subcutaneous administration.

TABLE 9.13　Follow-up of Patients with Cushing's Disease after Pituitary Surgery

HPAA	• Start glucocorticoid replacement therapy in the postoperative period • A postoperative pituitary MRI 1–3 months after surgery may be useful as comparison in case of future recurrence • Periodic[a] clinical control • Periodic[a] biochemical control: morning serum cortisol and plasma ACTH • Establish HPAA recovery with ACTH stimulation test or other provocative tests if morning cortisol level is not diagnostic (Table 9.11) • Stop hydrocortisone if HPAA has recovered
Hypopituitarism and diabetes insipidus	Monitor patient for the risk of hypopituitarism and diabetes insipidus: • Control serum sodium levels several times during the first 1–2 weeks after surgery • Assess free T_4 about 4 weeks after surgery • Assess for central hypogonadism weeks to months after curative surgery • Assess for GH deficiency 1–2 years after successful neurosurgery.
Disease relapse	• If relapse of Cushing's disease is suspected: 　• Biochemical assessment (e.g., plasma ACTH, 24-h UFC, cortisol circadian rhythm, midnight salivary cortisol, and low-dose DST) 　• Pituitary MRI • If relapse of Cushing's disease is not confirmed or results are conflicting: wait-and-see (especially if the clinical picture is mild) • If relapse of Cushing's disease is confirmed: evaluate other therapeutic approaches

ACTH, Adrenocorticotropic hormone; GH, growth hormone; HPAA, hypothalamic-pituitary-adrenal axis; DST, dexamethasone suppression test; MRI, magnetic resonance imaging; T4, thyroxine; and UFC, urinary free cortisol.

[a]*Timing clinical and biochemical controls depends on several factors, including the patient's personal history, the clinical picture, the response to and monitoring of replacement therapy, and suspicion of relapse of Cushing's disease during follow-up. Immediately after surgery closer controls may be required. In stabilized patients a 6–12 month reevaluation can be a feasible option. Patients should be advised to consult with their physicians if specific signs and symptoms emerge (e.g., signs and symptoms suggestive of hypercortisolism, adrenal insufficiency, or hypopituitarism).*

surgery (we do it every 8 weeks): if serum cortisol is 7.4 µg/dL (200 nmol/L) or more, HPAA recovery is likely, and a confirmation ACTH test for cortisol should be performed. Postcosyntropin serum cortisol values of 18 µg/dL (500 nmol/L) or more are diagnostic for HPAA recovery and allow the discontinuation of glucocorticoid replacement therapy. The use of the more sensitive insulin-induced hypoglycemia test, which provides a better picture of the HPAA response to stress, could be considered an option for unclear laboratory and clinical findings, given the patient has no contraindications to this test. Finally, a morning pre-hydrocortisone serum cortisol level more than 15 µg/dL (414 nmol/L) is diagnostic for HPAA recovery, making dynamic testing unnecessary (Table 9.11) [62]. It should be noted that cutoffs for basal and stimulated serum cortisol values considered predictive of HPAA recovery do vary among studies.

Pituitary surgery harbors a substantial risk of hypopituitarism (0.9–93.3%, mean 29.6%, for primary surgery; 9–78.5%, mean 38%, for repeated surgery) [1]. It is worth noting, however, that Cushing's disease can cause hypopituitarism per se (e.g., central hypothyroidism, central hypogonadism, and growth hormone [GH] deficiency) [63,64]. Therefore, patients should be re-evaluated in the months to years following curative surgery to confirm pituitary hormone deficiencies and the need for replacement therapy.

4.2 After Radiotherapy and Radiosurgery

4.2.1 *Pituitary Insufficiency*

A high risk of late-onset hypopituitarism follows RT, with significant differences in the incidence among clinical studies; the risk seems to be slightly smaller for RS (ranges: 21–78% for conventional RT; 0–69% for RS) [1]. Not surprisingly, the incidence and severity of hypopituitarism are higher in clinical studies with longer follow-up [65–69]. Table 9.14 outlines the management of pituitary insufficiency in adults in terms of diagnosis, treatment, and follow-up [70–73].

The secretion of GH is generally the first and more commonly involved axis followed, in descending order of frequency, by gonadotroph deficiency, thyrotroph deficiency, and corticotroph deficiency [69].

As already stated, it is worth noting that hypercortisolism alone can cause pituitary insufficiency. Therefore, we advise retesting patients during follow-up and after disease remission to confirm the diagnosis and the actual need for replacement therapy [63].

TABLE 9.14 Management of Hypopituitarism in Adults

Screening	• Serum levels of TSH, free T$_4$, IGF-1; LH, FSH, total testosterone (in men), and estradiol (in premenopausal women) should be measured to exclude hypopituitarism. TSH, LH, and FSH are low or inappropriately normal • Normal menses in a premenopausal woman exclude hypogonadism

Confirmatory testing	If central hypothyroidism is suspected
	• The TRH stimulation test for TSH may help to confirm the diagnosis (optional). TRH is not available in the United States
	If central hypogonadism is suspected
	• Exclude hyperprolactinemia
	• For men: only basal FSH, LH, and total testosterone are sufficient to confirm central hypogonadism. Measurement of free testosterone or SHBG may be useful in selected cases
	• Medroxyprogesterone testing (optional) may be used to confirm estradiol deficiency in premenopausal women. Medroxyprogesterone (10 mg) is given for 10 days to demonstrate vaginal bleeding at the end of the cycle
	If GH deficiency is suspected
	• Exclude hypothyroidism, which may lead to a blunted GH response to dynamic testing
	• The presence of deficiencies in three or more pituitary axes strongly suggests the presence of GH deficiency, making dynamic testing optional
	• The GHRH plus arginine stimulation test for GH: A pathological response is considered when peak GH is < 9 µg/L. Cutoffs related to BMIs have been proposed:
	  1. BMI < 25 kg/m^2 → peak GH < 11.5 µg/L;
	  2. BMI 25–30 kg/m^2 → peak GH < 8 µg/L; and
	  3. BMI > 30 kg/m^2 → peak GH < 4.2 µg/L
	Note that results of GHRH plus arginine testing may be misleading within 10 years of pituitary irradiation; however, other provocative tests may be considered, such insulin-induced hypoglycemia and the glucagon test (presently, GHRH not available in the United States).
	• The insulin-induced hypoglycemia test: A pathological response is considered when peak GH is < 5.1 µg/L
	• Glucagon test: A pathological response is considered when peak GH is < 3 µg/L
	• All GH stimulation tests are influenced by BMI. The higher the BMI, the lower the GH peak

(Continued)

TABLE 9.14   Management of Hypopituitarism in Adults (*cont.*)

Treatment and follow-up	**If Central Hypothyroidism Is Confirmed**
	• Look for adrenal insufficiency before correcting hypothyroidism, and start glucocorticoid treatment, if needed
	• Start LT$_4$ and titrate up to a maintenance dose of approximately 1.6 µg/kg of body weight
	• Periodic clinical and biochemical control: free T$_4$ should be maintained in the middle to upper half of the reference range
	If central hypogonadism is confirmed
	• Treat hypogonadal men who are not interested in fertility with testosterone
	• Treat hypogonadal women who are not interested in fertility with estrogen, preferably given by a nonoral route, because it is more physiological and because GH requirements will not be reduced in case of concomitant therapy. Add progestins in the presence of an intact uterus to prevent endometrial hyperplasia. Sex steroid replacement after the time of normal menopause should be based on current recommendations for the general population
	• Treat with gonadotropins if the patient wishes to become fertile.
	• Periodic clinical and biochemical control:
	  1. For men: Monitor morning serum total testosterone, PSA, and blood count (hematocrit)
	  2. For women: Monitor menses and late-follicular serum estradiol (optional)
	If GH deficiency is confirmed
	• Treat only when other concomitant pituitary hormone deficiencies are corrected:
	  1. The rhGH may reduce serum free T$_4$ and might lead to higher LT$_4$ requirements in hypothyroid patients. Moreover, starting rhGH may unmask a latent central hypothyroidism
	  2. Estrogen given orally impairs rhGH action, leading to higher dose requirements
	  3. Starting rhGH in patients taking cortisone acetate or prednisone may lead to an adrenal crisis because GH inhibits the action of 11β-HSD-1, which converts cortisone to cortisol. Moreover, starting rhGH may unmask a latent central adrenal insufficiency
	• Proposed rhGH starting doses: 0.2 mg/day (women); 0.3 mg/day (men); and 0.1 mg/day (older individuals). Titrate rhGH, according to age, gender, estrogen status (in women), clinical response, IGF-1 levels, and side effects (usually 0.1–1 mg rhGH/day)
	• Periodic clinical and biochemical control: IGF-1, liver function tests, lipid profile, blood count, blood glucose, thyroid and adrenal function tests, BMI, waist circumference, blood pressure

11β-HSD-1, 11β-hydroxysteroid dehydrogenase type I; BMI, body mass index; FSH, follicle-stimulating hormone; GH, growth hormone; GHRH, growth hormone–releasing hormone; GnRH, gonadotropin-releasing hormone; IGF-1, insulin-like growth factor 1; LH, luteinizing hormone; LT4, levothyroxine; PSA, prostatic-specific antigen; rhGH, recombinant human growth hormone; SC, subcutaneous administration; SHBG, sex hormone-binding globulin; T3, triiodothyronine; T4, thyroxine; TRH, thyrotropin-releasing hormone; TSH, thyroid-stimulating hormone.

4.2.2 Follow-Up

Long-term follow-up of patients undergoing RT or RS for Cushing's disease includes four main clinical issues: starting cortisol-lowering medications after external radiation, while awaiting for disease remission; establishing disease remission and HPAA recovery; monitoring for the risk of late-onset hypopituitarism; and early diagnosis and management of potential disease relapse (Table 9.15).

TABLE 9.15 Follow-up for Patients with Cushing's Disease after RT and RS

HPAA	<ul><li>Start medical therapy to control hypercortisolism while waiting for RT to work</li><li>Periodic[a] clinical control</li><li>Monitor patient to assess Cushing's disease cure with periodic[a] biochemical control. Measure serum cortisol and 24-h UFC at 6–12-month intervals to assess the efficacy of RT. There is no consensus about the use of low-dose DST and bedtime salivary cortisol to establish Cushing's disease remission after RT. These laboratory tests must be done while holding medical therapy for a variable period of time, depending on the medical therapy used</li><li>Look for signs and symptoms of adrenal insufficiency. Some side effects of drugs used to control hypercortisolism can resemble adrenal insufficiency. Drugs should be withheld or doses reduced if hypoadrenalism is suspected. Test the patient with provocative tests, if needed (Table 9.11)</li><li>Start hydrocortisone replacement therapy if a diagnosis of hypoadrenalism is made (Table 9.9)</li></ul>
Hypopituitarism	Periodic[a] clinical and biochemical control (Table 9.14)
Disease relapse	If relapse of Cushing's disease is suspected<ul><li>Biochemical assessment (e.g., plasma ACTH; 24-h UFC, cortisol circadian rhythm, bedtime salivary cortisol, and low-dose DST)</li><li>Pituitary MRI</li></ul>If relapse of Cushing's disease is not confirmed or results are conflicting<ul><li>Wait and see, especially if the clinical picture is mild</li></ul>If relapse of Cushing's disease is confirmed<ul><li>Evaluate other therapeutic approaches</li></ul>

ACTH, Adrenocorticotropic hormone; DST, dexamethasone suppression test; MRI, magnetic resonance imaging; RT, radiotherapy; RS, radiosurgery; UFC, urinary free cortisol.

[a]*Timing clinical and biochemical controls depends on several factors, including the patient's personal history, clinical picture, monitoring of cortisol-lowering therapies, and suspicion of Cushing's disease relapse during follow-up. Patients should be advised to consult with their physician if specific signs and symptoms emerge (e.g., signs and symptoms suggestive of hypercortisolism, adrenal insufficiency, hypopituitarism, or adverse drug reactions).*

4.3 After Bilateral Adrenalectomy

4.3.1 Primary Adrenal Insufficiency

A lifelong need of glucocorticoid and mineralocorticoid replacement therapy is expected after BLA. Differences exist in the management of primary and central adrenal insufficiency (Tables 9.9, 9.10, and 9.16) [42].

4.3.2 Follow-Up

Follow-up of patients who undergo BLA includes three main clinical issues: evaluating the adequacy of medical replacement therapy, early diagnosis of NS, and diagnosis of hypercortisolism in the unlikely event of disease relapse (Table 9.17).

The 10-year mortality after BLA for Cushing's disease is approximately 3%, but it is worth noting that approximately 50% of deaths occur during the first year after surgery [8]. These data highlight the importance of close monitoring soon after surgery to prevent, to detect early, and to treat hypercortisolism-related sequelae and comorbidities (e.g., thromboembolic events).

The risk of Cushing's disease recurrence after BLA is estimated around 2% (range: 0–12%), but only 1–2% of patients develop clinically evident hypercortisolism [1]. This might be

TABLE 9.16   Medical Treatment of Primary Adrenal Insufficiency in Adults

---

Short-acting glucocorticoids and modified-release hydrocortisone

Hydrocortisone: Usually 20–25 mg orally/day in two or three divided doses.
Cortisone acetate: Usually 25–37.5 mg orally/day in two divided doses
Modified-release hydrocortisone: One dose on awakening (usually 20–30 mg orally/day).

Long-acting glucocorticoids

Dexamethasone: 0.25–0.75 mg orally at bedtime. Evaluate adding 5–10 mg of oral hydrocortisone during the afternoon, according to the clinical picture. Its use is discouraged because of the long half-life and increased risk of excess exposure.
Prednisone: 3–5 mg orally once in the morning. Evaluate adding 5–10 mg of oral hydrocortisone in the afternoon, according to the clinical picture.
When to consider?
Long-acting glucocorticoids (alone or in combination with immediate-release hydrocortisone) can be considered in:
- Patients with morning or late-evening disabling symptoms, which are not controlled by a standard 3-times daily hydrocortisone regimen
- Patients with persistent hyperpigmentation (melanodermia) and persistent high plasma ACTH morning levels (usually > 400 pg/mL)

Mineralocorticoids

Fludrocortisone: 0.05–0.2 mg orally at awakening.
- Hydrocortisone has a mineralocorticoid potency (20 mg of hydrocortisone are equivalent to approximately 0.1 mg of fludrocortisone). Some patients show a higher sensitivity to the mineralocorticoid activity of hydrocortisone and may not require fludrocortisone.
- If the hydrocortisone dose is ≥50 mg/day, fludrocortisone is usually not required.

ACTH, Adrenocorticotropic hormone.

attributed to the presence of adrenal gland remnants after surgery, accessory adrenal glands, or ectopic adrenal tissue that is overstimulated by chronic ACTH secretion by normal and pathological corticotroph cells [7].

4.3.3 Corticotroph Tumor Progression

Corticotroph tumor progression (or NS) is the most important complication when BLA is used to control hypercortisolism in Cushing's disease and is characterized by the triad of

TABLE 9.17   Follow-up for Patients with Cushing's Disease after BLA

Proposed follow-up

- Periodic[a] clinical evaluation
- Periodic[a] biochemical evaluation: morning preglucocorticoid plasma ACTH, plasma renin activity assay or direct renin assay, serum potassium and sodium levels, or serum cortisol (if recurrence is suspected)
- Periodic[a] pituitary MRI for the risk of NS: soon after bilateral adrenalectomy (3–6 months) and at annual intervals (with a decrease in frequency based on previous radiological findings and biochemical data)

ACTH, Adrenocorticotropic hormone; BLA, bilateral adrenalectomy; MRI, magnetic resonance imaging; and NS, Nelson's syndrome.

[a]*Timing of clinical, biochemical, and radiological controls depends on several factors, including a patient's personal history, clinical picture, monitoring of replacement therapy, and suspicion of relapse of Cushing's disease during follow-up. Immediately after surgery, closer controls may be required. In stabilized patients, a 6–12 month reevaluation is a feasible option. Patients should be advised to refer to their clinician if specific signs and symptoms emerge (e.g., signs and symptoms suggestive of hypercortisolism, adrenal insufficiency, or NS).*

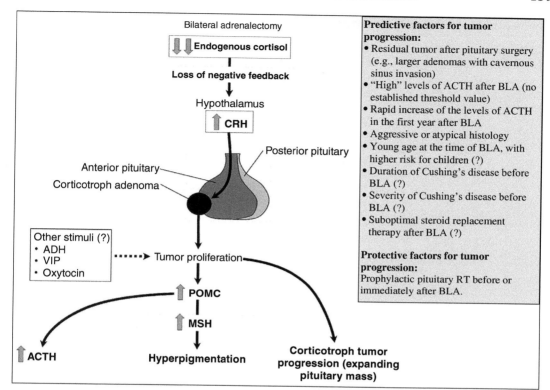

FIGURE 9.1   **Corticotroph tumor progression: pathophysiology.** Corticotroph tumor progression is characterized by the concomitant presence of an expanding pituitary mass and POMC overproduction, leading to hyperpigmentation and very high levels of plasma ACTH. The exact mechanisms leading to NS are not fully understood. The loss of the negative feedback of endogenous hypercortisolism after BLA is probably the triggering factor, which results in CRH overproduction and chronic stimulation of pituitary tumoral cells [79]. The concomitant development of atypical signaling within corticotroph cells may contribute to tumor aggressiveness [80]. Medical therapy with exogenous cortisol consists of adequate control of signs and symptoms of adrenal insufficiency, but it may not be sufficient to inhibit hypothalamic CRH secretion and ACTH production by the pituitary tumor. A contributing factor might be the potential presence of intratumoral somatic mutations in the glucocorticoid receptor, leading to lower responsiveness to exogenous glucocorticoids [81]. Moreover, a possible role of other stimuli, such as ADH, VIP, and oxytocin, has been advocated. For example, the ADH V3 receptor (also known as ADH V1b receptor) is frequently overexpressed in corticotroph adenomas and plays a role in corticotroph proliferation and ACTH secretion [82]. *ACTH*, Adrenocorticotropic hormone; *ADH*, antidiuretic hormone; *BLA*, bilateral adrenocorticotropic hormone; *CRH*, corticotropin-releasing hormone; *NS*, Nelson's syndrome; *MSH*, melanocyte-stimulating hormone; *POMC*, proopiomelanocortin; *RT*, radiotherapy; and *VIP*, vasoactive intestinal peptide.

an expanding pituitary mass, hyperpigmentation, and very high levels of plasma ACTH. The corticotroph tumor may demonstrate locally aggressive behavior. It rarely progresses to a pituitary carcinoma [74], is associated with significant morbidity, and may result in life-threatening complications (Fig. 9.1) [75–82].

The incidence of NS after BLA is 0–47% (median 21%), depending on the case series [1,8,83]. The onset of NS is usually observed 1–4 years after BLA, but it has been reported

TABLE 9.18 Corticotroph Tumor Progression: Features and Management

Diagnosis	Clinical Presentation	Biochemical Presentation	Imaging
	• Hyperpigmentation • Signs and symptoms of local tumor invasiveness: headache, optic chiasm involvement, involvement of cranial nerves within the cavernous sinus (III; IV; V1; V2; VI), and CSF fistula (discharge from nose or ears) • Signs and symptoms of new-onset hypopituitarism	• "High" levels of morning ACTH measured before steroid administration (usually > 500 pg/mL) • Rapid increase of the levels of ACTH (>30% on at least three consecutive occasions)	• Tumor progression at neuroradiological imaging (expanding mass in comparison to imaging performed before BLA) • Extrasellar extension is observed in ~30% of cases
Surgery	• Surgery should be the treatment of choice, especially if optic chiasm involvement is present • A transsphenoidal approach is usually preferred. Transcranial approaches can be considered in the case of extrasellar extension • Success rate: 10%–70%. Smaller tumors with less local invasiveness and no extrasellar extension have better surgical outcomes • Complications: panhypopituitarism (69%), permanent diabetes insipidus (38%), CSF fistula (15%), meningitis (8%), cranial nerve palsy (5%), and death (5%)		
Radiotherapy	• RT can be an adjuvant therapy to surgery in case of recurrent disease and tumors with extrasellar involvement • RT can be the first-line treatment if surgery is contraindicated • Weeks to months are necessary to control tumor progression and ACTH levels • Success rate for conventional RT: ~70% for ACTH level reduction and ~90% for tumor growth control • Success rate for gamma-knife RS: ~70–100% for ACTH level reduction and 14–93% for tumor growth control • Complications: hypopituitarism and involvement of the cranial nerve and optic chiasm		
Medical Therapy	• Medications can be an adjuvant therapy to surgery or RT • Proposed medications: sodium valproate, temozolomide, somatostatin analogues (octreotide, pasireotide), dopamine agonists, serotonin antagonist (cyproheptadine), and peroxisome proliferator-activated receptor γ agonist (rosiglitazone); none proven effective in large studies		
Observation	Observation and close, repeated imaging have been proposed in patients with limited tumor progression and no signs of local invasiveness; however, most patients are likely to progress (clinically, biochemically, or radiologically) during this wait-and-see period [85].		

ACTH, Adrenocorticotropic hormone; BLA, bilateral adrenalectomy; CSF, cerebrospinal fluid; RT, radiotherapy; and RS, radiosurgery.

acutely (2 months after surgery) and up to 24 years following adrenal surgery [76]. It has been suggested that prophylactic pituitary RT before or immediately after BLA may reduce the risk of developing NS or delaying its onset [78,84], but currently no consensus exists on the use of neoadjuvant RT [8]; a cautious balance between potential benefits and long-term risks of pituitary RT is required. Table 9.18 outlines the clinical, laboratory, and imaging criteria used for the diagnosis of NS and the proposed therapeutic options [85]. Modern accuracy of MRI imaging and of plasma ACTH measurement allow the timely diagnosis of corticotroph tumor growth before it is clinically obvious, a key to improving patients' outcomes [78].

The first-line therapy of NS is surgical resection, especially if there is evidence of optic chiasm involvement [75]. Radiotherapy may be considered as adjuvant therapy or primary therapy if neurosurgery is contraindicated, but weeks to months are necessary to obtain disease control. Both conventional RT and gamma-knife RS have been used successfully, and gamma-knife RS is expected to be more effective if used early after BLA and for small, well-defined tumors [86–88]. Data regarding the use of linear accelerator SRT and particle radiation therapy for NS are scarce. Several medications (alone or in combination) have been used in an attempt to control tumor progression in patients with NS after ineffective neurosurgery or while waiting for the effects of RT. Sodium valproate, dopamine agonists, and cyproheptadine have been shown to reduce ACTH secretion in NS, but none of these agents is able to normalize ACTH in the long-term [89], although case reports show that cabergoline can be effective in controlling both ACTH secretion and tumor progression [90,91]. Temozolomide is an alkylating agent used to treat several types of brain tumors and can be an effective therapeutic tool for the treatment of refractory NS [92]. Finally, reports of the use of somatostatin analogues to treat persistent ACTH excess and improve clinical status in NS are scarce, but the multireceptor-targeted somatostatin analogue, pasireotide, might be expected to offer good outcomes in this setting [93,94]. Additional studies are warranted to validate the use of pasireotide as a treatment for NS.

5 LONG-TERM EFFECTS OF HYPERCORTISOLISM IN CURED PATIENTS

A history of Cushing's disease is associated with long-term detrimental effects, which may persist for years after normalization of cortisol secretion: the longer the diagnosis is delayed, the higher the risk. Evaluation and management of the long-standing effects of hypercortisolism in patients who go into remission after treatment for Cushing's disease are reviewed in Chapter 10.

5.1 Cardiovascular Risk

A history of previous hypercortisolism presages a persistent and long-standing increase in cardiovascular risk. The degree of cardiovascular impairment differs among patients: on one hand, this is related to the duration and severity of the disease; on the other hand, the possible presence of polymorphisms of the glucocorticoid receptor can lead to variable inter- and intra-individual sensitivities to cortisol [95,96].

Markers of increased cardiovascular risk (e.g., increased carotid intima-media thickness, atherosclerotic plaques, and high homocysteine levels), as well as clinical and laboratory abnormalities of the metabolic syndrome can be observed for at least 5 years after disease remission [97–99]. Colao and colleagues reported that after 5 years of cortisol normalization, a body mass index (BMI) over 25 kg/m^2 was observed in 73% of patients, impaired glucose tolerance in 60%, hypertension in 40%, and dyslipidemia in 26.7%. The prevalence of these disorders, although lower than what is observed during active hypercortisolism, is still significantly higher when compared to controls [97].

After a demonstrated cure of hypercortisolism, normalization of cardiac function can be observed in terms of echocardiographic parameters (e.g., left ventricular hypertrophy, diastolic dysfunction, and subclinical left ventricular systolic dysfunction) [100]. An increased long-standing risk of myocardial infarction persists, however, after normalization of cortisol secretion, probably because of the persistence of the metabolic syndrome [101]. Similarly, the long-term effects of cortisol on blood pressure are complex, and diurnal arterial hypertension, as well as an alteration of the nocturnal dipping in blood pressure, can be detected after long-standing cure [97,102]. Children with cured hypercortisolism could be more sensitive to this detrimental effect on blood pressure, secondary to a cortisol-induced endothelial "programming" (Chapter 11) [103]. Conversely, adults may experience persistent arterial hypertension after hypercortisolism correction because of preexisting high blood pressure or cortisol-induced damage to microvessels, obesity, and insulin resistance [104].

5.2 Thromboembolic Events

Hypercortisolism causes a hypercoagulable state that is reflected by an increased incidence of venous thromboembolism. Patients with Cushing's syndrome have been reported to have a more than 10-fold increased risk of developing venous thromboembolism. Accordingly, the incidence of postoperative thrombosis is high, comparable to the risk after major orthopedic surgery, lasting at least 3 months after surgery [101]. Because of this, some authors have advocated that patients with active Cushing's disease need thromboprophylaxis [105].

5.3 Osteoporosis

The negative effect of hypercortisolism on bone, especially trabecular bone, is well-known and mediated by several direct and indirect mechanisms (e.g. osteoblastic/osteoclastic activity alteration, reduced intestinal calcium absorption, increase urinary calcium excretion, and central hypogonadism) [106].

Bone mineral density improves after disease remission, but normalization may require a long period of time (up to 9 years) and the use of anti-osteoporosis medications [107–110]. There are conflicting data regarding the actual restoration of normal bone mineral density after cure of hypercortisolism, since some authors have shown incomplete recovery of bone mass, increased prevalence of vertebral fractures, and low levels of osteocalcin [111–113]. Patient inclusion criteria, duration and severity of previous hypercortisolism, menopausal status in women, duration of follow-up, and comorbidities (e.g., hypopituitarism, impaired glucose tolerance) may partially account for these differences among clinical studies. Moreover, it should be noted that even glucocorticoid replacement therapy can be a risk factor for low bone mineral density [113].

5.4 Neurocognitive Impairment

The central nervous system, and in particular the limbic system, is a key target for cortisol, considering the high density of glucocorticoid receptors [114]. Irreversible or long-term effects of excess cortisol on the central nervous system are a major clinical problem in patients after normalization of cortisol secretion.

Impaired cognitive functions (e.g., alteration in memory and executive functions) as well as a high prevalence of psychopathology and maladaptive behaviors are observed for several years after resolution of hypercortisolism [115,116]. This may account for the long-standing quality of life impairment seen in these patients after cure [117] and may be explained by the anatomical cerebral changes observed. In fact, brain volume may not normalize after resolution of hypercortisolism even after 4 years of follow-up, with only partial recovery of hippocampal, caudate nucleus, and amygdala volume (Chapter 4) [118–121]. Conversely, children with endogenous Cushing's syndrome show a decline of cognitive functions after the cure of hypercortisolism despite a rapid reversal of cerebral atrophy [121]. The reasons for this apparent paradox are unclear and suggest that the effects of glucocorticoid excess on the brain in children are different from the effects in adults (Chapter 11).

References

[1] Pivonello R, De Leo M, Cozzolino A, et al. The treatment of Cushing's disease. Endocr Rev 2015;36(4):385–486.

[2] Saeger W, Ludecke DK, Buchfelder M, et al. Pathohistological classification of pituitary tumors: 10 years of experience with the German Pituitary Tumor Registry. Eur J Endocrinol 2007;156(2):203–16.

[3] George DH, Scheithauer BW, Kovacs K, et al. Crooke's cell adenoma of the pituitary: an aggressive variant of corticotroph adenoma. Am J Surg Pathol 2003;27(10):1330–6.

[4] Rutkowski MJ, Flanigan PM, Aghi MK. Update on the management of recurrent Cushing's disease. Neurosurg Focus 2015;38(2):E16.

[5] Alexandraki KI, Kaltsas GA, Isidori AM, et al. Long-term remission and recurrence rates in Cushing's disease: predictive factors in a single-centre study. Eur J Endocrinol 2013;168(4):639–48.

[6] Yap LB, Turner HE, Adams CB, et al. Undetectable postoperative cortisol does not always predict long-term remission in Cushing's disease: a single centre audit. Clin Endocrinol (Oxf) 2002;56(1):25–31.

[7] Ren PT, Fu H, He XW. Ectopic adrenal cortical adenoma in the gastric wall: case report. World J Gastroenterol 2013;19(5):778–80.

[8] Nieman LK, Biller BM, Findling JW, et al. Treatment of Cushing's syndrome: an Endocrine Society Clinical Practice Guideline. J Clin Endocrinol Metab 2015;100(8):2807–31.

[9] Bochicchio D, Losa M, Buchfelder M. Factors influencing the immediate and late outcome of Cushing's disease treated by transsphenoidal surgery: a retrospective study by the European Cushing's disease Survey Group. J Clin Endocrinol Metab 1995;80(11):3114–20.

[10] Amlashi FG, Swearingen B, Faje AT, et al. Accuracy of late-night salivary cortisol in evaluating postoperative remission and recurrence in Cushing's disease. J Clin Endocrinol Metab 2015;100(10):3770–7.

[11] Krone N, Hughes BA, Lavery GG, et al. Gas chromatography/mass spectrometry (GC/MS) remains a preeminent discovery tool in clinical steroid investigations even in the era of fast liquid chromatography tandem mass spectrometry (LC/MS/MS). J Steroid Biochem Mol Biol 2010;121(3-5):496–504.

[12] Pendharkar AV, Sussman ES, Ho AL, et al. Cushing's disease: predicting long-term remission after surgical treatment. Neurosurg Focus 2015;38(2):E13.

[13] Kidambi S, Raff H, Findling JW. Limitations of nocturnal salivary cortisol and urine free cortisol in the diagnosis of mild Cushing's syndrome. Eur J Endocrinol 2007;157(6):725–31.

[14] Alexandraki KI, Grossman AB. Is urinary free cortisol of value in the diagnosis of Cushing's syndrome? Curr Opin Endocrinol Diabetes Obes 2011;18(4):259–63.

[15] Raff H, Auchus RJ, Findling JW, et al. Urine free cortisol in the diagnosis of Cushing's syndrome: is it worth doing and, if so, how? J Clin Endocrinol Metab 2015;100(2):395–7.

[16] Petersenn S, Newell-Price J, Findling JW, et al. High variability in baseline urinary free cortisol values in patients with Cushing's disease. Clin Endocrinol (Oxf) 2014;80(2):261–9.

[17] Barbot M, Albiger N, Koutroumpi S, et al. Predicting late recurrence in surgically treated patients with Cushing's disease. Clin Endocrinol (Oxf) 2013;79(3):394–401.

[18] Blevins LS Jr, Sanai N, Kunwar S, et al. An approach to the management of patients with residual Cushing's disease. J Neurooncol 2009;94(3):313–9.

[19] Wind JJ, Lonser RR, Nieman LK, et al. The lateralization accuracy of inferior petrosal sinus sampling in 501 patients with Cushing's disease. J Clin Endocrinol Metab 2013;98(6):2285–93.

[20] Hofmann BM, Hlavac M, Kreutzer J, et al. Surgical treatment of recurrent Cushing's disease. Neurosurgery 2006;58(6):1108–18.

[21] Valassi E, Biller BM, Swearingen B, et al. Delayed remission after transsphenoidal surgery in patients with Cushing's disease. J Clin Endocrinol Metab 2010;95(2):601–10.

[22] McLaughlin N, Kassam AB, Prevedello DM, et al. Management of Cushing's disease after failed surgery—a review. Can J Neurol Sci 2011;38(1):12–21.

[23] Biller BM, Grossman AB, Stewart PM, et al. Treatment of adrenocorticotropin-dependent Cushing's syndrome: a consensus statement. J Clin Endocrinol Metab 2008;93(7):2454–62.

[24] Lee CC, Chen CJ, Yen CP, et al. Whole-sellar stereotactic radiosurgery for functioning pituitary adenomas. Neurosurgery 2014;75(3):227–37.

[25] Castinetti F, Nagai M, Dufour H, et al. Gamma knife radiosurgery is a successful adjunctive treatment in Cushing's disease. Eur J Endocrinol 2007;156(1):91–8.

[26] Landolt AM, Haller D, Lomax N, et al. Octreotide may act as a radioprotective agent in acromegaly. J Clin Endocrinol Metab 2000;85(3):1287–9.

[27] Stalla GK, Stalla J, Huber M, et al. Ketoconazole inhibits corticotropic cell function in vitro. Endocrinology 1988;122(2):618–23.

[28] Scott HW Jr, Liddle GW, Mulherin JL Jr, et al. Surgical experience with Cushing's disease. Ann Surg 1977;185(5):524–34.

[29] Colao A, Petersenn S, Newell-Price J, et al. A 12-month phase 3 study of pasireotide in Cushing's disease. N Engl J Med 2012;366(10):914–24.

[30] Pivonello R, De Martino MC, Cappabianca P, et al. The medical treatment of Cushing's disease: effectiveness of chronic treatment with the dopamine agonist cabergoline in patients unsuccessfully treated by surgery. J Clin Endocrinol Metab 2009;94(1):223–30.

[31] Castinetti F, Morange I, Jaquet P, et al. Ketoconazole revisited: a preoperative or postoperative treatment in Cushing's disease. Eur J Endocrinol 2008;158(1):91–9.

[32] Bademci G. Pitfalls in the management of Cushing's disease. J Clin Neurosci 2007;14(5):401–8.

[33] Morris LF, Harris RS, Milton DR, et al. Impact and timing of bilateral adrenalectomy for refractory adrenocorticotropic hormone-dependent Cushing's syndrome. Surgery 2013;154(6):1174–83.

[34] Wong A, Eloy JA, Liu JK. The role of bilateral adrenalectomy in the treatment of refractory Cushing's disease. Neurosurg Focus 2015;38(2):E9.

[35] Fitzgerald PA, Aron DC, Findling JW, et al. Cushing's disease: transient secondary adrenal insufficiency after selective removal of pituitary microadenomas; evidence for a pituitary origin. J Clin Endocrinol Metab 1982;54(2):413–22.

[36] Hermus AR, Pieters GF, Pesman GJ, et al. Coexistence of hypothalamic and pituitary failure after successful pituitary surgery in Cushing's disease? J Endocrinol Invest 1987;10(4):365–9.

[37] Berr CM, Di Dalmazi G, Osswald A, et al. Time to recovery of adrenal function after curative surgery for Cushing's syndrome depends on etiology. J Clin Endocrinol Metab 2015;100(4):1300–8.

[38] Flitsch J, Ludecke DK, Knappe UJ, et al. Correlates of long-term hypocortisolism after transsphenoidal microsurgery for Cushing's disease. Exp Clin Endocrinol Diabetes 1999;107(3):183–9.

[39] Ciric I, Zhao JC, Du H, et al. Transsphenoidal surgery for Cushing disease: experience with 136 patients. Neurosurgery 2012;70(1):70–80.

[40] Costenaro F, Rodrigues TC, Rollin GA, et al. Evaluation of Cushing's disease remission after transsphenoidal surgery based on early serum cortisol dynamics. Clin Endocrinol (Oxf) 2014;80(3):411–8.

[41] Aranda G, Ensenat J, Mora M, et al. Long-term remission and recurrence rate in a cohort of Cushing's disease: the need for long-term follow-up. Pituitary 2015;18(1):142–9.

[42] Grossman A, Johannsson G, Quinkler M, et al. Therapy of endocrine disease: perspectives on the management of adrenal insufficiency: clinical insights from across Europe. Eur J Endocrinol 2013;169(6):R165–75.

[43] Dorin RI, Qualls CR, Crapo LM. Diagnosis of adrenal insufficiency. Ann Intern Med 2003;139(3):194–204.

[44] Dokmetas HS, Colak R, Kelestimur F, et al. A comparison between the 1-microg adrenocorticotropin (ACTH) test, the short ACTH (250 microg) test, and the insulin tolerance test in the assessment of hypothalamic-pituitary-adrenal axis immediately after pituitary surgery. J Clin Endocrinol Metab 2000;85(10):3713–9.

[45] Soule SG, Fahie-Wilson M, Tomlinson S. Failure of the short ACTH test to unequivocally diagnose long-standing symptomatic secondary hypoadrenalism. Clin Endocrinol (Oxf) 1996;44(2):137–40.

[46] Tordjman K, Jaffe A, Grazas N, et al. The role of the low dose (1 microgram) adrenocorticotropin test in the evaluation of patients with pituitary diseases. J Clin Endocrinol Metab 1995;80(4):1301–5.

[47] Fiad TM, Kirby JM, Cunningham SK, et al. The overnight single-dose metyrapone test is a simple and reliable index of the hypothalamic-pituitary-adrenal axis. Clin Endocrinol (Oxf) 1994;40(5):603–9.

[48] Spark RF. Simplified assessment of pituitary-adrenal reserve. Measurement of serum 11-deoxycortisol and cortisol after metyrapone. Ann Intern Med 1971;75(5):717–23.

[49] de Miguel Novoa P, Vela ET, Garcia NP, et al. Guidelines for the diagnosis and treatment of adrenal insufficiency in the adult. Endocrinol Nutr 2014;61(Suppl. 1):1–35.

[50] Ospina NS, Al Nofal A, Bancos I, et al. ACTH stimulation tests for the diagnosis of adrenal insufficiency: systematic review and meta-analysis. J Clin Endocrinol Metab 2016;101(2):427–34.

[51] Bhattacharyya A, Kaushal K, Tymms DJ, et al. Steroid withdrawal syndrome after successful treatment of Cushing's syndrome: a reminder. Eur J Endocrinol 2005;153(2):207–10.

[52] Hochberg Z, Pacak K, Chrousos GP. Endocrine withdrawal syndromes. Endocr Rev 2003;24(4):523–38.

[53] Papanicolaou DA, Tsigos C, Oldfield EH, et al. Acute glucocorticoid deficiency is associated with plasma elevations of interleukin-6: does the latter participate in the symptomatology of the steroid withdrawal syndrome and adrenal insufficiency? J Clin Endocrinol Metab 1996;81(6):2303–6.

[54] da Mota F, Murray C, Ezzat S. Overt immune dysfunction after Cushing's syndrome remission: a consecutive case series and review of the literature. J Clin Endocrinol Metab 2011;96(10):E1670–4.

[55] Fenske W, Allolio B. Clinical review: current state and future perspectives in the diagnosis of diabetes insipidus: a clinical review. J Clin Endocrinol Metab 2012;97(10):3426–37.

[56] Loh JA, Verbalis JG. Diabetes insipidus as a complication after pituitary surgery. Nat Clin Pract Endocrinol Metab 2007;3(6):489–94.

[57] Smith TR, Hulou MM, Huang KT, et al. Complications after transsphenoidal surgery for patients with Cushing's disease and silent corticotroph adenomas. Neurosurg Focus 2015;38(2):E12.

[58] Oiso Y, Robertson GL, Norgaard JP, et al. Clinical review: treatment of neurohypophyseal diabetes insipidus. J Clin Endocrinol Metab 2013;98(10):3958–67.

[59] Verbalis JG, Goldsmith SR, Greenberg A, et al. Diagnosis, evaluation, and treatment of hyponatremia: expert panel recommendations. Am J Med 2013;126(10 Suppl. 1):S1–S42.

[60] Juul KV, Schroeder M, Rittig S, et al. National surveillance of central diabetes insipidus (Cushing's disease) in Denmark: results from 5 years registration of 9309 prescriptions of desmopressin to 1285 Cushing's disease patients. J Clin Endocrinol Metab 2014;99(6):2181–7.

[61] Olson BR, Rubino D, Gumowski J, et al. Isolated hyponatremia after transsphenoidal pituitary surgery. J Clin Endocrinol Metab 1995;80(1):85–91.

[62] Santhanam P, Saleem SF, Saleem TF. Diagnostic predicament of secondary adrenal insufficiency. Endocr Pract 2010;16(4):686–91.

[63] Sherlock M, Ayuk J, Tomlinson JW, et al. Mortality in patients with pituitary disease. Endocr Rev 2010;31(3):301–42.

[64] Mathioudakis N, Thapa S, Wand GS, et al. ACTH-secreting pituitary microadenomas are associated with a higher prevalence of central hypothyroidism compared to other microadenoma types. Clin Endocrinol (Oxf) 2012;77(6):871–6.

[65] Sharpe GF, Kendall-Taylor P, Prescott RW, et al. Pituitary function following megavoltage therapy for Cushing's disease: long term follow up. Clin Endocrinol (Oxf) 1985;22(2):169–77.

[66] Murayama M, Yasuda K, Minamori Y, et al. Long-term follow-up of Cushing's disease treated with reserpine and pituitary irradiation. J Clin Endocrinol Metab 1992;75(3):935–42.

[67] Martinez R, Bravo G, Burzaco J, et al. Pituitary tumors and gamma knife surgery. Clinical experience with more than two years of follow-up. Stereotact Funct Neurosurg 1998;70(Suppl 1):110–8.

[68] Hoybye C, Grenback E, Rahn T, et al. Adrenocorticotropic hormone-producing pituitary tumors: 12- to 22-year follow-up after treatment with stereotactic radiosurgery. Neurosurgery 2001;49(2):284–91.

[69] Cohen-Inbar O, Ramesh A, Xu Z, et al. Gamma knife radiosurgery in patients with persistent acromegaly or Cushing's disease: long-term risk of hypopituitarism. Clin Endocrinol (Oxf) 2016;84(4):524–31.

[70] Molitch ME, Clemmons DR, Malozowski S, et al. Evaluation and treatment of adult growth hormone deficiency: an Endocrine Society clinical practice guideline. J Clin Endocrinol Metab 2011;96(6):1587–609.

[71] Ho KK. GHDCWorkshop Participants. Consensus guidelines for the diagnosis and treatment of adults with GH deficiency II: a statement of the GH Research Society in association with the European Society for Pediatric Endocrinology, Lawson Wilkins Society, European Society of Endocrinology, Japan Endocrine Society, and Endocrine Society of Australia. Eur J Endocrinol 2007;157(6):695–700.

[72] Bhasin S, Cunningham GR, Hayes FJ, et al. Testosterone therapy in adult men with androgen deficiency syndromes: an endocrine society clinical practice guideline. J Clin Endocrinol Metab 2006;91(6):1995–2010.

[73] Hartoft-Nielsen ML, Lange M, Rasmussen AK, et al. Thyrotropin-releasing hormone stimulation test in patients with pituitary pathology. Horm Res 2004;61(2):53–7.

[74] Kemink SA, Wesseling P, Pieters GF, et al. Progression of a Nelson's adenoma to pituitary carcinoma; a case report and review of the literature. J Endocrinol Invest 1999;22(1):70–5.

[75] Patel J, Eloy JA, Liu JK. Nelson's syndrome: a review of the clinical manifestations, pathophysiology, and treatment strategies. Neurosurg Focus 2015;38(2):E14.

[76] Azad TD, Veeravagu A, Kumar S, et al. Nelson syndrome: update on therapeutic approaches. World Neurosurg 2015;83(6):1135–40.

[77] Shibasaki T, Masui H. Effects of various neuropeptides on the secretion of proopiomelanocortin-derived peptides by a cultured pituitary adenoma causing Nelson's syndrome. J Clin Endocrinol Metab 1982;55(5):872–6.

[78] Barber TM, Adams E, Ansorge O, et al. Nelson's syndrome. Eur J Endocrinol 2010;163(4):495–507.

[79] McNicol AM, Carbajo-Perez E. Aspects of anterior pituitary growth, with special reference to corticotrophs. Pituitary 1999;1(3-4):257–68.

[80] Dworakowska D, Grossman AB. The molecular pathogenesis of corticotroph tumours. Eur J Clin Invest 2012;42(6):665–76.

[81] Karl M, Von Wichert G, Kempter E, et al. Nelson's syndrome associated with a somatic frame shift mutation in the glucocorticoid receptor gene. J Clin Endocrinol Metab 1996;81(1):124–9.

[82] El Ghorayeb N, Bourdeau I, Lacroix A. Multiple aberrant hormone receptors in Cushing's syndrome. Eur J Endocrinol 2015;173(4):M45–60.

[83] Ritzel K, Beuschlein F, Mickisch A, et al. Clinical review: outcome of bilateral adrenalectomy in Cushing's syndrome: a systematic review. J Clin Endocrinol Metab 2013;98(10):3939–48.

[84] Jenkins PJ, Trainer PJ, Plowman PN, et al. The long-term outcome after adrenalectomy and prophylactic pituitary radiotherapy in adrenocorticotropin-dependent Cushing's syndrome. J Clin Endocrinol Metab 1995;80(1):165–71.

[85] Kemink SA, Grotenhuis JA, De Vries J, et al. Management of Nelson's syndrome: observations in fifteen patients. Clin Endocrinol (Oxf) 2001;54(1):45–52.

[86] Marek J, Jezkova J, Hana V, et al. Gamma knife radiosurgery for Cushing's disease and Nelson's syndrome. Pituitary 2015;18(3):376–84.

[87] Mauermann WJ, Sheehan JP, Chernavvsky DR, et al. Gamma knife surgery for adrenocorticotropic hormone-producing pituitary adenomas after bilateral adrenalectomy. J Neurosurg 2007;106(6):988–93.

[88] Vik-Mo EO, Oksnes M, Pedersen PH, et al. Gamma knife stereotactic radiosurgery of Nelson syndrome. Eur J Endocrinol 2009;160(2):143–8.

[89] Mercado-Asis LB, Yanovski JA, Tracer HL, et al. Acute effects of bromocriptine, cyproheptadine, and valproic acid on plasma adrenocorticotropin secretion in Nelson's syndrome. J Clin Endocrinol Metab 1997;82(2):514–7.

[90] Casulari LA, Naves LA, Mello PA, et al. Nelson's syndrome: complete remission with cabergoline but not with bromocriptine or cyproheptadine treatment. Horm Res 2004;62(6):300–5.

[91] Shraga-Slutzky I, Shimon I, Weinshtein R. Clinical and biochemical stabilization of Nelson's syndrome with long-term low-dose cabergoline treatment. Pituitary 2006;9(2):151–4.

[92] Moyes VJ, Alusi G, Sabin HI, et al. Treatment of Nelson's syndrome with temozolomide. Eur J Endocrinol 2009;160(1):115–9.

[93] Arregger AL, Cardoso EM, Sandoval OB, et al. Hormonal secretion and quality of life in Nelson syndrome and Cushing disease after long-acting repeatable octreotide: a short series and update. Am J Ther 2014;21(4):e110–6.

[94] Katznelson L. Sustained improvements in plasma ACTH and clinical status in a patient with Nelson's syndrome treated with pasireotide LAR, a multireceptor somatostatin analog. J Clin Endocrinol Metab 2013;98(5):1803–7.

[95] Huizenga NA, Koper JW, De Lange P, et al. A polymorphism in the glucocorticoid receptor gene may be associated with and increased sensitivity to glucocorticoids in vivo. J Clin Endocrinol Metab 1998;83(1):144–51.

[96] van Rossum EF, Koper JW, van den Beld AW, et al. Identification of the BclI polymorphism in the glucocorticoid receptor gene: association with sensitivity to glucocorticoids in vivo and body mass index. Clin Endocrinol (Oxf) 2003;59(5):585–92.

[97] Colao A, Pivonello R, Spiezia S, et al. Persistence of increased cardiovascular risk in patients with Cushing's disease after five years of successful cure. J Clin Endocrinol Metab 1999;84(8):2664–72.

[98] Faggiano A, Pivonello R, Spiezia S, et al. Cardiovascular risk factors and common carotid artery caliber and stiffness in patients with Cushing's disease during active disease and 1 year after disease remission. J Clin Endocrinol Metab 2003;88(6):2527–33.

[99] Terzolo M, Allasino B, Bosio S, et al. Hyperhomocysteinemia in patients with Cushing's syndrome. J Clin Endocrinol Metab 2004;89(8):3745–51.

[100] Pereira AM, Delgado V, Romijn JA, et al. Cardiac dysfunction is reversed upon successful treatment of Cushing's syndrome. Eur J Endocrinol 2010;162(2):331–40.

[101] Dekkers OM, Horvath-Puho E, Jorgensen JO, et al. Multisystem morbidity and mortality in Cushing's syndrome: a cohort study. J Clin Endocrinol Metab 2013;98(6):2277–84.

[102] Pecori Giraldi F, Toja PM, De Martin M, et al. Circadian blood pressure profile in patients with active Cushing's disease and after long-term cure. Horm Metab Res 2007;39(12):908–14.

[103] Lodish MB, Sinaii N, Patronas N, et al. Blood pressure in pediatric patients with Cushing syndrome. J Clin Endocrinol Metab 2009;94(6):2002–8.

[104] Pivonello R, Faggiano A, Lombardi G, et al. The metabolic syndrome and cardiovascular risk in Cushing's syndrome. Endocrinol Metab Clin North Am 2005;34(2):327–39.

[105] van der Pas R, Leebeek FW, Hofland LJ, et al. Hypercoagulability in Cushing's syndrome: prevalence, pathogenesis and treatment. Clin Endocrinol (Oxf) 2013;78(4):481–8.

[106] Chiodini I, Torlontano M, Carnevale V, et al. Skeletal involvement in adult patients with endogenous hypercortisolism. J Endocrinol Invest 2008;31(3):267–76.

[107] Pivonello R, De Martino MC, De Leo M, et al. Cushing's syndrome: aftermath of the cure. Arq Bras Endocrinol Metabol 2007;51(8):1381–91.

[108] Futo L, Toke J, Patocs A, et al. Skeletal differences in bone mineral area and content before and after cure of endogenous Cushing's syndrome. Osteoporos Int 2008;19(7):941–9.

[109] Kristo C, Jemtland R, Ueland T, et al. Restoration of the coupling process and normalization of bone mass following successful treatment of endogenous Cushing's syndrome: a prospective, long-term study. Eur J Endocrinol 2006;154(1):109–18.

[110] Manning PJ, Evans MC, Reid IR. Normal bone mineral density following cure of Cushing's syndrome. Clin Endocrinol (Oxf) 1992;36(3):229–234111.

[111] Hermus AR, Smals AG, Swinkels LM, et al. Bone mineral density and bone turnover before and after surgical cure of Cushing's syndrome. J Clin Endocrinol Metab 1995;80(10):2859–65.

[112] Faggiano A, Pivonello R, Filippella M, et al. Spine abnormalities and damage in patients cured from Cushing's disease. Pituitary 2001;4(3):153–61.

[113] Barahona MJ, Sucunza N, Resmini E, et al. Deleterious effects of glucocorticoid replacement on bone in women after long-term remission of Cushing's syndrome. J Bone Miner Res 2009;24(11):1841–6.

[114] Andela CD, van Haalen FM, Ragnarsson O, et al. Mechanisms in endocrinology: Cushing's syndrome causes irreversible effects on the human brain: a systematic review of structural and functional magnetic resonance imaging studies. Eur J Endocrinol 2015;173(1):R1–R14.

[115] Tiemensma J, Kokshoorn NE, Biermasz NR, et al. Subtle cognitive impairments in patients with long-term cure of Cushing's disease. J Clin Endocrinol Metab 2010;95(6):2699–714.

[116] Sonino N, Fava GA. Psychiatric disorders associated with Cushing's syndrome. Epidemiology, pathophysiology and treatment. CNS Drugs 2001;15(5):361–73.

[117] Webb SM, Badia X, Barahona MJ, et al. Evaluation of health-related quality of life in patients with Cushing's syndrome with a new questionnaire. Eur J Endocrinol 2008;158(5):623–30.

[118] Bourdeau I, Bard C, Forget H, et al. Cognitive function and cerebral assessment in patients who have Cushing's syndrome. Endocrinol Metab Clin North Am 2005;34(2):357–69.

[119] Starkman MN, Giordani B, Gebarski SS, et al. Improvement in learning associated with increase in hippocampal formation volume. Biol Psychiatry 2003;53(3):233–8.

[120] Starkman MN, Giordani B, Gebarski SS, et al. Improvement in mood and ideation associated with increase in right caudate volume. J Affect Disord 2007;101(1–3):139–47.

[121] Merke DP, Giedd JN, Keil MF, et al. Children experience cognitive decline despite reversal of brain atrophy one year after resolution of Cushing syndrome. J Clin Endocrinol Metab 2005;90(5):2531–6.

Coping with Cushing's Disease: the Patients' Perspectives

A. Santos, MPsy, PhD, S.M. Webb, MD, PhD

Endocrinology/Medicine Department, Centro de Investigación Biomédica en Red de Enfermedades Raras (CIBERER, Unidad 747), ISCIII, Research Center for Pituitary Diseases, Hospital Sant Pau, IIB-Sant Pau, and Universitat Autònoma de Barcelona (UAB), Barcelona, Spain

OUTLINE

1 INTRODUCTION

Cushing's syndrome, including pituitary-dependent Cushing's disease, adrenal causes, and ectopic adrenocorticotropic hormone (ACTH) secretion (all of which present as endogenous hypercortisolism and are included in Cushing's syndrome), can have significant effects on patients' lives. Most patients report that Cushing's syndrome has had some effect on their lives (20%), while others report that it has greatly affected their lives (71%) [1]. This disease presents as a series of symptoms, as well as physical and psychological changes, which may lead to a compromised health-related quality of life. It is important to note, however, that not all patients experience the same symptoms. Some patients are diagnosed by chance in the early stages of the disease after experiencing almost no major symptoms. Others may not be diagnosed for years, despite feeling that something is very wrong. When symptoms are more pronounced and include troublesome features, such as fatigue, depression, or anxiety, they often have a more obvious effect on daily life, particularly affecting work, family, and social relationships. Some patients may be unable to work, which can affect their economic well-being. This is especially important when working freelance or being on sick leave, which translates into little or no income and perhaps no health insurance.

The recovery time after successful treatment also differs from patient to patient. After surgery, most patients complain of feeling worse than when their disease was active, and their cortisol was high. This is the result of the sudden fall in cortisol levels. It often takes a long time to recover, perhaps months or even years. Even if there is information for patients during the diagnostic period, little information is available that covers the recovery phase or the long-term sequelae of Cushing's syndrome; patients often complain about not receiving enough information about their disease and the recovery period.

This chapter covers the patients' perspectives when coping with Cushing's syndrome, a topic on which few scientific studies are available; therefore, the authors have included information taken from the Cushing's Support and Research Foundation (CSRF) and from clinical practice when treating Cushing's syndrome patients.

2 COPING WITH A RARE DISEASE

An important problem when dealing with a rare disorder like Cushing's disease is often the long delay before the correct diagnosis is made. Most of the symptoms are nonspecific for the disease, so it often goes unnoticed for months to years. A study involving a large cohort of 481 patients found that the median delay to diagnosis was 2 years [2]; others have reported a mean delay of 3.5–5 years [3–5]. Clinical experience shows that it may take just a few months, or it may take more than 20 years to be diagnosed with Cushing's.

According to data from the European Register on Cushing's syndrome and other large cohort studies, most patients (77–83%) consult a general practitioner before obtaining a correct diagnosis [2,4]. Physician consultation may differ, depending on the cause of Cushing's syndrome. For instance, diabetologists are more frequently consulted by patients with ectopic ACTH secretion than by patients with an adrenal origin of Cushing's syndrome; gynecologists, on the other hand, are consulted more often by patients with pituitary or adrenal Cushing's syndrome than by patients with an ectopic origin [2]. This highlights the varying prevalence of clinical complaints among the different causes of Cushing's syndrome; these complaints unfortunately are most often considered in isolation while the syndrome itself is missed. It has been reported that only 6.3% of general practitioners make a definitive diagnosis of Cushing's syndrome, which is most frequently made by an endocrinologist (69.9% of cases) [4]. In order to shorten the diagnostic delay, guidelines for general practitioners have been developed and are available online (brochure available from: http://www.lb.de/ercusyn/wMedia/pdf/brochure/cushingsEN.pdf); this brochure has been translated into several languages. Patients with Cushing's syndrome (as well as their friends and relatives) have reported distributing this brochure to their general practitioners, hoping to help future patients to be diagnosed promptly.

The long delay to diagnosis is exhausting, as well as troubling. A questionnaire completed by 176 German patients with Cushing's disease showed that patients consulted a mean of 4.6 doctors (ranging from 1–30 specialists) during the diagnostic process [4]. In most cases, the symptom onset was recognized by the patients rather than by the physician. Another American cohort found similar data on the number of physicians consulted, a median of 4 physicians, with a range from 1–40 physicians [5]. However, 76% stated that the diagnosis had been first suggested by a physician [5]. In the German study, women recognized the disease more often than men (81.3% vs. 59.4%) [4]. Table 10.1 summarizes the reasons for which select patients sought a consultation before the correct diagnosis was established.

3 HEALTH COMPLAINTS IN THE ACTIVE PHASE

During the active phase of hypercortisolism patients have to contend with a number of health problems that accompany Cushing's syndrome, all of which have a profound effect on their lives.

3.1 Quality of Life

Poor quality of life is described by patients with active Cushing's syndrome as compared to healthy controls or patients with other pituitary adenomas [6–8]. A diminished quality of life, both physically and mentally, is reported, reflecting potentially significant physical and psychological impairments [6,7].

Quality of life can be affected by many factors. Specifically, Cushing's syndrome is marked by muscle weakness (leading to fatigue), sleeping difficulties, and psychological disturbances. Depression is one of the main predictors of quality of life when considered with age, gender, diagnosis, delay to diagnosis, body mass index, diabetes, and hypertension [2]. This is important, since depression can be treated, leading to improvement in the patient's well-being. Some patients benefit from psychological support or taking psychiatric medication during the active disease phase and even during recovery.

A negative correlation between the number of physicians consulted before diagnosis and quality of life has been found, indicating that patients who see more physicians to obtain a correct diagnosis show more serious quality-of-life impairments. It may be that experiencing greater discomfort leads to more physician visits, or it could simply indicate a longer duration of symptoms. By comparison, patients who are treated by a physician who specializes in Cushing's syndrome report having a better quality of life [5].

TABLE 10.1   Reasons for Consultation Before the Correct Diagnosis of Cushing's Disease was Established and Specialists Consulted

Physicians consulted and symptoms that led to the consultation	Percentage
Family physician	83.0
Weight gain	33.6
High blood pressure	26.5
Cushing's disease–related symptoms	19.8
Poor general condition	12.0
Endocrinologist	49.4
Clarification of hormone levels	13.8
Referral by other physicians	10.2
Weight gain	7.2
Suspicion of hormonal disease other than Cushing's disease	6.6
Suspicion of Cushing's disease	6.6
Gynecologist	46.0
Menstrual dysfunction	32.2
Weight gain	6.3
Clarification of hormone levels	4.9
Infertility	3.5
Loss of libido	2.1
Internist	33.0
Menstrual dysfunction	32.2
Weight gain	6.3
Clarification of hormone levels	4.9
Infertility	3.5
Loss of libido	2.1
Orthopedist	31.3
Pain (joints, muscles)	19.8
Fractures/osteoporosis	9.6
Joint inflammation	1.8
Muscle atrophy/buffalo hump	1.2
Neurologist	27.8
Pain	8.4
Neurological deficits	7.8
Mental symptoms	7.2
Dermatologist	26.1
General skin changes	11.4
Alopecia/hair growth	5.4
Acne/abscesses	2.4
Mycosis	1.8
Thin/dry skin	1.8
Cardiologist	19.3
High blood pressure	12.0
Heart complaints	6.0
Edema/vascular problems	4.2
Psychiatrist	16.5
Depression	9.0
Psychosis	3.5
Anxiety	1.8
Sleeping disorders	1.2

Adapted from Kreitschmann-Sandemahr I, Psaras T, Tsiogka M, et al. From first symptoms to final diagnosis of Cushing's disease: experiences of 176 patients. Eur J Endocrinol 2015;172:285–289.

Low quality of life can influence working status. In a large patient cohort, 9% of patients were on sick leave, and 14% were unemployed, at a mean age of 44 ± 14 years [2]. This can have major economic consequences for patients and their families. Furthermore, long waiting lists for surgery may prolong sick leave or the inability to work. A total of 56% of patients reported that having Cushing's syndrome affected their work/school performance [1]. In one study, two patients had been fired from their jobs as a result of so-called "rudeness" and the occurrence of "mental health issues." Four other patients were not able to work because the demands of their jobs were overwhelming. Some mothers reported that they were unable to perform their family duties. One patient stated, "My inability to think clearly interfered with my performance at my job" [1]. No differences in quality of life have been found among patients with different origins of Cushing's syndrome (i.e., pituitary, adrenal, or ectopic ACTH secretion), suggesting that hypercortisolism and not the location of the tumor determines quality-of-life impairment [2].

3.2 Physical Appearance

Obesity or weight gain is found in 81–95% of patients with active Cushing's disease (Fig. 10.1) [2,9]. Most patients are self-conscious about this weight gain, reporting that it affects their self-esteem. One patient stated: "I hated myself because I did not know what was wrong with me. I looked like a monster" [1]. Furthermore, many people (even physicians)

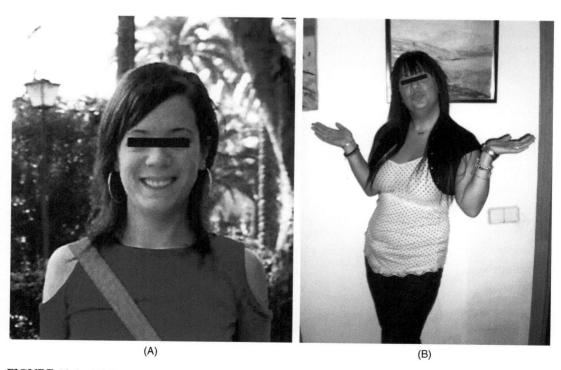

(A)   (B)

FIGURE 10.1   (A) Patient at age 19 in remission 2 years after successful pituitary surgery, and (B) patient 4 years later with a recurrence. *Source: Reprinted with permission from the patient.*

assume that the weight gain of Cushing's patients is due to overeating. Patients become frustrated when physicians, family, and friends do not believe that anything is wrong and continuously recommend diet and exercise, which many patients are already trying. In some cases, patients report being called names because of their weight, which makes them even more miserable: "It was summer, the people stared at me; some laughed, and some said that I looked like the Goodyear blimp." [1]. In a study where patients drew pictures of themselves during active Cushing's disease, most drew fat accumulations (98%), a moon face (87%), and increased abdominal fat (87%) [10].

Some patients also experience an increase in facial hair, which also negatively affects body image and self-esteem. In the study cited earlier where drawings were analyzed [10], 27% of the patients drew skin lesions, including bruises; red cheeks; and striae or acne, and 37% drew hirsutism or changes in their hair [10]. One patient reported, "Cushing's syndrome made me feel fat and ugly with facial hair, a ruddy complexion, and thin skin that bruised easily" [1]. Some patients reported not wanting to look at themselves in the mirror and, if they did, not recognizing themselves. They often expressed dislike for themselves, which has a negative effect on social and family relationships, as they may not want to socialize or be intimate with their partners.

3.3 Psychological and Cognitive Aspects

Most patients experience psychological alterations. The most common complaint is depression, which is found in approximately 50% of patients, although anxiety and emotional instability are also common [8,11–14]. Less frequently, patients experience panic attacks, hypomania (excited mood state or irritability), or suicidal thoughts [11,15,16].

In a patient survey, 61% of patients reported emotional instability, and 49% cognitive impairment, both of which affected their daily lives [1]. One patient reported, "I cried all of the time and had overwhelming feelings of hopelessness. It was hard sometimes to explain to friends and family that I thought I was losing my mind." Another patient stated "I, for no apparent reason, became somewhat violent and on edge" [1].

Cognitive deficits, including lack of memory, poor attention, or difficulty finding the correct word are also common complaints in Cushing's syndrome. Studies have confirmed the presence of neuropsychological deficits, cognitive decline, and memory impairment, which may improve after disease remission (Chapter 4) [17–25]. This can have consequences in everyday life, such as making it difficult to complete tasks (e.g., reading, studying); it may also make patients forgetful and thereby prone to making mistakes. A patient reported, "Cushing's slowed my thought processes and drastically affected my concentration. As a result, I had to recheck everything I did, to catch any errors that I may have made" [1].

3.4 Dealing with Comorbidities

Coping with comorbidities can be difficult for patients. Fatigue and weakness are very common. One patient stated: "At this time, I feel like a prisoner in my own home. I am unable to walk, climb stairs, or even shower by myself. To be able to go out and drive away in the car would be a major triumph" [1].

Pain and discomfort during the active phase of the disease are also frequent [26]. Patients with active Cushing's syndrome have reported more intense bodily pain as compared to healthy controls [27]. Furthermore, patients with osteoporosis may be afraid of fractures. One patient reported, "Although I did not realize that my bones had become very brittle, I broke several bones without knowing why. I then stopped being active because of my fear of hurting myself" [1].

When patients were asked which interventions they identified as helpful to cope with Cushing's syndrome, they cited patient education; maintenance of hope; prompt diagnosis; family involvement; support from family, friends, and physicians; peer counselor/support; support groups; mental health referrals; exercise; resting; completing activities considered normal before the onset of Cushing's syndrome; pain relief; religion; and entertainment [1,28].

Information about Cushing's syndrome is an important way in which to deal with any of its comorbidities. Information for patients is currently available online, including the guidelines on Cushing's syndrome developed by the Pituitary Society (https://pituitarysociety.org/sites/all/pdfs/Pituitary_Society_Cushings_brochure.pdf), which are available in different languages.

In order to deal with the comorbidities, patient education is also essential. Patients request that leading investigators and their teams develop patient education materials [1]. A recent prospective nursing study evaluated educational needs of Cushing's syndrome patients in reference to their disease. Patients reported having received proper information (i.e., > 5 on a scale of 0–10) on the following topics: their disease in general (88%), signs and symptoms (65%), complications (60%), treatment (80%), and medical tests (87%). Most, however, were not satisfied (< 5 on a scale of 0–10) when asked about information received on cardiovascular risk factors (76%), healthy lifestyle (82%), good eating habits (78%), physical activity (93%), resting habits (97%), sexual activity (100%), and psychological and cognitive alterations (94%) [29]; all of these topics are very important for a good quality of life, and patients should be questioned about these. A set of guidelines to accompany the aforementioned educational nursing program is currently available in Spanish (http://www.lb.de/ercusyn/wMedia/pdf/brochure/Guia_educativa_para_pacientes_con_sindrome_de_Cushing_.pdf). After using the educational modules over a 9-month period, patients showed improvement in healthy lifestyle, physical activity, sleep patterns, and pain, all of which positively benefited the patient's quality of life [30].

3.5 Family and Social Support

Social support and family support are important when coping with any disease. Understanding what Cushing's implies is not only complicated for the patients but also for the people close to them. Some patients prefer to avoid contact with friends or to socialize. Others have problems because of their mood swings. Social isolation when the disease is active is regularly reported, which can also negatively affect mood [8]. Both contact with other people and performing pleasurable activities are important for well-being and can help patients to avoid or ameliorate depression.

During the active phase of Cushing's syndrome, family relationships suffer in 80% of patients' families [1]. The most common problems are interpersonal conflicts (usually patients' irritable moods) and feelings of being "left out" of family life, because of their fatigue and weakness. Patients also report that their marital life is affected, and a few believed that the disease played an important role in their divorce [1]. Other patients were concerned about the impact of the disease on their children, whom they felt were unattended or very worried because it was difficult for them to understand Cushing's syndrome.

There are, however, ways to improve family situations. One patient stated, "You must let your family know everything about Cushing's. Have them talk with the physician. Cushing's is a living nightmare; you need to talk about it" [1]. It is also important to look for family support and to communicate one's feelings with them; while loved ones may not completely understand what is happening to the patient, most want to help; thus, communication of one's needs and feelings is essential. The feedback received from those closest to the patient is important too, so that patients understand better how they are perceived, allowing them to self-regulate if necessary. Some patients reported not noticing their angry outbursts until their relatives pointed them out.

Some patients find great relief when contacting and sharing their histories with other people who have suffered from Cushing's syndrome. Support groups can be very helpful at diagnosis but also during the recovery process. Patient associations may not be available in every country, but usually chats, Facebook pages, or even Whatsapp groups exist. For many, contacting a patient group has been very important for keeping hope alive and feeling understood.

4 DIAGNOSIS

Diagnosis is an important moment in the disease process. Before the diagnosis, many patients experience fear, anxiety, and uncertainty; they almost always feel that they are not understood. After the diagnosis, they usually feel great relief to know that a disease can finally explain their symptoms. Many are happy to find that the problems they have experienced, such as weight gain or mood swings, are not their fault (Table 10.2).

TABLE 10.2 Psychological Issues with Cushing's Syndrome in Different Phases

Before diagnosis
- Fear, anxiety, uncertainty, and not feeling understood or listened to

At diagnosis
- Relief
- New anxieties and needs: expert professionals; access to these professionals, to required tests, and to therapies; reliable information (e.g., therapies, legal issues); and support beyond endocrine care (confront quality-of-life issues)

After diagnosis
- Confronting the situation of living with Cushing's syndrome is necessary.
- Understanding by the family and social contacts is important.
- Sharing experiences with other patients, including support groups can help (and make one feel not alone).
- Being positive helps. Some tips for patients:
  - Take the reins of your life.
  - Don't blame yourself or others.
  - You can't always get what you want or avoid all pain and suffering.
  - Keep an open attitude toward change.
  - Avoid unrealistic expectations and decisions.
  - Get involved in new projects.

Diagnosis also has other implications: if there is a disease, then perhaps it can be treated. Many emotions may emerge, including hope to finally feel better but also fear and doubt about the next treatment steps.

Patients may also feel upset and angry with the health care providers who missed the diagnosis. In fact, this anger may last for years. The period before diagnosis can be very disturbing, since most Cushing's patients are sure that something is wrong but feel their physicians do not understand them. Up to a third of patients have feelings of frustration and anger about the inadequacies of medicine to reach a prompt diagnosis [1].

It is important to mention that once Cushing's syndrome is diagnosed, the differential diagnosis to establish the cause of the disease is essential to determine the correct treatment. In some cases, the delay in localizing the tumor can be an upsetting process. Pituitary tumors may be very small and are not always visible on a magnetic resonance imaging; in these cases, a inferior petrosal sinus sampling study may be necessary. Some patients may be eager to finish the process as soon as possible; they feel anxious and even exhausted by all the tests that must be performed to make a definitive diagnosis.

However, it should be explained that a definitive diagnosis may sometimes be very difficult and requires time and repetition of tests to confirm the best treatment. If the diagnosis is wrong and inadequate treatment is prescribed, consequences can be life-threatening. Furthermore, patients should be warned about the consequences of steroid withdrawal after successful surgery (after which cortisol production falls dramatically), a situation that can make them feel worse than when they were hypercortisolemic. In this case, small doses of steroids are necessary to prevent adrenal insufficiency and an acute adrenal crisis, a life-threatening situation. Guidance on the progressive steroid dose reduction should be given, as well as indications of what to do in case of intercurrent illness or complications when higher steroid levels are needed, since postoperative inhibition of the hypothalamic-pituitary-adrenal axis may last for months or even years in some patients.

5 TREATMENT

Patients are usually interested in learning about treatment options and their sequelae, as well as getting an idea about the time to recovery [1]. Treatment options include medications, surgery, and radiotherapy.

5.1 Medications

In some countries, it is common to take cortisol-lowering medications before surgery to improve symptoms. Most patients tolerate the drugs well, although adverse effects or intolerances may occur; thus, alternative drugs and combinations of several drugs might be used. If surgery cannot be performed because of contraindications or if the tumor has not been identified, cortisol-lowering medications may be prescribed for a longer time than simply preoperatively.

Additional drug therapy to deal with comorbidities is often required; this includes medications for high cholesterol or triglycerides, hypertension, diabetes mellitus, depression, or anxiety. Some patients object to taking so many different medications, and they often have difficulty remembering to take the doses as prescribed. Compliance is important, since Cushing's syndrome entails higher cardiovascular risk for which adequate control is essential. Organization may help patients to avoid forgetting their doses, like preparing pills daily in boxes with divisions for different times of the day and using alarms or apps to remember when to take each dose.

5.2 Surgery

Many patients have concerns regarding surgery. Anxiety often increases as the time for surgery approaches. Patients are often anxious about possible postoperative complications. It is also important that patients know that the best results of pituitary/adrenal surgery are obtained by experienced neurosurgeons/adrenal surgeons (Chapter 8). If patients have questions about surgery and want more information, they should definitely consult their physicians; however, if they prefer not to know further details, this should be respected.

Most patients do not dwell on the surgery or its consequences postoperatively. It appears that only when patients experience complications related to surgery, like infections, do they report their experience as annoying or even traumatic in some cases. Some patients complain about losing their sense of taste or smell for a long time after pituitary surgery or the frequent need to go to the toilet because of diabetes insipidus.

5.3 Radiotherapy

Radiotherapy is sometimes necessary for treating pituitary-dependent Cushing's disease, if it is not controlled by surgery or in cases of recurrence of Cushing's disease. Although effective in reducing ACTH secretion, its effect is slow and may take years, during which time medical therapy may be prescribed to normalize cortisol levels. Since all of the pituitary area is irradiated, other pituitary hormones may become deficient, such as growth hormone, thyrotropin, and gonadotropic hormones.

Any kind of radiotherapy requires immobilization of the head to ensure treatment of only the desired pituitary area. The most recent radiosurgery techniques use a metal fixing frame, which is applied to the head with screws. This can be a painful experience for some patients. Whether radiotherapy is given in one session (as with radiosurgery) or daily over several weeks (as with conventional radiotherapy or fractionated stereotactic radiosurgery), most patients report being tired and require some rest to recover once it is over; other common complaints are nonspecific abdominal symptoms (e.g., nausea, discomfort) and skin irritations (e.g., transient loss of hair in irradiated areas, skin irritation, or burns). The most common complaint of patients who undergo radiosurgery is that they would have appreciated more information on how the treatment is administered.

6 RECOVERY AND LONG-TERM COMORBIDITIES

6.1 Quality of Life

Quality of life is impaired in active Cushing's syndrome and usually improves after successful treatment [7,26,31–33]. However, immediately after surgery, patients often feel worse for a while because of the sudden decrease in cortisol. The recovery process may take months,

TABLE 10.3   Ways to Improve Quality of Life and Perception of the Disease

- Knowing there may be limitations and why they persist helps.
- Being realistic is encouraging, as knowledge can make a positive difference in coping with post-Cushing's issues.
- Not blaming oneself.
- Remembering that no "magic formula" works for everybody.
- Seeking psychological assistance if necessary, which may be helpful to identify and treat the psychological problems that may exist (i.e., depression, anxiety, attentional deficit, memory disturbances).
- Taking selective serotonin reuptake inhibitor drugs, such as fluoxetine, which may be a good option for depression; however, there have been no clinical trials that have identified the best drug.

even years, and often a certain degree of discomfort persists. In patients who undergo adrenalectomy, 78% stated that their quality of life improved after surgery (68% described a dramatic improvement), while 14% described no change, and 8.3% found it had worsened [34]. Using the SF-36 questionnaire, it has been found that all quality-of-life scores improve after transsphenoidal surgery. However, scores may not always equal those of the normal population [7,35]. This illustrates that the recovery process may not be optimal. In fact, patients usually complain of not being the same person as before they suffered the disease, either physically or psychologically. Table 10.3 summarizes some key issues that may be helpful to improve quality of life.

After remission, physical quality-of-life scores and "energy" subscores, are usually better in men than in women. Younger age and established disease remission are also related to better physical quality-of-life scores [7,35]. Quality of life seems to be independent of the kind of treatment received, the severity of disease, the number of pituitary operations, and the need for postsurgery steroids [5,7,35,36].

Impairment of quality of life may have significant economic consequences for the patients. A survey showed that only 38% of the patients reported feeling much better after treatment; 20% said they felt similar to the period before treatment; and 20% felt somewhat worse. The most prevalent symptoms described were fatigue (41.3%), forgetfulness (35.7%), trouble sleeping (33.3%), depression (31.2%), weight gain (30.4%), decreased muscle strength and weakness (30.4%), a bulging abdomen (39.3%), and anxiety (28.4%); see Lindslay et al. [7] for a comprehensive symptom list. Patients spend a mean of 3.8 months postoperatively on sick leave, and only 81% are able to return to work [37]. Several months after surgery, patients often report having difficulties at work or not feeling able to work.

In patients who did not undergo surgery but were treated with medical therapy, no clear quality-of-life improvement has been found after 80 days for most of the dimensions studied. The only improvement found was for the category "emotional reaction" [8]. After surgical treatment, quality-of-life improvement is seen 3–6 months after treatment, so possibly a longer follow-up may be needed to improve quality-of-life scores after medical treatment [26,33]. In addition, 3 months after treatment some patients experienced more pain than before treatment, possibly reflecting a glucocorticoid withdrawal effect, after cortisol levels fall to normal or subnormal values [8]. Patients often report an increase in pain after cortisol levels are normalized, as their bodies have become accustomed to hypercortisolism. Reducing stress, relaxation practices, and mild exercise, as well as physical therapy and social and family support have been found to help patients deal with all of these changes.

6.2 Physical Aspects

Patients usually complain of changes in physical appearance after disease remission; approximately 63% reported that Cushing's syndrome had affected their lives because of the changes in physical appearance [1]. Most complain of their big abdomen or the red striae, which may persist. Others manage to lose weight, but are upset by the consequences of losing weight rapidly, such as flaccid skin on their arms, legs, or abdomen. Some women also experience sagging breasts after weight loss, which can be very disappointing. The changes in physical appearance can be quite disturbing, especially for young women.

A study where patients were asked to draw themselves before, during, and after disease remission showed that after remission 60% of the patients still drew fat accumulation, a moon face (29%), and increased abdominal fat (36%). A total of 19% drew hirsutism or hair changes, and 2% drew skin lesions. Several patients were unhappy with their bodies after remission, reporting: "Reasonable in proportion but could always be thinner"; "Slender with 'apple' abdomen"; "I now have to accept that I am the way that I am; luckily I am still alive!" [10]. Questionnaires also reveal that patients in remission have less satisfaction with their body than normal controls [27].

Even if the body has objectively changed, there are some issues that can modify a patient's perception of body changes. Patients with depression have a worse body image and satisfaction with their body than those who are not depressed, despite similar weight and body mass index [27].

Fatigue is still present after remisssion as compared to healthy controls [35] for all fatigue subscales (measured by the Multidimensional Fatigue Index). A total of 85% of the patients reported experiencing fatigue, often the worst problem in their daily lives [1], since it interferes with usual activities, such as housekeeping or shopping, and requires frequent stops to rest between one task and another. Although more evident immediately after surgery, these effects can last for years.

6.3 Psychological and Cognitive Aspects

Persistent depression and anxiety are common in Cushing's disease patients despite disease remission as compared to healthy controls, although the level of depression after remission is less than in active patients [3,27,33,35]. Psychopathology reported at baseline in 66% of patients progressively improves after treatment (e.g., 53.4% at 3 months, 36% at 6 months, and 24.1% at 12 months) [16].

Cognitive performance also improves after treatment, but it may not improve to pre-Cushing levels. Patients often complain of poor memory, often associated with difficulties in attention and concentration [20,23–25]. Patients may find it helpful to keep their brains "working," with activities like reading, completing Sudokus, puzzles, or labyrinths. In fact, brain exercises are important to keep the mind healthy.

Experiencing a disease like Cushing's syndrome will require going through a grief process, which ends finally in adaptation (Table 10.4). Some patients may still feel angry or sad for all the years it took to be diagnosed, all the pain they felt, and all of the problems they experienced during the disease. Not infrequently, the patient's life may change dramatically during

TABLE 10.4   Psychological Phases of Adaptation

First phase: Uncertainty and confusion
Second phase: Bewilderment and negation
Third phase: Opposition and isolation
Fourth phase: Rage
Fifth phase: Sadness

      Depression   **Adaptation**
          (easier when one is positive!)

the disease, leading to changes in the family, jobs, or even themselves. Grief is essential before adaptation to the new situation and the ability to get on with one's life. Compromises may be necessary, like accepting that one's physical health prevents one from working the same job as before or for the same number of hours. However, being positive and not giving up hope are essential, and it is worth remembering that even if it takes time, most patients improve and are happy with the changes achieved.

Adopting proper coping strategies is essential after long-term remission of the disease. Less active coping, more avoidance coping, and seeking less social support have been reported after a diagnosis of Cushing's disease compared to healthy controls [38]. Optimism and adopting an active role in the recovery process are associated with a better quality of life and health status. Activities, such as staying involved in the recovery process, taking care of oneself, going out, eating a healthy diet, exercising, resting properly, and performing activities considered "normal" before the onset of the disease, as well as support by family, friends, physicians, and support groups can help Cushing's patients to feel better. Considering physical or occupational therapy, if necessary, and seeking psychological or psychiatric support in case of a depressed mood or other emotional disturbances are important [28]. Improvement is possible; it just takes time and effort. The top five most helpful resources during recovery may differ when asking patients or physicians. For physicians, they are: (1) family and friends, (2) exercise, (3) activities, (4) work, and (5) support groups. For patients, they are: (1) family and friends, (2) rest, (3) education, (4) exercise, and (5) activities [39].

Negative illness perceptions may persist in patients in remission, and this is correlated with a worse quality of life [40]. Compared to patients with acute pain, Cushing's syndrome patients reported more complaints related to illness and more chronicity and fluctuations of the disease; they perceived more negative consequences of the disease and less treatment and personal control. However, when compared to patients with chronic pain, Cushing's disease patients attributed fewer symptoms to their disease and had a better understanding of the disease when compared to both acute and chronic pain patients. It is important to mention that patients' perceptions do not necessarily represent the medical status of the disease, and there is a relationship between illness perceptions and quality of life; thus, one might speculate that if illness perceptions improve, quality of life may improve in parallel.

The psychological issues discussed by patients with Cushing's syndrome differ in the different phases of the disease. Table 10.2 summarizes these and gives some tips on how to deal with the disease after diagnosis.

6.4 Dealing with Long-term Consequences: The Aftermath of Cushing's Syndrome

It is important to remember that physical and psychological recovery after successful treatment may be slow. A patient stated: "Between 12–18 months after surgery, I realized that I enjoyed working hard and was doing fun things again" [1]. On average, it takes about 1 year to experience a significant improvement. However, "physical" and "emotional" recovery can differ, as reported by one patient: "I had surgery in June, and it felt that from the time the tumor was removed, I had recovered; however, it wasn't until I started to lose weight (September) and felt stronger, that I felt I recovered emotionally" [1]. Differences between the estimated recovery times as evaluated by physicians' judgment and patients' feedback have been observed (12 vs. 16 months) [39], as well variability in the recovery process from one patient to another. Feedback from participants in a recent CSRF-organized patient webinar (October 2015, https://csrf.net/conference-reports/patient-webinars/quality-of-life-webinar-2015/) showed how important it is to consider quality-of-life issues after endocrine cure of Cushing's syndrome. Some patients reported: "I have been in remission for 25 years and have struggled with quality-of-life issues. I am told that I am cured and my blood tests are normal, so I feel like a hypochondriac. Today (at the webinar), finding a physician who 'spoke my language' gave me a sense of relief and confirmed that my feelings are real and not imaginary." Another patient noted, "The discussion of how challenging it is after surgery helps to normalize this very difficult journey. Just to know that someone understands what we are going through is very therapeutic."

After Cushing's syndrome, it may be necessary to take medications for life, like antihypertensive drugs, medications to reduce cholesterol and triglycerides, and glucocorticoid or growth hormone replacement in cases of deficiencies. Furthermore, patients need to attend regular medical appointments, even after remission. During the active phase, patients are eager to finish the treatment process and forget about the long-term consequences or comorbidities of having suffered Cushing's syndrome. The long-term therapies may come as a shock, leading to low self-esteem and emotional distress [41]. Again, it may be necessary to go through a grieving process to readapt and accept the new situation, something that is not always easy to do (Table 10.4).

On the other hand, patients who require glucocorticoid substitution need to remember to take extra doses in case of intercurrent disease to prevent symptoms of adrenal insufficiency (i.e., vomiting, diarrhea, low blood pressure, or sudden penetrating pain in the abdomen, lower back, or legs). Information about what to do in case of an emergency or intercurrent process is essential for both the patient and family. Having an emergency kit of injectable hydrocortisone or some other glucocorticoid to be administered subcutaneously, intramuscularly, or intravenously may be life-saving.

After bilateral adrenalectomy (after which no cortisol is produced), the time until symptoms resolve varies among patients; most symptoms resolve between 7 and 9 months after surgery (i.e., menstrual problems, purple striae, hypertension, moon facies, easy bruising, facial plethora and central obesity), while others take 9–12 months (i.e., buffalo hump, depression, hirsutism, diabetes), 12–18 months (i.e., weakness, hyperpigmentation, acne), or more than 2 years [34].

Most patients report the need for more support information after "cure." Information is available on the Internet, but it is mostly in English and rather limited. An educational program, including guidelines to deal with comorbidities, has been developed in Spanish [30]. In case of doubts when dealing with comorbidities, asking health care providers or support groups is helpful.

6.5 Family, Background, and Social Support

After remission, patients can still experience psychosocial functioning problems. There is higher impairment than with other pituitary adenomas, both self-reported by patients and reported by relatives or friends [41]. Family support and encouragement to start going out again, perform activities, and keep in contact with friends are important to enhance recovery. This can also positively influence mood, although in some cases, it may take some time. Even seemingly insignificant activities, like walking or sitting outside and feeling the warm sun on the skin, can be helpful.

Spending some time working on family relationships may not be easy when the patient does not feel well. It is important to inform family members about how one feels, since the more they know, the more they can understand and help. Calmly sharing feelings and avoiding reproaches can be helpful to avoid dissension. Family support is important, and making time for family is very worthwhile.

Marital relations and sexuality are often still impaired during the recovery period. Patients may feel awkward because of their body changes and lack of libido, all of which may lead to feelings of sadness or guilt. Communication with partners is important. It can also be helpful to report these problems to the health provider to find a way to cope with them. They may resolve over time or persist in some cases if no help is sought.

In this recovery phase, support groups can still be helpful. Sharing experiences with others who have or have had Cushing's syndrome may be a source of relief, as well as finding someone to ask unresolved questions. For others, helping newly diagnosed patients may be rewarding and satisfying.

6.6 Relapses

Even if treatment is successful, Cushing's syndrome may relapse after many years. This may result in fear and anxiety of having to go through the same process again [42]. On the whole, patients who do have a recurrence report subtle body or psychological changes that appear before the tests are abnormal. This is why it is important to maintain regular checkups after remission to detect any possible relapse as soon as possible. However, being excessively worried about the possibility of a recurrence of the tumor may increase anxiety or depression and affect one's quality of life. It is important to keep going on with one's life, following healthy habits; however, if a relapse does occur, patients should learn to live and cope with it. Patients may feel like they have lost the battle, but it is important to know that the war is not lost, because other therapeutic options are available. Even though this period can be very tough, family support, social support, and professional support are all essential. A message of hope certainly helps patients to deal better with the process.

7 CONCLUSIONS

Dealing with Cushing's syndrome can be a difficult and exhausting process, since the disease can have serious psychological and physical consequences. However, it is essential to remember that improvement is possible and coping is essential. Accepting the disease and its aftermath is necessary, next to taking care of oneself to feel better. It is recommended that patients follow a healthy diet and get regular exercise; follow the physicians' recommendations regarding treatment; stay in contact with friends and family, looking for their support when necessary; and undertake pleasurable activities. Encouragement is important. While many things in one's life may change after Cushing's syndrome, it may be necessary to accept that while life may be different, it is still possible to be happy if one works at it.

References

[1] Gotch PM. Cushing's syndrome from the patient perspective. Endocrinol Metab Clin North Am 1994;23:607–17.

[2] Valassi E, Santos A, Yaneva M, et al. The European Registry on Cushing's syndrome: 2-year experience. baseline demographic and clinical characteristics. Eur J Endocrinol 2011;165:383–92.

[3] Santos A, Resmini E, Crespo I, et al. Small cerebellar cortex volume in patients with active Cushing's syndrome. Eur J Endocrinol 2014;171:461–9.

[4] Kreitschmann-Andermahr I, Psaras T, Tsiogka M, et al. From first symptoms to final diagnosis of Cushing's disease: experiences of 176 patients. Eur J Endocrinol 2015;172:285–9.

[5] Papoian, Biller BM, Webb SM, et al. Patients' perception on clinical outcome and quality of life after a diagnosis of Cushing's syndrome. Endocr Pract 2016;22:51–67.

[6] Johnson MD, Woodburn CJ, Vance ML. Quality of life in patients with a pituitary adenoma. Pituitary 2003;6:81–7.

[7] Lindslay JR, Nansel T, Baid S, et al. Long-term impaired quality of life in Cushing's syndrome despite initial improvement after surgical remission. J Clin Endocrinol Metab 2006;91:447–53.

[8] Van der Pas R, de Bruin C, Pereira AM, et al. Cortisol diurnal rhythm and QoL after successful medical treatment of Cushing's disease. Pituitary 2013;16:536–44.

[9] Newell-Price J, Bertagna X, Grossman AB, et al. Cushing's syndrome. Lancet 2006;367:1605–17.

[10] Tiemensma J, Daskalakis NP, van der Veen EM, et al. Drawings reflect a new dimension of the psychological impact of long-term remission of Cushing's syndrome. J Clin Endocrinol Metab 2012;97:3123–31.

[11] Dorn LD, Burgess ES, Dubbert B, et al. Psychopathology in patients with endogenous Cushing's syndrome: 'atypical' or melancholic features. Clin Endocrinol 1995;434:33–42.

[12] Kelly WF. Psychiatric aspects of Cushing's syndrome. QJM 1996;89:543–51.

[13] Sonino N, Fava GA, Raffi AR, et al. Clinical correlates of major depression in Cushing's disease. Psychopathology 1998;31:302–6.

[14] Santos A, Resmini E, Crespo I, et al. Cardiovascular risk and white matter lesions after endocrine control of Cushing's syndrome. Eur J Endocrinol 2015;173:765–75.

[15] Starkman MN, Schteingart DE. Neuropsychiatric manifestations of patients with Cushing's syndrome. Relationship to cortisol and adrenocorticotropic hormone levels. Arch Intern Med 1981;141:215–9.

[16] Dorn LD, Burgess ES, Friedman TC, et al. The longitudinal course of psychopathology in Cushing's syndrome after correction of hypercortisolism. J Clin Endocrinol Metab 1997;82:912–9.

[17] Whelan TB, Schteingart DE, Starkman MN, et al. Neuropsychological deficits in Cushing's syndrome. J Nerv Ment Dis 1980;168:753–7.

[18] Forget H, Lacroix A, Somma M, et al. Cognitive decline in patients with Cushing's syndrome. J Int Neuropsychol Soc 2000;6:20–9.

[19] León-Carrión J, Atutxa AM, Mangas MA. A clinical profile of memory impairment in humans due to endogenous glucocorticoid excess. Clin Endocrinol 2009;70:192–200.

[20] Mauri M, Sinforiani E, Bono G, et al. Memory impairment in Cushing's disease. Acta Neurol Scand 1993;87:52–5.

[21] Starkman MN, Giordani B, Berent S, et al. Elevated cortisol levels in Cushing's disease are associated with cognitive decrements. Psychosom Med 2001;63:985–93.

[22] Michaud K, Forget H, Cohen H. Chronic glucocorticoid hypersecretion in Cushing's syndrome exacerbates cognitive aging. Brain Cogn 2009;71:1–8.

[23] Martignoni E, Costa A, Sinforiani E, et al. The brain as a target for adrenocortical steroids: cognitive implications. Psychoneuroendocrinology 1992;17:343–54.

[24] Starkman MN, Giordani B, Gebarski SS, et al. Improvement in learning associated with increase in hippocampal formation volume. Biol Psychiatry 2003;53:233–8.

[25] Hook JN, Giordani B, Schteingart DE, et al. Patterns of cognitive change over time and relationship to age following successful treatment of Cushing's disease. J Int Neuropsychol Soc 2007;13:21–9.

[26] Santos A, Resmini E, Martínez-Momblán MA, et al. Psychometric performance of the Cushing QoL questionnaire in conditions of real clinical practice. Eur J Endocrinol 2012;167:337–42.

[27] Alcalar N, Ozkan S, Kadioglu P, et al. Evaluation of depression, quality of life and body image in patients with Cushing's disease. Pituitary 2013;16:333–40.

[28] Abel B. Post-surgical recovery in patients with Cushing's: results from an open-ended survey. Published on: Sep 12, 2012. Available from: http://csrf.net/doctors-articles/recovery/post-surgical-recovery-in-patients-with-cushings-results-of-an-open-ended-survey/

[29] Martínez MA, Gómez C, Santos A, et al. Quina informació van rebre els malalts amb síndrome de Cushing i risc cardiovascular? Ag Inf 2012;16:17–22.

[30] Martínez-Momblán MA, Gómez C, Santos A, et al. A specific nursing educational program in patients with Cushing's syndrome. Endocrine 2016;53(1):199–209.

[31] Lindholm J, Juul S, Jorgensen JO, et al. Incidence and late prognosis of Cushing's syndrome: a population-based study. J Clin Endocrinol Metab 2001;86:117–23.

[32] Webb SM, Badia X, Barahona MJ, et al. Evaluation of health-related quality of life in patients with Cushing's syndrome with a new questionnaire. Eur J Endocrinol 2008;158:623–30.

[33] Milian M, Honegger J, Gerlach C, et al. Health-related QoL and psychiatric symptoms improve effectively within a short time in patients surgically treated for pituitary tumors—a longitudinal study of 106 patients. Acta Neurochir (Wien) 2013;155:1637–45.

[34] Sippel RS, Elaraj DM, Kebebew E. Waiting for a change: symptom resolution after adrenalectomy for Cushing's syndrome. Surgery 2008;144:1054–60.

[35] Van Aken MO, Pereira AM, Biermasz NR, et al. Quality of life in patients after long-term biochemical cure of Cushing's disease. J Clin Endocrinol Metab 2005;90:3279–86.

[36] Wahenmakers MN, Netea-Maier RT, Prins JB, et al. Impaired quality of life in patients in long-term remission of Cushing's syndrome of both adrenal and pituitary origin: a remaining effect of long-standing hypercortisolism? Eur J Endocrinol 2012;167:687–9.

[37] Pikkarainen L, Sane T, Reunanen A. The survival and well-being of patients treated for Cushing's syndrome. J Intern Med 1999;245:463–8.

[38] Tiemensma J, Kaptein AA, Pereira AM, et al. Coping strategies in patients after treatment for functioning or nonfunctioning pituitary adenomas. J Clin Endocrinol Metab 2011;96:964–71.

[39] Abel B, Neary NM, Kampbell K, et al. Post-surgical recovery in patients with Cushing's syndrome: comparison of patient perceptions and endocrinology perspectives. Published on: Sep 12, 2012. Available from: http://csrf.net/doctors-articles/recovery/post-surgical-recovery-in-patients-with-cushings-syndrome-comparison-of-patient-perceptions-and-endocrinology-perspectives/

[40] Tiemensma J, Kaptein AA, Pereira AM, et al. Negative illness perceptions are associated with impaired quality of life in patients after long-term remission of Cushing's syndrome. Eur J Endocrinol 2011;165:527–35.

[41] Heald AH, Ghosh S, Bray S, et al. Long-term negative impact on quality of life in patients with successfully treated Cushing's disease. Clin Endocrinol 2004;61:458–65.

[42] Andela CD, Van Haalen FM, Ragnarsson O, et al. Mechanisms in endocrinology: Cushing's syndrome causes irreversible effects on the human brain: a systematic review of structural and functional magnetic resonance imaging studies. Eur J Endocrinol 2015;173:R1–R14.

Cushing's Disease in Children and Adolescents: Diagnosis and Management

E.J. Richmond, MD, MSc*, A.D. Rogol, MD, PhD**

*Pediatric Endocrinology, National Children's Hospital, San Jose, Costa Rica; **Emeritus,
Department of Pediatrics, University of Virginia, Charlottesville, VA, United States

OUTLINE

Cushing's Disease. http://dx.doi.org/10.1016/B978-0-12-804340-0.00011-5

1 INTRODUCTION

Cushing's syndrome is caused by prolonged exposure to high levels of cortisol (hydrocortisone) from any source: exogenous (often iatrogenic) or endogenous. A minor subset of patients with Cushing's syndrome has an adrenocorticotropic hormone (ACTH)–producing anterior pituitary tumor, which is considered Cushing's disease or secondary hypercortisolism. This chapter begins with a description of Cushing's syndrome and then focuses on Cushing's disease in infants, children, and adolescents.

Cushing's syndrome comprises a large group of signs and symptoms as a result of prolonged exposure of all body tissues to inappropriate levels of cortisol. These may be excessive at all times of the day or so mild as to merely abrogate the daily rhythm of circulating cortisol concentrations (high in early morning but cycling downward to very low levels late in the evening). The greatest number of diagnoses is due to medically prescribed corticosteroids (iatrogenic); however, endogenous Cushing's syndrome is quite uncommon, with an incidence of 2–5 cases per 1 million people per year [1].

With significantly high levels of cortisol for a long enough period of time, patients are likely to present with easy bruising; facial plethora; proximal muscle weakness or myopathy; striae, especially over 1 cm in width; and as described in detail later for children, continuing weight gain as height velocity diminishes to very much below the normal range (the key sign).

Several other diseases and conditions may mimic Cushing's syndrome and are collectively recognized as pseudo-Cushing's syndrome [1]. All are more common than Cushing's syndrome in adults but are rarely confused with Cushing's syndrome in children.

2 EPIDEMIOLOGY

Given that Cushing's syndrome is rare in adults, it should be noted that only 10% of new cases each year are diagnosed in children. While adult Cushing's disease affects women more frequently than men, recent studies in children and adolescents document that the incidence in boys and girls before and during puberty is equal, with an increasing predominance in postpubertal girls [2,3]. Male pediatric patients may have more aggressive disease with an elevated body mass index, shorter height, and higher ACTH levels as compared with female patients [3].

3 ETIOLOGY AND PATHOGENESIS

The most common pathophysiology of endogenous Cushing's syndrome in children is ACTH overproduction from a pituitary adenoma, which is designated as Cushing's disease. Ectopic secretion of ACTH [or corticotropin-releasing hormone (CRH)] as a cause of Cushing's syndrome is exceedingly rare in children. In children older than 7 years Cushing's disease accounts for 75% of the diagnoses [4]. In younger children adrenal causes of Cushing's syndrome [i.e., adrenal adenoma or carcinoma or bilateral adrenal hyperplasia, predominantly primary pigmented nodular adrenocortical disease (PPNAD)] are more frequent [5]. Primary pigmented nodular adrenocortical disease is a genetic disorder [PPNAD 4; Online

Mendelian Inheritance in Man (OMIM) 615830] and may be associated with the Carney complex of several genetic causes (OMIM 160980 and 605244; autosomal dominant multiple neoplasia syndrome with cardiac, endocrine, cutaneous, and neural myxomatous tumors, as well as a variety of pigmented lesions of the skin and mucosae) [5]. As it may simultaneously involve multiple endocrine glands, it has certain similarities to classical multiple endocrine neoplasia (MEN) syndromes (MEN 1, OMIM 13100; MEN 2, OMIM 171400; and to the McCune-Albright syndrome, OMIM 174800). All of these conditions are more prevalent after adolescence, except for the McCune-Albright syndrome. The cutaneous and endocrine manifestations appear in the adult. Cushing's syndrome in young children with the McCune-Albright syndrome is usually adrenal in origin from a somatic (nongermline) mutation of the *GNAS1* gene, leading to a constitutively active GSα subunit and continuous non–ACTH-dependent cortisol production by the adrenal or parts of the adrenal cortex [6].

In childhood functional pituitary tumors are quite uncommon and are most often ACTH-producing, causing Cushing's disease. The majority are less than 5 mm in diameter. While macroadenomas (>1 cm in diameter) account for approximately 10% of tumors in adults with Cushing's disease, they are extremely uncommon in children [7]. These seem to be sporadic and even less commonly part of a MEN 1 syndrome [5,8].

4 CLINICAL PRESENTATION

4.1 Age and Gender Distribution

The rarity of pediatric Cushing's disease underlies the fact that the diagnosis may be overlooked. Early recognition of typical features of Cushing's disease is crucial to permit a prompt diagnosis and effective treatment. Presenting signs and symptoms in children and adolescents with Cushing's disease are often less typical than those of their adult counterparts. The mean interval from initial symptoms to surgery is 2–3 years, which is less than the period reported in adults [9,10]. The median age of presentation in large studies is between 10 and 14 years [11,12].

4.2 Growth and Puberty in Pediatric Cushing's Disease

In the pediatric population detailed evaluation of the growth trajectory is key because diminished linear growth and increased weight gain are the hallmarks of this disease in children [13]. This auxological feature distinguishes hypercortisolemia from patients with simple obesity, where most children are tall and often have a height velocity greater than average for age [14]. Glucocorticoids suppress growth by increasing secretion of somatostatin; by suppressing growth hormone (GH) secretion and insulin-like growth factor-1 (IGF-1) production; and by acting directly on the epiphyses of long bones to inhibit sulfation of cartilage, mineralization, and cell proliferation.

By contrast, children with dietary obesity often grow more rapidly and are tall, which is likely due to chronic exposure to high levels of insulin and other growth factors. Thus, any overweight child who ceases growing within the normal range should be evaluated for hypercortisolism. A typical cushingoid appearance and growth chart for a child with Cushing's disease are shown in Figs. 11.1A–B and 11.2.

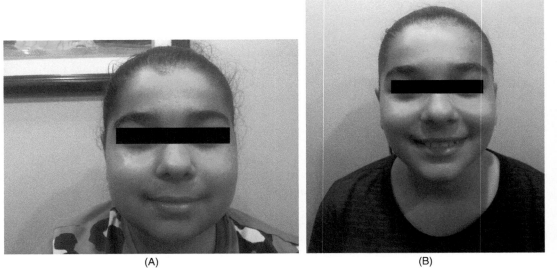

(A)   (B)

FIGURE 11.1   (A) A child with Cushing's disease before treatment. (B) The child after treatment.

Careful examination of secondary sexual maturation is also important because most children with Cushing's disease show signs of abnormal virilization with advanced pubic hair and penile growth in boys in association with prepubertal testicular volume or pubic hair growth in girls without breast development. It is crucial to remember that hypercortisolism not only impairs growth but also delays pubertal maturation. Virilization and hirsutism are also well recognized in the adult female with Cushing's disease as a result of excessive androgen secretion, but they appear to be more common in childhood [15].

4.3 Signs and Symptoms

There are some striking differences in the clinical presentation of Cushing's disease among children and adults. Adults usually present with signs and features of prolonged exposure to hypercortisolemia. When annual photographs of such patients are reviewed, it is often apparent that these features can take 5 years or longer to develop. The classic cushingoid appearance is usually not the initial presentation seen in the child with Cushing's disease. The earliest, most reliable indicator of hypercortisolism in children is the combination of excessive weight gain and growth failure [11].

Hypertension, glucose intolerance, and diabetes are more common in adult patients with Cushing's disease than in children [7,16]. Other findings associated with hypercortisolism that may be present in pediatric and adolescent patients with Cushing's disease include: moon-shaped facies, central obesity, dorsal cervical or supraclavicular fat pad, striae, acne, fatigue, headaches, depression, anxiety, and emotional liability [16].

Most lesions in pediatric Cushing's disease patients are microadenomas (≤10 mm in diameter) located in the anterior lobe, with a mean diameter of 6.9 ± 4.3 mm. Macroadenomas in

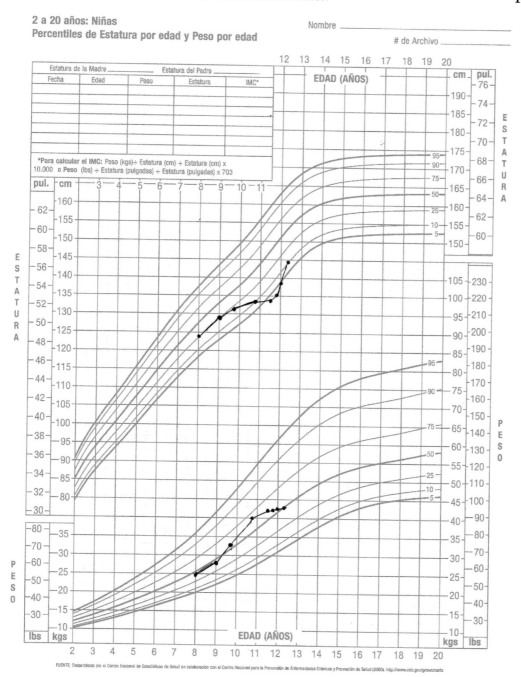

FIGURE 11.2   Growth chart of the child with Cushing's disease pictured in Fig. 11.1A–B.

pediatric patients with Cushing's disease are rare (<10%). Evaluation by magnetic resonance imaging (MRI) identifies only 50% of ACTH pituitary adenomas in the pediatric population, perhaps because of the small size of the lesions as compared to those in adults [16].

The prognosis of Cushing's disease in children has improved dramatically over the last decades. In specialized centers with experienced neurosurgeons remission after surgery is greater than 90%, and complications are infrequent with almost no mortality [16].

4.4 Body Composition

An underappreciated aspect of pediatric Cushing's disease is the substantial degree of bone loss and undermineralization in these patients and the negative impact on other aspects of body composition. There are few studies of the long-term effects on bone and fat mass in children with Cushing's disease. A well-designed study showed that despite remission of Cushing's disease, children and adolescents have alterations in body composition that result in a small but significant decrease in bone mass and an increase in visceral adiposity. Although bone mass largely recovers after Cushing's disease remission, changes in total and visceral fat suggest that these children and adolescents are at increased risk for some of the various aspects of the metabolic syndrome [17].

5 DIAGNOSTIC GUIDELINES AND CONFIRMATION OF THE DIAGNOSIS OF CUSHING'S DISEASE

5.1 When to Screen

Before conducting biochemical testing for Cushing's disease, it is important to exclude exogenous glucocorticoid exposure, including oral, nasal, inhaled, and topical corticoid treatments, as exogenous Cushing's syndrome is far more common than endogenous Cushing's syndrome.

When Cushing's syndrome is suspected in children, the best screening approach is to perform a detailed evaluation of the growth trajectory. Children with hypercortisolism usually present with the typical combination of reduced linear growth and increased weight gain. Tests for Cushing's syndrome are not indicated in obese children unless their height velocity has slowed [18].

5.2 How to Screen

The first step in the diagnosis of Cushing syndrome is to document hypercortisolism, which is typically done in the outpatient setting. Due to the circadian nature of cortisol and ACTH release, isolated cortisol and ACTH concentration measurements are not of great clinical value. Once the diagnosis of Cushing's syndrome is confirmed, there are several tests to distinguish ACTH-dependent disease (Cushing's disease) from ACTH-independent causes.

There are five tests that are used for the confirmation of Cushing's syndrome: urinary free cortisol (UFC), late-night salivary cortisol, sleeping midnight serum cortisol, 1-mg overnight dexamethasone suppression test (DST), and the 48-h, 2 mg/day DST.

Measurement of cortisol (urinary cortisol or salivary cortisol) is the end point for each of the recommended tests. As with all hormone assays, the physician must be aware that several collection and assay methods are available for the measurement of cortisol, and results for a single sample measured in various assays may be quite different [19]. As the hypercortisolism of Cushing's syndrome can be variable, it is recommended that at least two measurements of urine or salivary cortisol be obtained. This strategy increases confidence in the test results if consistently normal or abnormal results are obtained.

Variable absorption and metabolism of dexamethasone may influence the results of both the overnight 1-mg DST and the 48-h, 2 mg/day low-dose DST. Drugs, such as phenytoin, phenobarbital, carbamazepine, rifampicin, and alcohol, induce hepatic enzymatic clearance of dexamethasone, thereby reducing the plasma dexamethasone concentration [20]. Conversely, dexamethasone clearance may be reduced in patients with liver or renal failure.

Estrogens increase the cortisol-binding globulin concentration in the circulation. As serum assays measure total cortisol, false-positive rates for the overnight DST are obtained in 50% of women taking oral contraceptive pills [21]. Wherever possible, estrogen-containing drugs should be withdrawn for 6 weeks before testing [22].

5.2.1 Urinary Free Cortisol

One excellent screening test for hypercortisolism is a 24-h UFC excretion (corrected for body surface area), with a reported sensitivity of 88% and a specificity of 90% in children [18,23]. The diagnostic cut-off for a 24-h UFC is 70 $\mu g/m^2$; values above this level are considered abnormal.

It is important to ensure that patients provide a complete 24-h urine collection with appropriate total volume and urinary creatinine levels. The first morning void is discarded so that the collection begins with an empty bladder. All subsequent voids throughout the day and night are included in the collection, which is kept refrigerated, up to and including the first morning void on the second day. Once the bladder has been emptied into the collection on the second morning, the sample is complete.

False-positive results of UFC may be reported in several conditions. High-fluid intake significantly alters UFC [24]. Any physiological or pathological condition that increases cortisol production raises UFC, including depression, physical and emotional stress, severe obesity, intense chronic exercise, pregnancy, alcoholism, poor diabetes control, anorexia nervosa, and malnutrition. In patients with these conditions, a normal result is more reliable than an abnormal one. False-negative results for UFC may be reported in several conditions. As UFC reflects renal filtration, values are significantly lower in patients with renal failure [25]. The UFC may be normal in the rare patient with cyclic disease, if the urine collection is performed when the disease is inactive.

5.2.2 Late-night Salivary Cortisol

The loss of circadian rhythm with absence of a late-night cortisol nadir is a consistent biochemical abnormality in patients with Cushing's syndrome [26]. This difference in physiology forms the basis for measurement of a midnight serum or late-night salivary cortisol.

Biologically active free cortisol in the general circulation is in equilibrium with cortisol in the saliva, and the concentration of salivary cortisol does not appear to be affected by the rate of salivary production. Furthermore, an increase in blood cortisol is reflected by a change in the salivary cortisol concentration within a few minutes [27].

Saliva is collected either by passive drooling into a plastic tube or by placing a cotton pledget (salivette) in the mouth and chewing for 1–2 min; consequently, this test may not be appropriate for small children.

Late-night salivary cortisol has been evaluated in obese children, and high sensitivity (100%) and high specificity (95%) for Cushing's syndrome have been reported [28]; however, the influences of age, gender, and coexisting medical conditions have not been fully characterized.

Nocturnal salivary cortisol levels may be transiently abnormal in individuals crossing widely different time zones. Stress immediately before the collection also may increase salivary cortisol concentration physiologically; therefore, ideally, samples should be collected on a quiet evening at home [29].

5.2.3 Sleeping Midnight Serum Cortisol

The evidence of the accuracy of sleeping midnight serum cortisol values in the screening for hypercortisolism in children is limited. One study of 105 children with Cushing's syndrome demonstrated that midnight cortisol levels in the sleeping child give the highest sensitivity and specificity for the diagnosis of Cushing's syndrome (99 and 100%, respectively) [18].

This, however, is a cumbersome test to perform. The sleeping midnight serum cortisol in children requires catheterization and inpatient admission for a period of 48 h or longer to avoid false-positive responses as a result of the stress of hospitalization; this approach may not be possible in some practice settings.

Where there is a low clinical index of suspicion, such as in simple obesity, but lack of suppression on dexamethasone testing and mildly elevated UFC, a sleeping midnight serum cortisol less than 1.8 µg/dL effectively excludes Cushing's syndrome [30].

5.2.4 The 1-mg Overnight DST

In normal subjects, the administration of a supraphysiological dose of glucocorticoid results in suppression of ACTH and cortisol secretion. In endogenous Cushing's syndrome of any cause, there is a failure of this suppression when low doses of dexamethasone are given [31].

This low-dose DST involves giving 1 mg of dexamethasone between 2300 and 2400 h and measuring a serum cortisol level the following morning between 0800 and 0900. If the serum morning cortisol level is greater than 1.8 µg/dL, further evaluation is necessary. At the 1.8 µg/dL cutoff, sensitivity is greater than 95%, but specificity is 80% [32].

Although the 1-mg overnight DST is used as a screening test for pediatric patients, there are no specific data regarding its interpretation or performance in this population.

5.2.5 The 48-h (2-mg/day) Low-dose DST

In this test, dexamethasone is given in doses of 0.5 mg for 48 h, beginning at 0900 on day 1, at 6-h intervals. Serum cortisol is measured at 0900 h, 6 h after the last dose of dexamethasone.

For pediatric patients weighing more than 40 kg, the adult protocol described earlier and the adult threshold for normal suppression (1.8 µg/dL) are used. For patients weighing less than 40 kg, the dose is adjusted to 30 µg/kg/day (in divided doses) [4]. With a cutoff of

1.8 μg/dL, the sensitivity for Cushing's syndrome in 36 pediatric patients was 94% [4] and is considered a useful screening test for pediatric patients in an outpatient setting.

5.3 Confirmation of Causes of Cushing's Syndrome

After confirmation of hypercortisolism, the priority is to determine its cause. The most common cause is iatrogenic from medically prescribed corticosteroids as endogenous Cushing's syndrome is an uncommon disorder. Endogenous Cushing's syndrome may be caused by either excess ACTH secretion (from a pituitary or other ectopic tumor) or independent adrenal overproduction of cortisol. In all patients with Cushing's disease, ACTH is detectable, and using a cutoff value of 29 ng/dL, sensitivity and specificity are reported as 70 and 100%, respectively [18]. In ACTH-independent Cushing's syndrome, ACTH is always low and usually undetectable.

The standard high-dose DST (Liddle's test) and the CRH-stimulation test are used to differentiate Cushing's disease from ectopic ACTH secretion and adrenal causes of Cushing's syndrome [33]. Ectopic ACTH syndrome is so rare in children that the need for either of these two tests is questionable. In the standard high-dose DST, dexamethasone (120 μg/kg/dose; maximum 2 mg/dose) is given every 6 h for eight doses. A 20% cortisol suppression from baseline has a sensitivity and specificity of 97.5 and 100%, respectively, with the high-dose DST used for differentiating patients with Cushing's disease from those with adrenal tumors [18]. Approximately 85% of patients with Cushing's disease respond to CRH stimulation with increased plasma ACTH and cortisol concentrations, but patients with ectopic ACTH production do not respond to the administration of CRH. The criterion for diagnosis of Cushing's disease is a mean increase of 20% above baseline for cortisol values at 30 and 45 min and an increase in the mean ACTH concentration of 35% (at least) over a basal value at 15 and 30 min after CRH administration.

5.4 Imaging

The most important initial imaging when Cushing's disease is suspected is pituitary MRI. The MRI should be done with thin sections with high resolution and always with contrast (gadolinium). The latter is relevant, since only macroadenomas are detectable without contrast. A T2-weighted imaging offers additional identification of cystic components, with postcontrast sequences improving the visualization of small lesions. Pituitary adenomas are generally hypointense compared with the adjacent gland and take up contrast less avidly and in a more delayed fashion and, therefore, fail to enhance with gadolinium. On pituitary postcontrast MRI scanning, 63 and 55% of ACTH adenomas were identified in two large pediatric series [13,34].

Bilateral simultaneous inferior petrosal sinus sampling (IPSS) was initially used in adults to enable the distinction between Cushing's disease and ectopic ACTH secretion, as well as to identify a lateral versus a central source of ACTH secretion within the pituitary [31]. It has now become routine in adult practice unless the MRI unequivocally shows a pituitary adenoma. In children, ectopic ACTH secretion is extremely rare, and so the primary aim of bilateral simultaneous IPSS is to contribute to the localization of the microadenoma by demonstrating lateral or midline ACTH secretion.

A recent study described the experience of bilateral simultaneous IPSS in 94 pediatric patients and reported that localization of ACTH secretion concurred with the site of the adenoma at surgery in 58% of cases, concluding that the technique was not an essential part of a pediatric investigation protocol [35].

6 THERAPY

6.1 Goals

To treat children and adolescents with Cushing's disease optimally, the circulating cortisol levels should be normalized, usually by selective pituitary adenomectomy, to eliminate the associated signs and symptoms of Cushing's syndrome and to treat the comorbidities, including diminished quality of life.

6.2 Primary Therapy

First-line therapeutic options focus on the resection of the causal pituitary adenoma. Transsphenoidal adenomectomy is the preferred surgical procedure. The success rate to induce a remission is usually above 90% at comprehensive pituitary disease centers. Although a more recent addition, the endonasal endoscopic transsphenoidal adenomectomy is available, neurosurgeons have less experience with this technique, especially in children and adolescents. The initial results, however, are promising and appear at least as successful as the older transsphenoidal technique [36]. Advantages to the endonasal endoscopic technique appear to include a shorter hospital stay, decreased patient discomfort, and a virtually equivalent complication rate. However, given that the adenomas in children are so small, the transsphenoidal approach with its enhanced magnification may offer additional benefit (E. Oldfield, personal communication March 30, 2016).

Results for children have been reported recently [12,13]. A very large series (200 children and adolescents) was reported from the National Institutes of Health in Bethesda, Maryland. These investigators reported remission following the transsphenoidal approach in more than 98% of patients, the majority of whom were hypocortisolemic immediately postoperatively. It should be noted that a maximal morning serum cortisol level of less than 1 μg/dL within a few days of surgical excision had a positive predictive value for a lasting remission of 96%. Further analysis indicated that the following factors were associated with an initial remission: identification of an adenoma at surgery, immunohistochemical indication of an ACTH-producing adenoma on pathological examination, and the surgical finding of a noninvasive adenoma.

Proper postoperative evaluation permitted physicians to assess remission after the procedure. All children and adolescents received dexamethasone, 0.5 mg every 6 h for 5 or 6 doses, beginning on the day of surgery. Plasma cortisol levels and UFC concentrations were obtained from postoperative day 3 until hypocortisolemia was achieved. Complications were uncommon but included: diabetes insipidus (at hospital discharge), 5%; and hyponatremia with seizures, 1.5% (all recovered without incident). The investigators were able to follow and reevaluate 90% of their patients for a mean of almost 7 years. Overall 14 patients (8%) had a recurrence after surgery but on average at almost 5 years later. Despite most having immediate hypocortisolemia, those factors associated with later recurrence included cavernous sinus and contiguous dural invasion, macroadenoma noted at surgery, and an inability to locate an adenoma, leading to partial hypophysectomy.

Those late "recurrences" could include new tumors arising from the same conditions that led to the original tumor. The reappearance of Cushing's disease years following the successful treatment of the first tumor makes life-long surveillance mandatory.

6.3 Secondary Therapy

Secondary modalities of therapy for Cushing's disease include repeat surgery; radiation, both of the "global" external variety and the more focused techniques of the gamma knife; bilateral adrenalectomy; and long-term medical therapy.

6.3.1 *Repeat Transsphenoidal Surgery and Radiation Therapy*

Repeat transsphenoidal surgery is used uncommonly in children when compared to adults and can be accomplished in the immediate postoperative period if hypocortisolemia is not induced or with a later recurrence. The success rate is usually below that of primary transsphenoidal surgery, but the numbers in children and adolescents are quite small [12].

External beam radiation therapy is apparently more successful than in the adult, but again the numbers of children and adolescents treated are quite small. There are few data on the more focused types of radiation therapy.

6.3.2 *Medical Therapy and Bilateral Adrenalectomy*

Long-term medical therapy has been used in increasing numbers of adults, but there are few data relevant to children and adolescents.

Bilateral adrenalectomy is usually a last resort because additional transsphenoidal surgery and radiation therapy are often successful. After bilateral adrenalectomy, physicians need to be alert to the presence of Nelson's syndrome for which radiation therapy is a viable option, especially in children and adolescents as compared to adults.

6.4 Follow-up

Irrespective of the secondary therapeutic option chosen, physicians must continue to be alert to secondary hypopituitarism. This requires regular surveillance, especially if the height velocity does not normalize, although catch-up growth is expected. In its absence physicians should investigate specifically for GH deficiency. For patients with GH deficiency, the physician would certainly treat with recombinant human GH. In some unusual cases with the bone age near to epiphyseal closure and a very short adolescent, physicians may consider the addition of gonadotropin-releasing hormone agonists or aromatase inhibitors to dampen pubertal maturation and to slow the process of epiphyseal closure.

Normal body composition is more difficult to achieve, and abnormalities may exist more than 7 years after remission [17,37]. Excess adipose tissue, especially in the deep visceral compartment, is the main issue and has major implications for later cardiovascular disease risk for these young patients with a projected long life.

In adults, long-term adverse events following Cushing's syndrome or Cushing's disease in addition to those of body composition include brain atrophy, cognitive impairment, and psychopathology, most commonly depression. In children, there are fewer data, but comprehensive studies 1 year after treatment have been done and note impaired health-related quality of life, especially as related to physical [38] and cognitive [39] function. These are more apparent for cognitive function in younger children.

7 CONCLUSIONS

Cushing's syndrome is an uncommon endogenous condition in children, although quite common following therapy with glucocorticoids for various medical conditions. In infants and preschool children, Cushing's syndrome is likely due to adrenal causes, but in school-children and adolescents, a pituitary adenoma (Cushing's disease) is the more common etiology. The clinical presentation, especially slowing and subnormal height velocity together with stable or increasing weight velocity, is key to suspecting this diagnosis and evaluating children. The other signs and symptoms, such as facial plethora, abnormal fat distribution, striae, and hypertension, are more common in adults although, some or all of these signs and symptoms may be present in children, especially in the more florid presentations.

Specific diagnostic tests are undertaken only after screening tests indicate hypercortisolism. Among the most critical is the hypothalamic/pituitary MRI examination to locate a pituitary adenoma should a pituitary disorder be confirmed on preliminary testing. A pituitary microadenoma is clearly present in 50% or more children.

Transsphenoidal surgery and increasingly endonasal endoscopic transsphenoidal surgery are the mainstays of primary treatment, although the former with its higher magnification may be more appropriate for the smaller tumors. Repeat surgery and various forms of radiation therapy are often applied in the relatively small percent of children who require a second procedure.

There are continuing concerns for patients in remission from Cushing's disease, and life-long surveillance for recurrence or new (secondary) tumors is mandatory.

References

[1] Nieman LK, Biller BM, Findling JW, et al. Treatment of Cushing's syndrome: an Endocrine Society clinical practice guideline. J Clin Endocrinol Metab 2015;100:2807–31.

[2] Storr HL, Isidori AM, Monson JP, et al. Prepubertal Cushing's disease is more common in males, but there is no increase in severity at diagnosis. J Clin Endocrinol Metab 2004;89:3818–20.

[3] Libuit LG, Karageorgiadis AS, Sinaii N, et al. A gender-dependent analysis of Cushing's disease in childhood: pre- and postoperative follow-up. Clin Endocrinol 2015;83:72–7.

[4] Magiakou MA, Mastorakos G, Oldfield EH, et al. Cushing's syndrome in children and adolescents. Presentation, diagnosis, and therapy. N Engl J Med 1994;331:629–36.

[5] Stratakis C. Cushing syndrome in pediatrics. Endocrinol Metab Clin North Am 2012;41:793–803.

[6] Collins MT, Singer FR, Eugster E. McCune-Albright syndrome and the extraskeletal manifestations of fibrous dysplasia. Orphanet J Rare Dis 2012;7(Suppl 1):S4.

[7] Storr HL, Savage MO. Management of endocrine disease: paediatric Cushing's disease. Eur J Endocrinol 2015;173:35–45.

[8] Marx SJ, Agarwal SK, Kester MB, et al. Multiple endocrine neoplasia type: 1 clinical and genetic of the heredi-tary endocrine neoplasias. Recent Prog Horm Res 1999;54:397–438.

[9] Kanter AS, Diallo AO, Jane JA, et al. Single-center experience with pediatric Cushing's disease. J Neurosurg 2005;103:413–30.

[10] Bochicchio D, Losa M, Buchfelder M. Factors influencing the immediate and late outcome of Cushing's disease treated by transsphenoidal surgery: a retrospective study by the European Cushing's Disease Survey Group. J Clin Endocrinol Metab 1995;80:3114–20.

[11] Chan LF, Storr HL, Grossman AB, et al. Pediatric Cushing's syndrome: clinical features, diagnosis, and treat-ment. Arq Bras Endocrinol Metabol 2007;51:1261–71.

[12] Lonser RR, Wind JJ, Nieman LK, et al. Outcome of surgical treatment of 200 children with Cushing's disease. J Clin Endocrinol Metab 2013;98:892–901.

[13] Storr HL, Alexandraki KI, Martin L, et al. Comparisons in the epidemiology, diagnostic features and cure rate by transsphenoidal surgery between paediatric and adult-onset Cushing's disease. Eur J Endocrinol 2011;164:667–74.

[14] Greening JE, Storr HL, McKenzie SA, et al. Linear growth and body mass index in pediatric patients with Cush-ing's disease or simple obesity. J Endocrinol Invest 2006;29:885–7.

[15] Newell-Price J, Trainer P, Besser M, et al. The diagnosis and differential diagnosis of Cushing's syndrome and pseudo-Cushing's states. Endocr Rev 1998;195:647–72.

[16] Lonser RR, Wind JJ, Nieman LK, et al. Outcome of surgical treatment of 200 children with Cushing's disease. J Clin Endocrinol Metab 2013;98:892–901.

[17] Leong GM, Abad V, Charmandari E, et al. Effects of child- and adolescent-onset endogenous Cushing syndrome on bone mass, body composition, and growth: a 7-year prospective study into young adulthood. J Bone Miner Res 2007;22:110–8.

[18] Batista DL, Riar J, Keil M, et al. Diagnostic tests for children who are referred for the investigation of Cushing syndrome. Pediatrics 2007;120:575–86.

[19] Klose M, Lange M, Rasmussen AK, et al. Factors influencing the adrenocorticotropin test: role of contemporary cortisol assays, body composition, and oral contraceptive agents. J Clin Endocrinol Metab 2007;92:1326–33.

[20] Kyriazopoulou V, Vagenakis AG. Abnormal overnight dexamethasone suppression test in subjects receiving rifampicin therapy. J Clin Endocrinol Metab 1992;75:315–7.

[21] Nickelsen T, Lissner W, Schöffling K. The dexamethasone suppression test and long-term contraceptive treat-ment: measurement of ACTH or salivary cortisol does not improve the reliability of the test. Exp Clin Endocri-nol 1989;94:275–80.

[22] Qureshi AC, Bahri A, Breen LA, et al. The influence of the route of oestrogen administration on serum levels of cortisol-binding globulin and total cortisol. Clin Endocrinol (Oxf) 2007;66:632–5.

[23] Crapo L. Cushing's syndrome: a review of diagnostic tests. Metabolism 1992;28:955–77.

[24] Mericq MV, Cutler GB Jr. High fluid intake increases urine free cortisol excretion in normal subjects. J Clin En-docrinol Metab 1998;83:682–4.

[25] Chan KC, Lit LC, Law EL, et al. Diminished urinary free cortisol excretion in patients with moderate and severe renal impairment. Clin Chem 2004;50:757–9.

[26] Glass AR, Zavadil AP, Halberg F, et al. Circadian rhythm of serum cortisol in Cushing's disease. J Clin Endocri-nol Metab 1984;59:161–5.

[27] Read GF, Walker RF, Wilson DW, et al. Steroid analysis in saliva for the assessment of endocrine function. Ann NY Acad Sci 1990;595:260–74.

[28] Martinelli CE Jr, Sader SL, Oliveira EB, et al. Salivary cortisol for screening of Cushing's syndrome in children. Clin Endocrinol (Oxf) 1999;51:67–71.

[29] Raff H, Raff JL, Findling JW. Late-night salivary cortisol as a screening test for Cushing's syndrome. J Clin En-docrinol Metab 1998;83:2681–6.

[30] Pecori Giraldi F, Pivonello R, Ambrogio AG, et al. The dexamethasone-suppressed corticotropin-releasing hor-mone stimulation test and the desmopressin test to distinguish Cushing's syndrome from pseudo-Cushing's states. Clin Endocrinol (Oxf) 2007;66:251–7.

[31] Newell-Price J, Trainer P, Besser M, et al. The diagnosis and differential diagnosis of Cushing's syndrome and pseudo-Cushing's states. Endocr Rev 1998;19:647–72.

[32] Wood PJ, Barth JH, Freedman DB, et al. Evidence for the low dose dexamethasone suppression test to screen for Cushing's syndrome—recommendations for a protocol for biochemistry laboratories. Ann Clin Biochem 1997;34:222–9.

[33] Chrousos GP, Schulte HM, Oldfield EH, et al. The corticotropin-releasing factor stimulation test. An aid in the evaluation of patients with Cushing's syndrome. N Engl J Med 1984;310:622–6.

[34] Batista DL, Oldfield EH, Keil MF, et al. Postoperative testing to predict recurrent Cushing disease in children. J Clin Endocrinol Metab 2009;94:2757–65.

[35] Batista D, Gennari M, Riar J, et al. An assessment of petrosal sinus sampling for localization of pituitary micro-adenomas in children with Cushing disease. J Clin Endocrinol Metab 2006;91:221–4.

[36] Storr HL, Drake WM, Evanson J, et al. Endonasal endoscopic transsphenoidal pituitary surgery: early experience and outcome in pediatric Cushing's disease. Clin Endocrinol 2013;80:270–6.

[37] Davies JS, Storr HL, Davies K, et al. Final height and body mass index after cure of paediatric Cushing's disease. Clin Endocrinol 2005;62:466–72.

[38] Keil MF, Merke DP, Gandhi R, et al. Quality of life in children and adolescents 1-year after cure of Cushing syndrome: a prospective study. Clin Endocrinol 2009;71:326–33.

[39] Merke DP, Giedd JN, Keil MF, et al. Children experience cognitive decline despite reversal of brain atrophy one year after resolution of Cushing syndrome. J Clin Endocrinol Metab 2005;90:2531–6.

Challenges and Future Developments for Improvement in the Diagnosis and Management of Cushing's Disease

E.R. Laws, Jr., MD, FACS

Harvard Medical School, Boston, MA, United States; Neuro-Endocrine/Pituitary Program, Department of Neurosurgery, Brigham and Women's Hospital, Boston, MA, United States

As we look to the future, perhaps it is wise to consider and to explore some of the mysteries that are associated with Cushing's disease, many of which remain largely unexplained. The abnormalities characteristic of Cushing's may provide a better understanding of this disease and its management (Table 12.1).

1 IMAGING

Since many of the tumors associated with Cushing's disease are small in size and are often below the accurate resolving capability of current imaging methods, a number of strategies have been used to improve the detection of these tumors. Previous attempts at dynamic magnetic resonance imaging (MRI) as contrast goes through the gland have produced suboptimal

Cushing's Disease. http://dx.doi.org/10.1016/B978-0-12-804340-0.00012-7

TABLE 12.1   Mysteries and Unexplained Aspects of Cushing's Disease

1. The tumors are much more common in women than men. Why?

2. Symptoms and signs are often precipitated by stress of various kinds, particularly pregnancy.

3. The disease is associated with cognitive, memory, emotional, and psychological problems.

4. There is a very high level of disease recurrence, even as late as 20+ years after surgery.

5. The pathology of ACTH-secreting tumors can demonstrate a spectrum, from hyperplasia to diffuse tumor cells to microadenomas to multiple adenomas to macroadenomas, both invasive and noninvasive.

6. Is recurrence of tumor related to a hypothalamic "drive" or simply to tumor cells remaining after surgery, or both?

7. Patients with Cushing's develop weight gain despite strict dieting and regular exercise.

8. Multiple comorbidities are common and can be difficult to manage: hypertension, which is often difficult to control; cardiomyopathy; diabetes mellitus, which is often difficult to control; sleep apnea and other sleep disturbances; facial rounding with rosy cheeks and an oily complexion; infections, both bacterial and fungal (e.g., acne, urinary tract, other); osteopenia and osteoporosis; edema and fluid retention; perspiration, which is sometimes odiferous; and profound fatigue with muscle weakness and atrophy.

9. Some patients have darkening of the skin on the knuckles, elbows, and neck, perhaps related to the melanocyte-stimulating effect of tumor hormone secretion.

ACTH, Adrenocorticotropic hormone.

results, as have a number of attempts to use different pulse sequences during MRI. There was hope that a 3T magnet would provide better resolution and improve detection of Cushing's disease tumors, but this has been disappointing as well. There is excitement about the use of a 7T MRI for the study of human patients, and we will have the opportunity to evaluate this new modality sometime in the fall of 2016.

Previous attempts at ultrasonic imaging of the pituitary for the detection of small tumors have been only partially successful. Ultrasonic probes have been developed that have a high resolution and also show associated structures around the pituitary, including the carotid arteries, the cavernous sinuses, and the optic chiasm. They have yet to be tested in clinical use.

Ocular computed tomography (OCT) has been quite useful in assessing the thickness of the retinal nerve fiber layer in the optic nerves, particularly when they are compressed or distorted by a pituitary tumor. The developments with this modality have led to additional possibilities for imaging of the pituitary gland, using a mini-OCT device that is under development at the Massachusetts Institute of Technology. Again, further development is necessary, and we eagerly await an opportunity to use this new technology.

Nuclear imaging, using 2-deoxyglucose positron emission tomography (PET) scans and radiolabeled octreotide scans, has been investigated, particularly for use in patients suspected of having ectopic sources of adrenocorticotropic hormone (ACTH) or corticotropin-releasing hormone (CRH). Results have been somewhat disappointing as well. A novel nuclear imaging isotope, namely ^{68}Ga-DOTATATE PET/CT, has been employed experimentally and appears to be useful in the detection of peripheral neuroendocrine tumors that can provide an ectopic source of ACTH or CRH, which mimics Cushing's disease [1].

2 INTRAOPERATIVE TECHNIQUES

MALDI mass spectroscopy is being developed to be used in the mapping of the exposed pituitary gland intraoperatively [2,3]. This methodology allows the gland to be geographically mapped for the location of clusters of the different types of hormone-expressing cells and also of tumors composed of these cells. Initial studies are very promising, and a probe that can identify the location of pituitary tumors is the next step.

The fact that most pituitary tumors are surrounded by a capsule of compressed normal pituitary gland has been known for some time. Recent attention, however, has focused on attempts to improve outcomes by doing what is called an extracapsular dissection of the lesion. Techniques to find the capsule and to keep it intact so that the tumor can be removed completely have been refined and have been successfully employed to improve results, particularly in Cushing's disease.

Many pituitary tumors have invasive components that go beyond the capsule and can actually invade the structures surrounding the pituitary gland, primarily the membrane called the dura. Microsurgical techniques and good visualization now allow for resection of the involved dura in some cases, again leading to improved long-term results.

3 GENETIC FACTORS AND POTENTIAL THERAPIES

The genetic basis of neoplasia within the pituitary gland is under continuous investigation. Familial hereditary syndromes have been recognized for some time, including the multiple endocrine neoplasia type 1 (MEN 1) correlation of several different types of endocrine tumors, including pituitary adenoma and the familial isolated pituitary adenoma syndrome (FIPA). Both MEN 1 and FIPA are rather uncommon; however, they do highlight pathways of genetic mutations that may be important for the basic concepts of tumor growth within the pituitary. Some of the genetic characteristics of particular pituitary tumors, including those associated with Cushing's disease, may be targets for potential therapy. Some pituitary tumors in Cushing's disease harbor *USP-8* mutations, which affect the epidermal growth factor receptor (EGFR) pathway, so that EGFR alterations might be potentially therapeutic.

Another potential therapeutic target is the programmed death receptor ligand 1 pathway associated with the programmed death of cells, which is a candidate for checkpoint mutation therapy [4]. For some time there has been interest in the retinoic acid pathway, which surely plays some role in the synthesis of ACTH, but effective agents have not yet been discovered [5,6]. Temolozolomide has been used for chemotherapy of refractory tumors of the pituitary, including those associated with Cushing's disease, particularly when they are highly aggressive or malignant. Although initial results appear promising, long-term curative results have not occurred often using this strategy.

References

[1] Susmeeta T, Sharma I, Millo CM, et al. Utility of 68Ga-Dotatate PET/CT in comparison to other imaging modalities for the detection of ACTH-secreting neuroendocrine tumors in ectopic Cushing's syndrome. Boston: Endocrine Society Abstracts; 2016, PP17-4.

[2] Feldman D, Vestal M, Calligaris D, et al. Mapping the concentrations of hormones in non-pathologic human pituitary samples using MALDI mass spectroscopy. Chicago: AANS Abstracts; 2016.

[3] Calligaris D, Feldman DR, Norton I, et al. MALDI mass spectrometry imaging analysis of pituitary adenomas for near-real-time tumor delineation. Proc Natl Acad Sci USA 2015;112(32):9978–83.

[4] Mei Y, Du Z, Agar NYR, et al. Elevated expression of programmed death ligand 1 in human pituitary tumors. Scottsdale: North American Skull Base Society; 2016.

[5] Bush ZM, Vance ML, Hussaini IM, et al. A unique retinoic acid signaling environment in corticotroph cells offers hope for a tumor-directed medical treatment for Cushing's disease. Endocrine Society Abstracts; 2005.

[6] Bush ZM, Lopes MB, Hussaini IM, et al. Immunohistochemistry of COUP-TFI: an adjuvant diagnostic tool for the identification of corticotroph microadenomas. Pituitary 2010;13(1):1–7.

Patients' Perspectives

CLASSIC FEATURES OF CUSHING'S SYNDROME

The classic features of Cushing's syndrome—truncal obesity, moon-shaped face with an oily complexion, and supraclavicular fat pads—develop insidiously in most cases (although in some cases there is rapid progression); thus, it is not uncommon for patients who have developed Cushing's syndrome to go for years without a diagnosis for their myriad symptoms. Such changes in physical appearance often go unrecognized by physicians (even when they know their patients well), spouses, family, and friends in a society where obesity is endemic and weight gain in middle age is perceived as normal.

In contrast, however, Cushing's patients are painfully aware of all of the physical changes, the knowledgeable among them often demanding to be tested in spite of the sometimes skeptical protests of their physicians. As one patient related, "I had only gained 30 pounds when I asked to be tested for Cushing's syndrome. My physician asked me if I knew what someone looked like who had the disease. I pulled out a picture from a textbook, and he said, 'It is an extremely rare disorder, and you do not look cushingoid.' I replied that I felt I was headed that way." A careful comparison with earlier photographs can help physicians distinguish these changes.

Patients with Cushing's syndrome experience a large number of seemingly unrelated symptoms, and these are variable both at the onset and throughout the progression of the disease. While all patients have the same disease, their reasons for seeking a medical evaluation are often entirely different. One patient recalled neglecting to mention weight gain even though she had gained 90 pounds, focusing instead on other body changes: "I felt like I was falling apart. I was growing hair where I had never had hair before. I had a huge hump between my shoulder blades (buffalo hump), and I had bruises all over my arms and legs. The shape of my face had changed; my hair was falling out; and I was very weak."

Virtually all Cushing's patients suffer from low self-esteem as physicians, friends, spouses, and partners simply do not believe that their weight gain is not self-induced. Dieting and exercise are futile. Thus, the frustration and emotional impact of the physical deterioration cannot be overestimated. One patient related her frustration: "I felt so embarrassed about being so ugly and so fat. I tried every diet imaginable. I even tried hypnosis, but never did lose weight. My husband was convinced that I was a closet eater and was not trying very hard."

Weakness, muscle pain, and low energy are common presentations, as are complaints of poor wound healing, cracking skin, shortness of breath, palpitations, and spontaneous

Cushing's Disease. http://dx.doi.org/10.1016/B978-0-12-804340-0.00013-9

fractures. One patient related, "While sitting back in a chair, I felt a jabbing sensation that took my breath away. After weeks of discomfort, I learned that I had spontaneously broken several ribs." Another patient recalled, "being so weak that I could not get up from a squatting position without difficulty, climb stairs without getting severely out of breath, or hold a glass of water without using both hands." Complaints of sleeping most of the day are common, as is exhaustion as a result of the insomnia.

Cushing's syndrome has many deleterious effects on emotional stability and cognitive function. Approximately 61% of patients report feelings of emotional lability, especially depression and suicidal ideation; 49% report cognitive difficulties, most commonly an inability to concentrate and memory loss; and 17% report at least one admission to a mental health facility before diagnosis. In fact, for some patients the emotional upheaval and psychological disruption caused by cortisol excess are the most difficult aspects of the disease. One patient reported "being uncontrollably changed, trying desperately to get a grip, but ultimately failing. I was perceived as a hypochondriac by family and friends. I cried for no apparent reason but was just as apt to become enraged for no reason. I had episodes of sheer panic and intense anxiety, which often kept me from my normal activities. I thought about suicide often. My husband was convinced that I was crazy and had me committed to the psychiatric unit of our local hospital. I felt betrayed, angry, and confused."

Cognitive difficulties often prevent patients from fulfilling their job responsibilities; approximately 56% report work or school difficulties. In some cases, bosses and coworkers are sympathetic and concerned; in other cases, the disease is devastating to professional pursuits. As one patient recalled, "I lacked my usually proficient verbal skills. I avoided my usual public-speaking responsibilities because I just could not remember the words and had a terrible time concentrating and completing a thought. I had to write everything down so that I would not forget it. I was once terribly embarrassed because I forgot that I had asked colleagues for dinner. I once got lost in a shopping center with which I was very familiar. It was very scary. I thought I was losing my mind." A lawyer wrote: "I had to stop practicing law because I was no longer able to concentrate or read what was required. I was physically uncoordinated and thus unable to write."

Financial hardships resulting from lost work may further strain social and family relationships already damaged by the psychiatric, cognitive, and physical changes wrought by the disease. Marriages dissolve, jobs are lost, professions deteriorate, and schoolwork is neglected, often resulting in repeated failures. Many patients recall being dropped by friends, spouses, and partners not only because of their changed appearance but also because of personality changes. Even outgoing patients may become reclusive and self-conscious. One Cushing's patient recalled: "I felt that I had robbed my children of the stable mother they deserved and my husband of the loving wife he had married. I cannot shake the guilt about being so ill that I destroyed my family. I could not cope with birthday parties, shopping, or just the normal demands put on a mother. My husband asked me, 'Where is the wife I married?' I was in the hospital recovering from surgery when my husband took me to court for a divorce and custody of the children."

Cushing's disease can be particularly devastating for adolescents, whose concern with physical appearance is exaggerated under the best of circumstances. One young woman, who started having symptoms at age 8 but was not diagnosed until she was 24 after surviving many suicide attempts recalls, "I was picked last for teams. I constantly avoided my friend's entreaties to be social and stayed home alone most weekends, eventually stopping the friendships altogether. I was very self-conscious about my appearance; I felt that I looked hideous."

DIAGNOSIS

There is not only tremendous relief once the diagnosis of Cushing's syndrome is finally made but also often tremendous anger that the correct diagnosis took so long to be made. One patient recalled feeling so happy to know that she was not crazy: "I felt frightened but also vindicated. All of the devastation in my life was not my fault! However, I soon experienced overwhelming anger and disgust that everyone, even my closest friends, had so readily dismissed my complaints and that no one had taken the time or shown enough interest to help me."

After elevated cortisol levels are demonstrated, it cannot be emphasized enough how important it is to find the correct cause, which then guides treatment. There are many very distressing cases of numerous surgeries and no cure.

If surgery is deemed the most appropriate treatment, then a surgeon with a lot of experience with Cushing's must be chosen. For example, if Cushing's disease, resulting from a pituitary tumor, is diagnosed, the patient should be referred to a neurosurgeon with extensive experience with the transsphenoidal procedure to remove the tumor. Not all neurosurgeons are trained appropriately to perform this surgery. A valid question to ask your surgeon is, "How many pituitary surgeries do you perform a year?" or "What is your success rate for these surgeries overall?" Patients are often sadly misled by eager but relatively inexperienced surgeons. Recurrences can be prevented and lifelong replacement medications avoided in the hands of a skilled and experienced surgeon who has performed hundreds if not thousands of these operations. Many of these surgeons are at medical centers that focus on pituitary tumors (Chapter 8).

No less care should be taken picking a surgeon for the other causes of Cushing's syndrome, where an adrenalectomy is necessary. Surgeons qualified to perform this surgery laparoscopically can often save patients the trauma of a standard open adrenalectomy, where muscles must be severed and ribs must be cut, thereby reducing pain and recovery time.

RECOVERY

After living with high cortisol levels for many years, many patients are unprepared for the effects of steroid withdrawal syndrome, which can accompany successful treatment of Cushing's syndrome. Physicians may have little experience treating Cushing's patients postoperatively, so it is important for patients to know that they need to be tapered back to physiological steroid levels slowly to avoid numerous trips to the emergency room with severe withdrawal symptoms. All patients should be advised to wear a MedicAlert bracelet, be taught how to increase their oral steroid dose during an intercurrent infection or other physical stress, and carry a syringe for injecting a glucocorticoid, such as hydrocortisone or dexamethasone, in a severe emergency. This advice should be supplemented by provision of a written leaflet making everything clear. This increase in steroid dosing is necessary for as long as it takes for adrenal function to be restored. While tapering too rapidly is dangerous, tapering too slowly or not tapering at all can lead to lifelong steroid dependence and a decreased quality of life. Patients' reactions to withdrawal are as variable as their presentations of the syndrome.

The reason for the slow recovery of the hypothalamic-pituitary-adrenal axis (HPAA) after the high-blood levels of hydrocortisone are lowered with successful treatment of Cushing's syndrome, whether the result of an adrenocorticotropic hormone (ACTH)–secreting tumor or an adrenal tumor, is because ACTH secretion from the normal pituitary is completely suppressed during the active phase of the disease. Recovery of this secretion is very variable from one person to another and may take years to occur; indeed, occasionally it never recovers. Endocrinologists generally agree that for the HPAA to recover, only short-acting steroids, such as prednisone, prednisolone, or hydrocortisone, should be used during the tapering process.

Even when an appropriate tapering protocol is followed, patients are often surprised by the duration of the recovery period. It can take years before patients are completely free of replacement therapy and feel more or less like themselves. While some patients experience few problems during this period, others are plagued by debilitating fatigue, muscle and joint pain, depression, and difficulty in concentrating. One patient related, "It took me 3 years to get on my feet. I could not work, clean my house, or do much of anything but sleep. The 'after' period was never discussed by my physician." Thus, returning to normal often means reducing work responsibilities and the number of hours spent working. Rest is essential. Physical therapy can help patients to rebuild strength and stamina, and occupational therapy can help patients regain lost skills. A nutritionist can help to provide an adequate diet, perhaps with added protein to help rebuild muscle strength. Psychiatric treatment should be sought for emotional difficulties.

Most patients, however, are extremely grateful to have their lives back once the recovery period is over. One patient's exuberance is unmistakable: "I lost 50 pounds, my hair grew back, and my blood pressure and blood sugar are normal. I feel strong and energized and have even gone back to nursing."

SUPPORT NETWORKS

A patient's personal support network can make an enormous difference in outcome. Family support or religion can be a key to preventing suicide. For example, family members should be encouraged to become involved with physician appointments in order to have a deeper understanding of the disease and its repercussions. Patients who have this support do well. One patient related: "My family and friends talked, listened, hugged, and held my hand through all of the stages of my disease and recovery. My husband held me, let me cry, and raced me to the emergency room when necessary. He often stood by helplessly, but he never gave up on me."

Patients should be encouraged to seek out support organizations (see later). Most Cushing's patients express extreme relief at being able to talk with other Cushing's patients: "No one can understand Cushing's like another person who has experienced it."

Jane Edwards
Conway, Massachusetts

Acknowledgments

Thank you to the board members of the Cushing's Support and Research Foundation, who are also Cushing's patients, for sharing their stories.

Reprinted with permission from Michael O. Thorner and G. Michael Besser. This article first appeared in Thorner MO, Besser GM. *Comprehensive Clinical Endocrinology*, 3rd ed. San Diego: Elsevier Publishers, 2002, pp 698–700.

Support Groups

For networking and support services specifically for Cushing's patients:
The Cushing's Support and Research Foundation
60 Robbins Road, No. 12
Plymouth, MA 02360
Phone: 617-723-3674
Email: Cushinfo@CSRF.net

For support for patients with all types of pituitary tumors:
The Pituitary Network Association
P.O. Box 1958
Thousand Oaks, CA 91358
Phone: (805) 499-9973
Email: info@pituitary.org

For support for patients with either Cushing's syndrome or Addison's disease:
The Dutch Federation Addison and Cushing Patients
P.O. Box 174
Nijkerk, 3860 AD The Netherlands
Phone: 31332471460
Email: bestuur@nvacp.nl

For information about all rare diseases:
National Organization for Rare Disorders National Headquarters
55 Kenosia Avenue
Danbury, CT 06810
Phone: 203-744-0100
Fax: 203-798-2291

Index

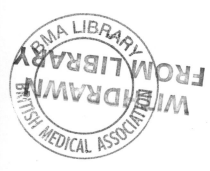

CPI Antony Rowe
Chippenham, UK
2018-01-05 17:44